PHYSICIAN-SOLDIERS AT THE FORKS

THE IMPACT OF THE MILITARY ON MEDICAL CARE IN PITTSBURGH (1754-1900)

ROBERT M. GROM

AMERICA THROUGH TIME®
ADDING COLOR TO AMERICAN HISTORY

America Through Time is an imprint of Fonthill Media LLC
www.through-time.com
office@through-time.com

Published by Arcadia Publishing by arrangement with Fonthill Media LLC
For all general information, please contact Arcadia Publishing:
Telephone: 843-853-2070
Fax: 843-853-0044
E-mail: sales@arcadiapublishing.com
For customer service and orders:
Toll-Free 1-888-313-2665

www.arcadiapublishing.com

First published 2019

ISBN 978-1-63499-106-3

Typeset in 10pt on 13pt Sabon
Printed and bound in England

Prologue

My interest in the history of military medicine and physician-soldiers in Pittsburgh began in the late 1980s while employed at Western Pennsylvania Hospital. I was always fascinated by history, but my attention centered primarily on politics and social activism. My focus changed when I was invited to participate in a new project at the hospital. The "Antiquity Project" grew out of several years of dialog between senior members of the hospital's medical staff and administration. The project's primary goal was to preserve the institution's history and artifacts since it was the first hospital chartered in Pittsburgh.

Charles R. Wilson, Jr., M.D. was the driving force among the medical staff. At the time, he served as Chief of Medicine, and it was his love of medical history and vision that drove the project. Vision was one thing, but it was not enough. Administrative sanction and internal political support were needed, as was funding and project management. Those things came together initially in the form of a small committee comprised of Dr. Wilson; Steven A. Caywood, hospital president and CEO; Frely Shea, president of The Western Pennsylvania Hospital Foundation; and John "Jack" P. Vetter, director of the hospital's Medical Media Department.

Collaboratively, the group defined the parameters of an initial project to assess the number and quality of historical assets and artifacts extant throughout the hospital. Through fortunate circumstance and the recommendation of Jack Vetter, I became a member of the Antiquity Committee. Jack was aware of my interest in history, so I seemed to fit a "volunteer" job description that had not yet been fully written.

Over the next several months, while maintaining my regular job, I spent several days a week after work and weekends searching the hospital. I visited every department, meeting with managers and supervisors to ask for their help. Questions like "what old records do you have?," "how far back do the records date?," and "where are your department's records stored?" became common refrains. I quickly learned the nuances involved in determining which staff members were most likely to know the details of their department's history and record keeping.

The hospital's medical records department and medical library seemed like logical places to explore. My visit with the director of medical records was unproductive. Old hospital records were destroyed or removed to offsite storage once mandatory retention periods were met. Conversely, my visit to the medical library was productive. There I discovered bound volumes of medical and surgical records from the late 1800s and early 1900s.

Recognizing the material I sought might be considered refuse if not covered by a policy or government regulation, the target of my next investigation became the hospital's housekeeping department. With the assistance of department supervisors, I was introduced to many of the hospital's obscure storage areas. In the deepest, darkest, dustiest recesses of the hospital, I uncovered dozens of old bronze plaques and commemorative tablets dating from the hospital's earliest days. In old buildings outside the main facility, I found trash barrels destined for disposal. Inside the barrels, I found historical photographs, vintage corporate documents, annual reports, handwritten correspondence between hospital Managers and Dorothea Dix dating from the 1850s, and a range of old hospital publications. Scattered around the buildings, I also found discarded medical equipment. Old blood pressure machines, an ancient EKG machine, and other instruments were there resting in their dusty glory.

Locating the photographs made me wonder what other images might be hidden in the hospital. Along with the day-to-day routine of capturing images of contemporary hospital events, the hospital's Medical Media Department was also responsible for taking photographs of medical procedures, and for producing artwork and illustrations for education and marketing. The thought there might be historic photographs buried in the files had escaped me until then. After a little searching, I was rewarded with a treasure trove of vintage images of old hospital buildings, medical procedures, physicians, board members, administrators, and events.

All of a sudden, the Antiquity Committee had enough material to serve as a basis for a larger project. Now all that was needed was money. In this regard, the timing was excellent. Dr. Wilson happened to have a philanthropically minded patient who was interested in the Antiquity Committee's work. A few days after a visit to his office, a check for $75,000 arrived. The donor suggested that we "stop talking about it and start doing it." That investment served as the nucleus for what would soon become a $750,000 multi-year project. The donation was placed in a restricted account at the Foundation and detailed project planning commenced. It was agreed subsequent project development and operations would now be the work of the Foundation. Frely Shea became the project administrator and I became the project director.

A visit to our nation's oldest hospital, Pennsylvania Hospital in Philadelphia, provided a framework for what form West Penn's project might take. Founded by Benjamin Franklin and Dr. Thomas Bond in 1751, Pennsylvania Hospital was not only 100 years older than West Penn, it also had a long tradition of preserving and displaying its history. Our team was impressed and decided to engage one of their administrators, Dolores Ziff, and one of the hospital's design consultants, Charles Schock, a senior designer with Berm Studios in Philadelphia, as advisors.

Back at West Penn, it was time to define the initial elements of the project. It was decided that permanent display panels would be created to highlight the hospital's early history and showcases would be constructed to hold rotating collections of artifacts. Thematically, the panels would offer a chronological timeline of the hospital's key achievements on a parallel track with the general development of medicine in Pittsburgh. They would also incorporate major milestones in the city's civic and industrial past as reference points. Recognizing we would likely need additional funds for the project, we thought it wise to incorporate some of the old donor plaques and commemorative tablets into the inaugural project. Once the initial elements of the project were defined, additional research was needed, and appropriate photographs and illustrations had to be collected. These were responsibilities I gladly accepted.

In a matter of weeks, all of the plaques and tablets were moved to a central location and cataloged. There was some impressive history memorialized in metal. Major events were evident, as were the names of many of the hospital's major donors, including members of the city's most celebrated families and a large number of Pittsburgh's prominent bankers, businessmen, and industrialists.

After cataloging, researching, and cleaning, the decision to incorporate the plaques and tablets proved an excellent idea. Important events and people in the hospital's history were already commemorated, so it made sense to include them. Doing so not only expanded the scope of visual displays incorporated into the "Antiquity Project" but also opened doors to new fundraising opportunities. Who better to approach for support than individuals and families who had already shown their interest and generosity?

Within a few months, we developed several permanent display panels describing the hospital's history and heritage in the context of the development of medicine in Pittsburgh. We incorporated dozens of plaques and commemorative tablets into the design as well as display cases filled with artifacts. A ribbon-cutting ceremony was held, and the project received glowing reviews. Our team was repeatedly asked: "what's next?" It did not take long for the question to be answered.

Like many of the city's older hospitals, over the years, West Penn had added new floors to existing buildings or built new structures to add space for patients and diagnostic equipment. As new floors were added skyward and structural footprints extended in all directions, moving patients and visitors from one department to another became a nagging issue. A directional signage system was needed to show the way. With the success of the initial project, it struck hospital leadership that history panels and displays might offer a solution by becoming an integral part of the hospital's wayfinding system. The idea was incorporated into the overall project design.

Financial support became easier to obtain as various groups in the hospital inquired about having the history of their respective services or departments incorporated. As a result, I took on a new role in addition to the project director. I became the project fundraiser, an event that soon changed my life and professional career.

During this period, the hospital and foundation embarked on a $7.9 million capital campaign to build a new Critical Care Tower. Due to my work with the "Antiquity Project", familiarity with the hospital and medical staff, and a growing number of project donors, I was asked to assist in the capital campaign.

Over a few years, panels covering the history of nursing, medical education, pioneering physicians, burn care, volunteers, and neonatology was researched, designed, and fabricated. As new panels were added, it seemed to ignite interest in the next group. Once completed, the panels were placed along the hospital's main corridors. As the Critical Care Tower was completed, panels were placed in elevator lobbies relevant to the department or services rendered on a particular floor. A pathway of history now tied the hospital together vertically and horizontally.

The next phase of the "Antiquity Project" went beyond anything the committee had originally contemplated. We expanded the project to create a new boardroom and a small history of medicine museum. New panels were developed for the boardroom to highlight early board members and Life Managers (early major donors). The museum was named the James I. McGuire Antiquity Center and was located in prime space on the second floor of the hospital's Mellon Pavilion outpatient and ambulatory care facility. Opened in January 1990, the Center was dedicated to the memory of James I. McGuire, who served the hospital as its Chief Executive Officer from 1952 to 1979.

Shortly before opening the McGuire Center, Frely Shea asked if I would be interested in leaving my position in the hospital to join the Foundation as Vice President of Development. I accepted, and as the saying goes, the rest is history. I now had the best of all worlds. I retained my position as director of the "Antiquity Project" and I joined Frely and the foundation team in completing the Critical Care Tower capital campaign. I was also invited to lead discussions on the foundation's next capital campaign to remodel the hospital's cafeteria and construct a medical education conference center. The conference center was something that had been sorely lacking for years.

Long before final plans for the conference center and cafeteria were complete, I presented an overview of the preliminary plans to a few groups, including the Women's Committee and Governing Board of the Hospitality Shops. That presentation quickly turned into a $2-million commitment. A short time later, a hospital employee campaign and major donor visits brought additional funding commitments, and we were soon more than half way toward completing a $5.5-million goal that had not been publicly revealed.

Today, many of the permanent panels remain on display in West Penn's central corridors, and the conference center hosts hundreds of lectures and medical education seminars each year. Unfortunately, the museum was dismantled and placed in storage in the late 1990s in order to make room for a new outpatient clinic.

I never lost sight of the nexus between history and fundraising. Over the years, I have used the knowledge gained at West Penn to navigate my career. During a period of administrative upheaval at West Penn, I resigned my position in 1994 to start a new fund development program at a community hospital located a short distance outside Pittsburgh. I spent the last quarter century using the lessons learned at West Penn to raise funds for a plethora of health-related programs and services. In practically every situation I found a way to weave in history.

Along the way, the number of military-related connections to medicine that I discovered amazed me. The legacy of the city's physician-soldiers was evident at every turn. This book is my attempt at offering tribute to their many contributions.

Acknowledgments

I will never forget the many gifts of time and knowledge that I received from Charles R. Wilson, Jr., M.D. He instilled the love of Pittsburgh medical history in me. His mentoring, friendship, and care as a personal physician will forever be part of me. Likewise, I am grateful to Frely Shea for offering me the opportunity to learn and grow personally and professionally. Her experience, grace, and wisdom had a profound impact on my life.

The volunteer spirit and giving nature of the leaders of West Penn Hospital's Governing Board of the Hospitality Shops and the Women's Committee were rewarding in numerous ways. Ruth Say, Norma Walter, June Davidson, and other members of both groups offered never-ending support and enthusiasm. Many important and lasting things have been accomplished at the hospital with their unwavering support and investment.

My colleagues in West Penn's Medical Media Department were likewise essential to the "Antiquity Project's" success. Through their efforts, many old and brittle photographs were salvaged, restored, and incorporated.

Early in my research on West Penn Hospital, Jack Krah, executive director of the Allegheny County Medical Society and his communications staff, opened the Society's old minute books and photo archives for my inspection and use. Their collegiality and support were highly valued, as was the recent assistance offered by the Society's new executive director, Jeremy Bonfini.

The knowledge and untiring efforts of the librarians and archivists at the Carnegie Library of Pittsburgh and the Historical Society of Western Pennsylvania (Heinz History Center) have long been a source of inspiration. In the past, they helped make the West Penn project a reality. Almost thirty years later, the staff of these two institutions continue to provide the research and reference support that helped make this book possible. In particular, I wish to thank Gilbert Pietrzak in the Pittsburgh Carnegie Library Pennsylvania Department, Pittsburgh Photographic Library for all of the time and resources he has devoted to assisting me in this work. At the Heinz History Center, I am grateful to Mary Jones for the special attention she gave to my many requests.

Many thanks are also extended to Wayne Winters, a good friend, college buddy, and the best man at my wedding who has carved out countless hours to read and edit this work. His support and that of his wife, Carol, cannot be understated.

I also owe a special note of gratitude to Diane Wuycheck. As Communications Director at the Allegheny County Medical Society, she opened the files of the Society to me on many occasions. This access informed my work at West Penn. More recently, Diane authored a new book recounting the history of the Society. While writing her book, *A Tradition of Leadership, Innovation and Caring: A History of Medicine in Allegheny County,* she asked me to read and comment on many of its chapters. Her work reignited my interest in finishing this book, which I had started over twenty-five years ago.

The resources made available through the United States National Library of Medicine, the Library of Congress, and the U.S. National Archives and Records Administration were incredibly important to me at West Penn and in writing this book. Over the years, I have spent many hours scouring their databases, reading their books and articles, and retrieving dozens of photographic images and illustrations that add important texture to this book.

Most importantly, I wish to recognize the love, patience, and support that I received from my wife, Carol. For more than forty years, she has stayed the course and put up with my countless hours of work, writing, and hobbies. Without her, there would be little reason for living or writing. My children, Adam and Jessica, have likewise been supportive of their father. Traipsing through libraries and museums was not always their idea of a great vacation, but they persevered. Time has certainly changed things for them, as they are now smarter and much better educated than their father. The days of dad helping with a term paper or report are now being repaid; the kids have now become my research assistants and editors. I am grateful for all of their love and devotion, and this book is dedicated to them.

Contents

Introduction

Most Pittsburgh historians agree the first trained medical practitioners in the city had their roots in military service. However, few researchers have studied the relationship between medicine and the military outside the colonial period. The involvement of military contingents, physicians serving with or being trained by the military, and the myriad organizations that were formed to respond to their exertions, played a significant role in the long-term development of healthcare in the city. Much of the current status held by the Pittsburgh medical establishment can be directly attributed to the foundations laid by these physician-soldiers during the eighteenth and nineteenth centuries.

Although records indicate the French may have established trading posts as early as 1730, the earliest recorded French excursion exploring the headwaters of the Ohio River occurred in 1739. The area lay between settlements they had established at the mouths of the St. Lawrence and Mississippi rivers.

The British began to counter the French interest in the region in 1748. That year, the King of England awarded a Royal Charter to the Ohio Land Company along with a grant of 500,000 acres of ground lying principally on the southern side of the land between the Monongahela and the Great Kanawha rivers. The King's charter mandated that 100 families settle on the land within seven years, and required the Ohio Land Company to build and maintain a fort sufficient to protect the settlers. With these requirements in place, it was not long before the military came to the area, bringing with them the first physician-soldiers.

During this period, it is estimated all the English colonies in America contained approximately and 1¼ million inhabitants. The French population was estimated at 80,000. Before the earliest explorers encountered the raw beauty of the lands around the three rivers, American Indians resided there. They had been present in the Ohio Valley for many hundreds of years before the first European explorer set foot in the area.

Over countless decades, American Indian culture developed. Unique tribes, differentiated principally by geography and language, formed and were transformed by the environment and through interactions with each other. While tribal customs and languages were a common differentiator, hunting, fishing, farming, pottery making, and curing illness served as a common bond. Tribes traded with each other, and at times, fought each other long before the first European explorers navigated the area. The ordinary trials of daily life and the often-harsh consequences of battle necessitated the development of medicine to treat illness and wounds from hunting or conflict.

The American Indian's nomadic lifestyle led to the development of numerous encampments and villages, typically located along rivers or streams. The transient nature of their existence also led to the creation of trails and pathways across the wilderness, many of which later became avenues of passage for early explorers and traders, surveying parties, military contingents, and, ultimately, the region's first settlers. These paths also brought the first physician-soldiers to the forks of the Ohio River.[1] Initially, the physician-soldiers came in the service of the British Army, later in answer to the burgeoning call of a population in need of protection from American Indians, and finally, for the provision of medical care. Physician-soldiers were not always there when needed by the pioneers, but their presence was highly valued when available. Their legacy lives on, and this is their story.

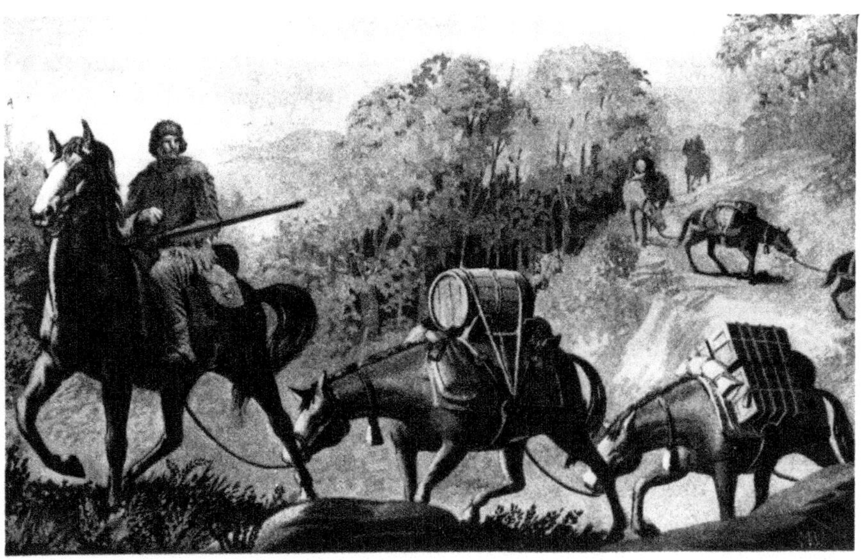

PACK-HORSE TRAIN, SHOWING VARIOUS METHODS OF PACKING BURDENS

Packhorse train carrying supplies over the mountains. (*Carnegie Library of Pittsburgh. All rights reserved. Unauthorized reproduction or usage prohibited*)

1

Health and Healthcare in Pioneer Pittsburgh

Before the arrival of any military in Western Pennsylvania, the local population—albeit a small, hardy, and widely dispersed group of explorers and traders—relied on themselves when it came to medical care. In the mid-1700s, there were no physicians to tend to the needs of a small population in such an untamed wilderness. Only the hardiest, or most foolhardy, settlers risked their lives to strike out from the civilized confines of the eastern cities to seek their fortunes in the area. Typically, these pioneers were able-bodied, rugged individuals with resilient constitutions honed over time. With few vices and easy access to pure water and natural food, they were skilled at living off the land. In his history of Western Pennsylvania's pioneer physicians, Thomas Davis commented about the generally healthy condition of the region's early inhabitants: "The pioneers of this section were exceedingly hardy. Their out-door life, simple food, pure water, long nights and few condiments and narcotics enabled them to resist disease and endure hardships impossible in these effeminate times."[1]

Medical historian John Duffy likewise noted:

> In the history of American colonial health a startling contrast exists between the descriptions of the early colonial environment and the stark picture, once the colonies were established, of recurrent pestilential epidemics and omnipresent endemic diseases. The early explorers and settlers were unanimous in their praise of the New World. They wrote of fresh bracing air, the vast acres of fertile land, forests full of game, and streams and lakes of pure water.[2]

Regarding the health status of the American Indian population, Duffy added: "The native inhabitants were described as strong and healthy and apparently having none of the common disorders of Europe."[3] While Duffy's assessment of the health situation was true and early settlers enjoyed a more healthful experience than what they left in Europe, things changed rapidly as the years progressed.

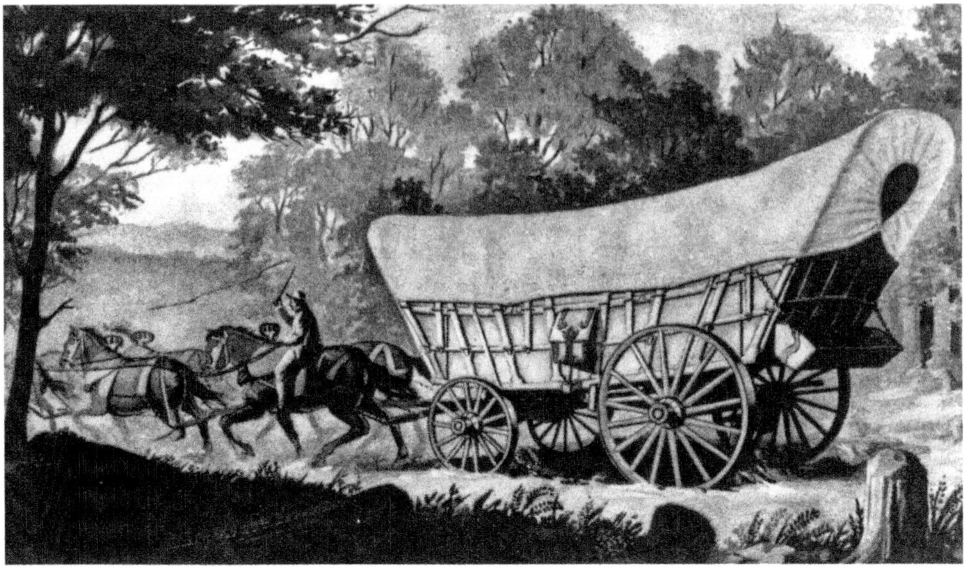

Conestoga wagon used to transport freight across the mountains. (*Carnegie Library of Pittsburgh.*)

The rampant epidemics that plagued Europe were not at all common during the early period of American colonization. Geographic distance and isolated living conditions initially offered respite from the contagions of Europe's large cities. To a large extent, the number of outbreaks of disease and the virulence of such epidemics was greatly reduced in the early colonies. As the population grew, however, "the common infectious disorders of Western Europeans—smallpox, malaria, diarrheas and dysenteries, respiratory complaints, measles, mumps, scarlet fever, diphtheria, and so forth—quickly established themselves."[4] When they did strike, they were highly destructive, and the absence of doctors and medicines proved to be a significant challenge.

The lack of American Indian experience with disease proved a boon for early settlers intent on displacing them from their lands. James Gibson in his biography of Bodo Otto wrote:

> Epidemics of various kinds appeared in a short time and on several occasions destroyed entire settlements. Smallpox was one of the scourges soon encountered, frequently devastating Indian villages as well as white settlements. The Pilgrims, while regretting the resulting mortality among the natives, often looked upon the Indian casualties as acts of Providence sent for the white man's protection.[5]

By the second decade of the 1700s, the benefits of smallpox inoculation were beginning to be recognized in England, Africa, the Middle East, and elsewhere. In America, beginning in 1721, Cotton Mather of Boston was among the country's earliest advocates for inoculation. However, there remained considerable debate over its use. Benjamin Franklin was an initial skeptic until the disease took his four-year-old son's life in 1736. After his son's death, Franklin became a vocal advocate. A little over two decades later, Franklin would write the introduction to a monograph written on the subject by Dr. William Heberden in London. A pamphlet was subsequently prepared and widely distributed throughout England and the colonies. Franklin became even more invested in healthcare in 1751 when he and Dr. Thomas Bond collaborated in founding Pennsylvania Hospital in Philadelphia, the first hospital developed in the colonies.

Some strides were made in the mid-1700s, although smallpox inoculation was still viewed with suspicion as it was commonly believed that contagion could still be spread through the practice. In 1796, Edward Jenner's discovery of a vaccine for smallpox offered a better—and safer—recourse to the prevention of the contagious disease. Smith's 1833 book, *The Indian doctor's dispensatory, or Every man his own physician*, described the introduction of smallpox inoculation, the precursor to vaccination when he wrote:

> This was discovered and introduced about the beginning of the present century, (i.e. the 19th) by some Doctors in England, who transmitted it to America. It has now been practised with, for about 12 years, to general satisfaction, and patronised by two of the honorable presidents of the United States of America, Jefferson and Madison.

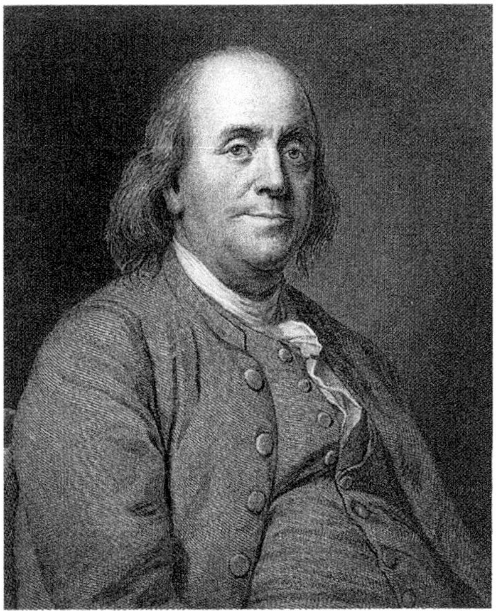

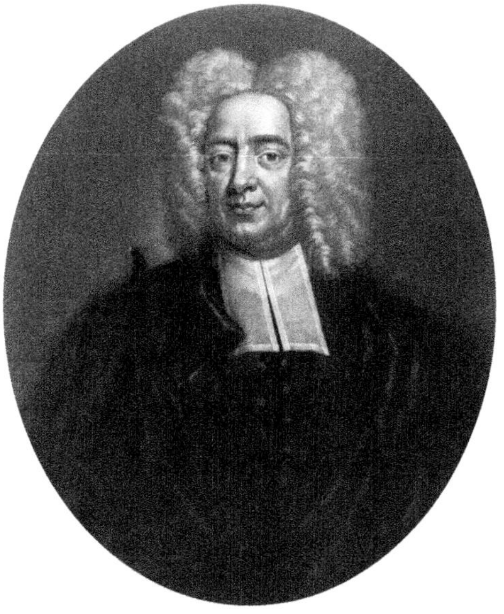

Above left: Benjamin Franklin. (*Library of Congress*)

Above right: Cotton Mather. (*Library of Congress*)

> The history, as near as we recollect, is as follows: Certain Milk-Maids in England being inoculated with the small-pox, it was found that the small-pox could not be communicated to them; and when the reason was sought, it was conceived that the said Milk-Maids had taken an infection from the Cow's bags or teats, on their hands, which has brought blisters and sores on them; and that in the instances where this had taken place, the small-pox could not be communicated.[6]

Smith added details about the actual process of inoculation, a practice that was soon routinely followed by the American physician-soldiers assigned to military contingents, and among physicians in cities and large settlements. He described the process:

> 1. Take the watery slime, at about the 6th or 8th day, from the arm of a healthy person who has been inoculated, while the blister is still in its clear state; for when it becomes yellow, it will be uncertain to give the infection.
> 2. Raise the cutis, or grain of the skin, about two inches above the knuckle bone of the wrist, with a lanset or needle, into a little cup, so deep that the water will just rise in it; then introduce a small drop of the above, such as you can carry on the point of your lanset or needle into the raised cup—and cover the inoculated cup, with a little lint or clean cotton, touched with spittle, or the white of an egg, to make it stick.
> 3. In a few hours the lint may be removed from the arm; and if the infection has taken, it will show a little inflammation in 48 hours. All excesses in eating, drinking and exercise, should be avoided, as the system will be thoroughly affected; and frequently the person will experience chills and a slight fever—and kernels in their groins and under their arms—and you may expect the sore on the arm to be considerable.[7]

When illness or disease struck early travelers, the only medical knowledge available was what they brought with them over the Allegheny Mountains, with most relying on instinct, folk medicine, or American Indian remedies instead of science. In his book series, *Tales of an Indian Camp*, James Athearn Jones offers insight into prevalent practices by observing:

> The priests of the Indians are at the same time their physicians, and their conjurors; whilst they heal their wounds, or cure their diseases, they interpret their dreams, give them protective charms, and satisfy that desire which is so prevalent among them, of searching into futurity. When any of the people are ill, the person who is invested with this triple character of doctor, priest, and magician, sits by the patient.[8]

In general, the pioneers took most ailments in stride for there was usually very little that could effectively counter most illnesses. Letting nature take its course was often the prevalent sentiment for many of the fevers or other contagious diseases. In children, such incidents were viewed as necessary stages in a child's development.

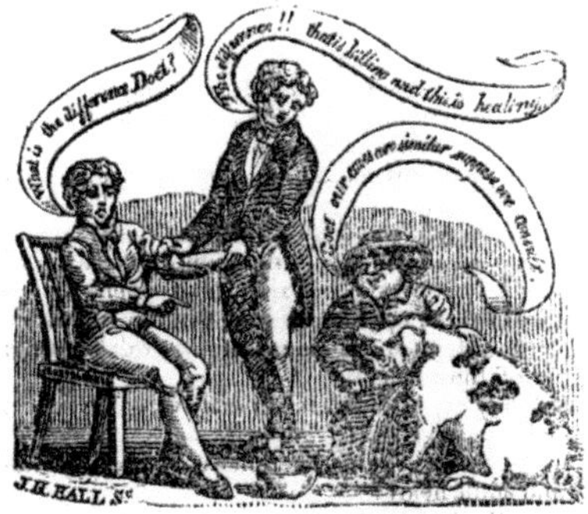
MEDICAL ANECDOTES.
What is the difference Doct?
The difference!! that is killing and this is healing.
The *Doctor* takes the *life* to *heal*,
The *Butcher* does the *same* to *kill*;
The first *designs* the *breath should stay*,
The next *direct* the other way.
Should proof of this you wish to know,
See *plate* above, and *scrip* below.
Now form your minds, which of the two,
If sickness press, the work shall do.
Ratsbane, zinc, and vitriol too,
And mercury, to physic through;
We know these poisons they do give,
Are not their patients tough to live.

Medical Anecdotes. (*National Library of Medicine*)

Superstition played a large role in both pioneer and American Indian life. Joseph Doddridge, in his history of Pennsylvania and Western Virginia, noted:

> The wilderness was a region of superstition. The adventurous hunter sought for ominous presages of his future good or bad luck in every thing about him. Say what you please about this, doctors, the first settlers of this country were seldom mistaken in this latter indication of the weather. The croaking of a raven, the howling of a dog, and the screech of an owl, were as prophetic of future misfortunes among the first adventurers into this country, as they were amongst the ancient pagans; but above all, their dreams were regarded as ominous of good or ill success.[9]

Gunn's Domestic Medicine, or, Poor Man's Friend was one of the earliest books covering popular treatments tailored specifically for frontiersmen and early settlers. First published in 1830, the book went through many successive updates into the early twentieth century. Gunn's book contained instructions on medical treatments and preventive measures, including notes on the best way to sleep in the wilderness:

> It is worthy of observation that most persons who sleep hard, are more healthy and lively than others: look at the Indians who sleep on deer and bear skins: look at soldiers who sleep on blankets; and at wagoners, who always on journeys, sleep on hard mattresses on the floors of houses, or on the hard ground in tents. And it is worthy of particular remark, that a hard bed promotes digestion, and prevents incubus or night-mare, that demon of

> indigestion which is a scourge of thousands. All asthmatic persons, or in other words, those who have the phthisic, should sleep hard, and in refreshing and pure air; feather beds in close rooms are murdering thousands of these people by inches.[10]

Christopher Gist, a colonial explorer, surveyor, and guide for the British, was one of the earliest travelers into the primal woods of Western Pennsylvania. During his 1750–1751 travels to the area under the employ of the Ohio Company, he noted several bouts of illness in his diary. In November 1750, he wrote: "I was very sick, and sweated myself according to the Indian Custom in a Sweathouse, which gave Me Ease, and my fever abated."[11] Several months later, on 22–23 March 1751, he noted, "I killed a fat Bear, and was taken sick that Night," the next day he wrote, "I stayed here, and sweated after the Indian Fashion, which helped me."[12] It is interesting to note his reliance on American Indian remedies. Gist is credited with providing the first detailed descriptions of the region to British colonists. At the beginning of the French and Indian War (1754), Gist escorted George Washington on missions into the area and is attributed with saving his life twice.

Around the same time, Benjamin Rush, a founding father of the United States and leading expert on medicine in general and military medicine specifically, reported on the poor state of affairs in 1751 when he wrote: "medical therapy than in use consisted of bloodletting, sweating, physicking, diuretics, vomiting and blisters."[13] That situation would soon change with the onset of the Revolutionary War.

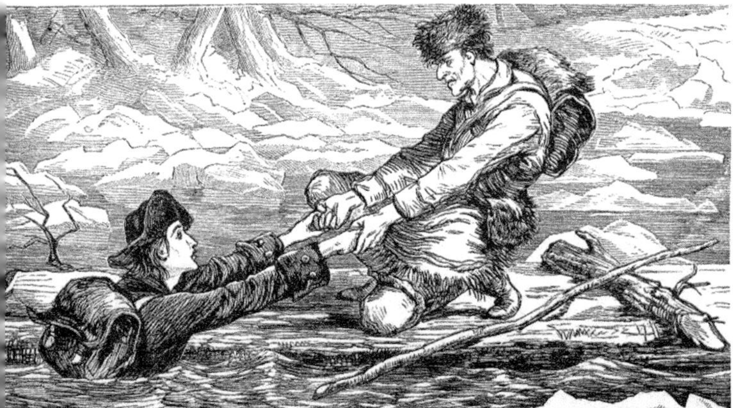

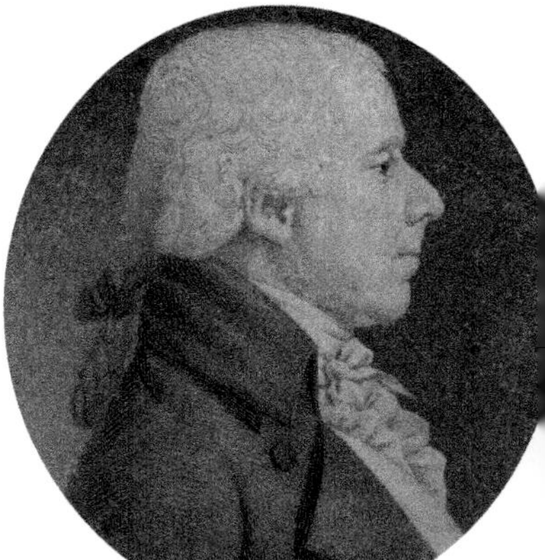

Above left: George Washington and Christopher Gist on the icy Allegheny River. (*Library of Congress*)

Above right: Dr. Benjamin Rush. (*Library of Congress*)

2

Pioneer Medical Practices and Medical Training

Dr. Bodo Otto, Senior Surgeon of the Continental Army during the American Revolution, wrote:

> The professional preparation of the Colonial physicians, compared to present-day requirements, seems woefully inadequate, for, prior to 1762 when Dr. William Shippen, Jr., introduced public medical lectures for students and young practitioners, the only available method of learning "the art and science of physic and chirurgery," was through apprenticeship with some local medical man whose training, in the great majority of cases, had been similarly obtained. Proud was the physician who possessed an institutional medical degree, or a technical library.[1]

Otto indicated there were only 3,500 practicing physicians in the Colonies at the outbreak of the Revolutionary War. Of those, he estimated fewer than 200 were university trained. The majority of physicians at the time were trained through apprenticeship, and most had never set foot in a hospital or participated in a dissection of a human body.

Though offered fewer opportunities to gain the higher levels of knowledge gleaned from university-based medical education, apprenticeship-trained physicians were nevertheless able to establish themselves as key members of the community. Typically, they served a preceptor for a period of three to seven years; their learning and engagement limited only by their competence and the scope of the preceptor's practice. For a fortunate few, principally those with sufficient support networks and adequate funding, subsequent study abroad would lead to a medical degree.

Apprenticeship in Pittsburgh was very much aligned with general practice throughout the colonies. Pittsburgh's first locally trained physician, Peter Mowry, began his service as an apprentice under British regimental surgeon Nathaniel Bedford. After resigning his commission to practice medicine in Pittsburgh, Bedford is recognized as the city's first "resident" physician. Thomas Davis, in an early review of local medical history, described Mowry's apprenticeship under Bedford in this way:

> The student of medicine in those days was certainly not carried to his profession "on flowery beds of ease!" As an apprentice his duties were manifold. He spread plasters, mixed ointments, picked lint and made decoctions. All medicines were purchased in their crude form and the grinding of them, in the great iron mortar, was no small job, while their odor and irritating qualities tried eyes, nose and lungs as well as patience. He learned to cup and bleed, and apply leeches, which he may have secured himself from the neighboring brook. Much of his work was more menial, attending the horse, chopping wood, running errands, and it is said, in Philadelphia, "they even had to help the doctor's good wife with the family washing." As he progressed he helped his master in surgery, often a physical task in those days before anesthetics. He drew teeth and performed other acts of minor surgery. He often accompanied the doctor, carrying the link or lantern at night and the saddle-bags by day, or sat at the patient's bed-side while his master slept. When adjudged fit he crossed the mountains to attend "a course of lectures" in some eastern school. Returning home he was dubbed "Doc." and was much sought after, as a desirable catch, by the neighboring young ladies. Opening a "shop" of his own, he sometimes, after a few years, made sufficient money to return east, secure his degree, and become a full-fledged doctor.[2]

John Duffy reported that American medicine assumed somewhat unique features compared to those in Europe. Degreed physicians from European universities, he noted, "were considered a class apart from surgeons, apothecaries, and other practitioners of medicine."[3] With relatively few physicians available in frontier America—whether university or apprenticeship trained—physician-class distinctions were greatly diminished. Only when there were choices between physicians did it make much of a difference, and that happened very infrequently the further removed one was from the larger cities. With few universities and no European-style guilds to foster or promote such differentials, early Americans were challenged to make a distinction between physicians, surgeons, apothecaries, or the many "quacks" that plied their trade in the colonies.

When all else failed, a physician would be summoned. In remote areas, the trip was long, and at times, cost prohibitive—whether taking the patient to the doctor or summoning the nearest doctor to attend to the patient. Duffy considered the situation when he noted that "America was a rural nation and for either the doctor or patient to travel several miles by horse back or buggy was expensive of time and effort."[4] It is interesting to note a typical fee schedule for physicians and surgeons in the late eighteenth century. Bodo Otto recorded that one of the first actions of a new medical society formed in New Brunswick, N.J., in 1776, was to set a common fee schedule: "Visits in town, whereby the physician and surgeon can be readily attending the patients without ridding, to be charged for, according to the duration of the ailment and degree of attendance."

> Per week:
> In other cases, requiring longer and daily care and attendance, in proportion for lesser or more time, exclusive of medicines—10 shillings (approximately $57 in U.S. currency today).
>
> Visits in the country:
> Under half a mile to be charged for as in town.
> Above half a mile and not more than one and one-half mile—1 shilling.
> Above one and a half miles and not exceeding fifteen miles, 1 shilling for each additional mile.
> Every visit above fifteen miles and not exceeding twenty-five miles 1 shilling for each additional mile.
> Above twenty-five miles, 2 shillings per mile.[5]

It was true physicians did have more heroic measures in their armamentarium. Bloodletting by cupping or leeches, the use of strong purgatives such as calomel, blistering by application of cantharides, or the incision and implanting of seton or pease would be enough to convince the uneducated pioneer of the professional prowess of the doctor. Surprisingly, many lived through these treatments to profess to the capabilities of the physician. Should the physician's treatment fail, he was expected to lead the funeral procession of the victim as Erasmus Wilson noted:

> During the first quarter of the century the burying-grounds of the town were in different churchyards, and, the distance rarely being great, the corpse was usually carried thither on a bier borne on the shoulders of the pallbearers. Custom demanded the presence of the physician at the funeral of his patient, and his place was usually at the head of the procession to the grave. If this habit were in vogue at present some of our busy physicians would be frequent visitors to the cemeteries.[6]

Even if a physician were available, they frequently would arrive too late since the terrain was rough and the traveling distance long. In reality, there was little a trained physician could do that would separate his actions from that of the pioneer since the physician had as few certain cures as did the family of the victim. Without the benefit of trained physicians, superstition, folk medicine, and herbal concoctions were mainstays of early medical care. By today's standards, many of the responses to illnesses that prevailed until after the Civil War are worthy of note since only those with staunch hearts would possess the fortitude required to partake in many of the remedies.

In summarizing the state of the relationship between receiving medical treatment by trained physician or reliance upon self-help, William Buchan opined in 1841:

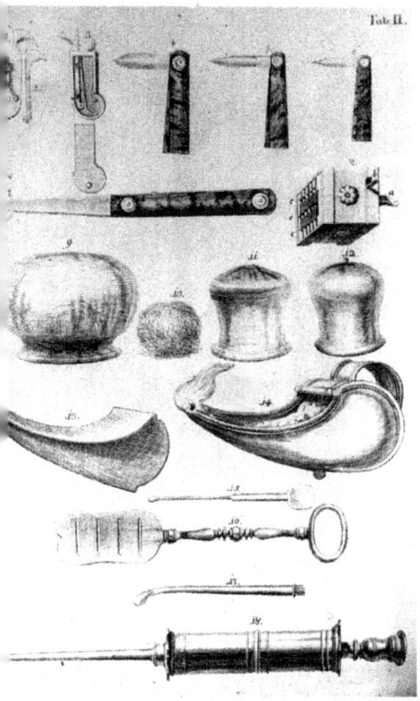

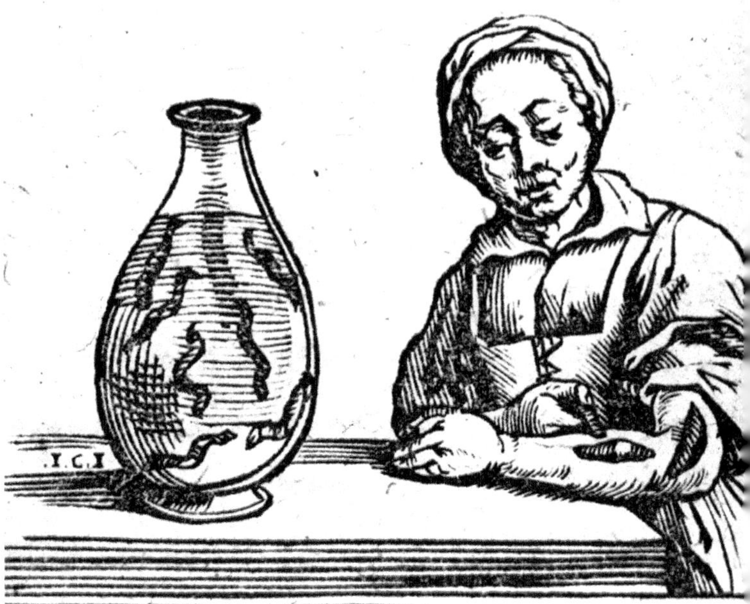

Above left: Various types of bloodletting instruments. (*National Library of Medicine*)

Above right: Woman applying a medicinal leech. (*National Library of Medicine*)

> It is the ignorance and credulity of the multitude with regard to medicine, which renders them such an easy prey to every pretender; nor can the evil be remedied by any other means but by making them wiser. Persons who have most knowledge in these matters, are commonly most ready both to ask and follow the advice of a physician, when it is necessary. The ignorant are always most apt to tamper with medicine, or consult quacks, and have the least confidence in physicians.[7]

Quacks, charlatans, midwives, and practitioners of folk, domestic, or American Indian medicine abounded, as did a growing group of "irregular" practitioners practicing homeopathy, phrenology, electrotherapy, botanical medicine, or other such movements. Whether university trained or apprenticed, regular physicians often competed unsuccessfully with the quacks. As Dr. Benjamin Rush observed: "... sickness deprives men of the means of acquiring money; that it increases all the expences of living; and that high charges often drive patients from regular-bred physicians to quacks."[8] Relative to American Indian medicine, John Duffy noted:

> In terms of the medical problems of the Native Americans, their medicine was quite satisfactory, and it did not compare too unfavorably with the medical practices of sixteenth- and seventeenth-century Europe. The major difference was that Western medicine had already begun the shift from a spiritual to a rational basis. In the clash

> of cultures, the most significant impact of Europeans upon Native American medicine was to transform it from a religious procedure with empirical overtones to an empirical procedure with religious overtones.[9]

In his study *Medical Inquiries in the Continental Army, 1775–1781*, Richard Blanco states:

> Most physicians had little formal education, and they usually had haphazard apprenticeships. Only a handful attended medical lectures. In an era when licensure for health services was not required, when only King's College in New York and the College of Philadelphia conferred medical degrees, when little regulatory legislation for medical practice existed, it was easy for quacks, the untutored, and for ill-trained apprentices to advertise themselves as qualified to heal a gullible public anxious for cures.[10]

We owe a debt of gratitude to Joseph Doddridge for describing some of the treatments that prevailed in early Pittsburgh. Examples include:

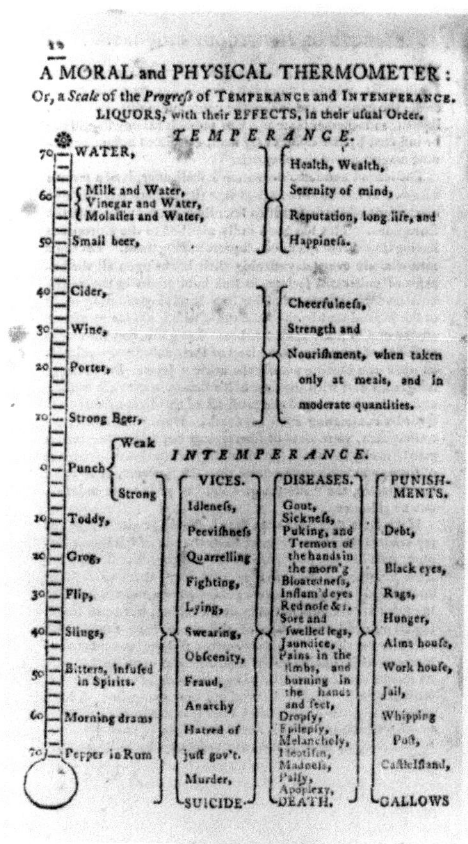

Benjamin Rush's Moral and Physical Thermometer measuring the effects of temperance and intemperance. (*National Library of Medicine*)

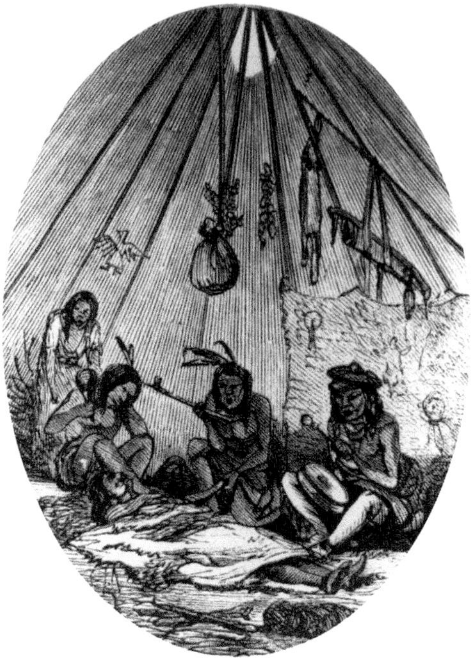

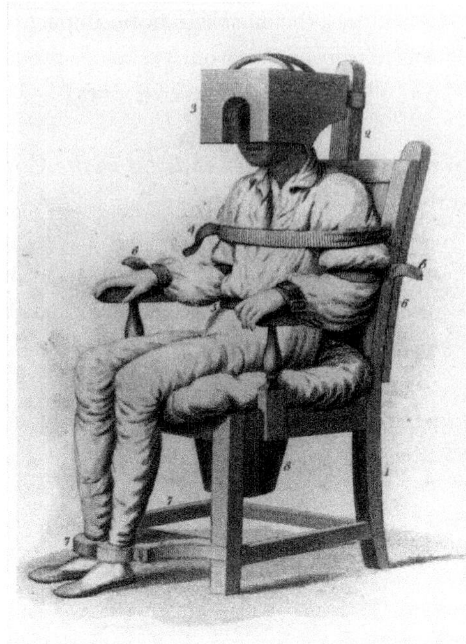

Above left: American Indian medicine lodge. (*National Library of Medicine*)

Above right: Tranquillizing chair for treating mental disorders, *c.* 1811. (*National Library of Medicine*)

Below: Metallic tractors would supposedly heal most ailments by simply touching skin with metal. (*National Library of Medicine*)

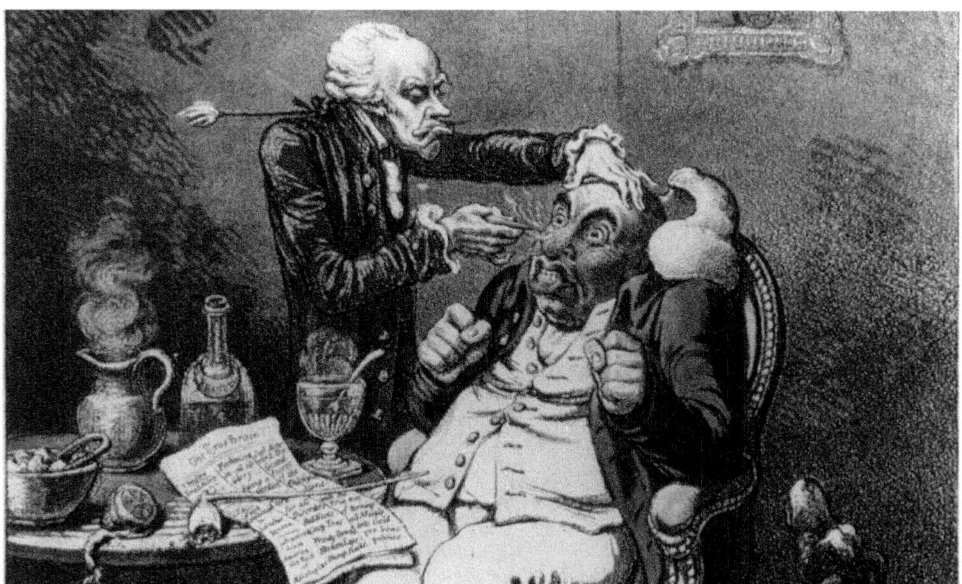

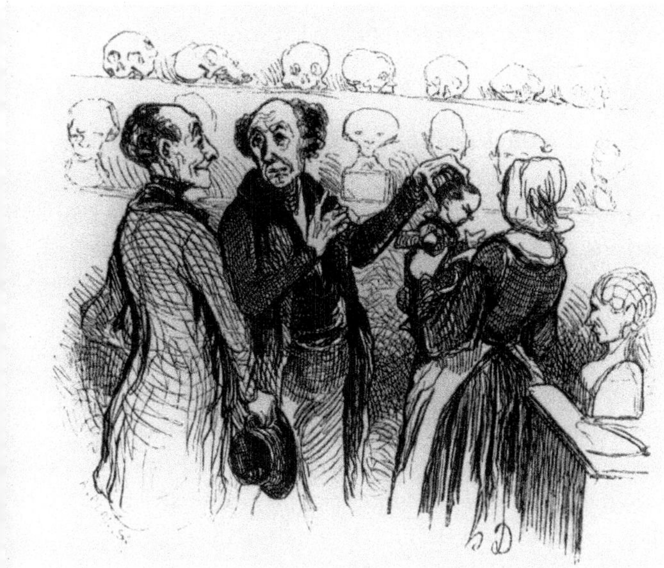

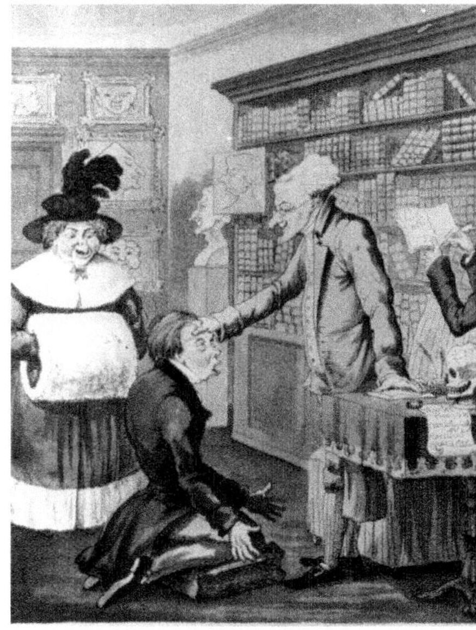

Above left: Phrenology: A mother brings her child to have his head read. (*National Library of Medicine*)

Above right: "Bumpology" was a derisive term used to describe phrenology. (*National Library of Medicine*)

Diseases of children—The diseases of children were mostly ascribed to worms, for the expulsion of which a solution of common salt was given. The dose was always large. I well remember, having been compelled to take half a tablespoon full, when quite small. To the best of my recollection, it generally answered the purpose.

The itch—The itch, which was a very common disease in early times, was commonly cured by an ointment made of brimstone and hog's lard.

Gun shot, and other wounds—Wounds were treated with slippery elm bark, flax seed and other such like poultices. Many lost their lives from wounds, which would now be considered trifling and easily cured. The use of the lancet and other means of depletion, in the treatment of wounds, constituted no part of their cure in this country in early times.

Rheumatism—Most of the early settlers of this country were affected with the rheumatism. For relief from this disease the hunters generally slept with their feet to the fire. From this practice they certainly derived much advantage. The oil of rattlesnakes, geese, wolves, bears, raccoons, ground-hogs and pole-cats, was applied to swelled joints and bathed in before the fire.

Erysipelas—Erysipelas, or St. Anthony's fire, was circumscribed by the blood of a black cat. Hence there was scarcely a black cat to be seen whose ears and tail had not been frequently cropped, for a contribution of blood.

Pleurisy—The pleurisy was the only disease, which was, in any considerable degree, understood by our people. A pain in the side called for the use of the lancet, if there was

> any to be had; but owing to its sparing use, the patient was apt to be left with a spitting of blood, which sometimes ended in consumption.[11]

Snakebites were a pervasive problem, and remedies abounded as snakes were often encountered on the frontier, on military excursions, or in the fields around the settlements. A seemingly endless number of "cures" were offered as folk remedies in extant self-help medical publications. Doddridge shared many observations on several of the practices. One of the most interesting was as follows:

> For the bite of a rattle, or copper snake, a great variety of specifics was used. I remember when a small boy to have seen a man bitten by a rattlesnake brought into the fort on a man's back. One of the company dragged the snake after him by a forked stick fastened in its head. The body of the snake was cut into pieces of about two inches in length, split open in succession, and laid on the wound to draw out the poison, as they expressed it. When this was over, a fire was kindled up in the fort yard and the whole of the serpent burned to ashes, by way of revenge for the injury he had done.[12]

Doddridge also described botanical and folk remedies then in vogue. Sucking venom from the wound, whether by mouth or through cupping, was another favorite treatment, as was cutting into the wound and filling it with gunpowder and salt. Mistakes nearly ended the lives of those treated. When the victim survived, there was great uncertainty as to whether they got well because of the treatment or as a result of nature taking its course. Commenting on snakebite treatments, Doddridge stated: "The truth is, the bite of a rattle or copper snake in a fleshy or tenderous part, where the blood vessels are neither numerous nor large, soon healed under any kind of treatment."[13]

In 1841, Dr. William Buchan offered advice for the treatment of intoxication, a situation that often occurred in both the settlements and on the frontier. He reported:

> I have seen repeated instances of persons being restored to perfect sobriety, and the complete use of their senses, from a state of most alarming intoxication, by taking away eight or ten ounces of blood from the nape of the neck, as near the head as possible, by means of cupping-glasses. The same effect is produced by taking blood from the arm, but the practice is not perhaps quite so safe; cupping certainly deserves the preference.[14]

Such treatment was considered "heroic," but he did add this caveat: "Most remedies in medicine are evils employed to counteract others of greater magnitude..."[15]

It is interesting to note intoxication had long been an issue in colonial America. Almost a century earlier, it was a bane to General Edward Braddock. Not long before the American Indians of southwestern Pennsylvania gave him something worse to consider:

> Heavy drinking was the curse of all walks of eighteenth-century life, and the arduous lot of the common soldier did not promote abstinence. General Braddock was eager to remove his troops from the seaport of Alexandria "as the greatest care and severest punishments could not prevent immoderate use of spirituous liquors."[16]

Geographic isolation, rugged individualism, and prerequisite self-reliance were required for colonial Americans to create and execute the terms of their survival. In the major settlements, early settlers sought to recreate many of the vestiges of the countries, communities, and homes they remembered. During periods of exploration, they made do with what could be created, gathered, or traded. In many instances, anyone who could both survive the frontier and read had the opportunity to become their own physician, lawyer, or minister.

It was not until after the Revolutionary War that medical schools began to form and medical societies organize. Together, they did their best to shape American medical training and promote "professional" credentials. Reacting to the ever-growing numbers of empirics, many large cities began to consider, or in some instances enact, laws regulating the "business" of medicine. As a result, allopathic or "orthodox" physicians as they were known were able to use these new laws to restrict competition.

It did not take long, however, for the disaffected groups of practitioners and the medical sects they represented to counter with increased political activity. With their reputations under siege and their incomes threatened, there was little to lose and much to gain through contradictive political action. They did not suffer long as public sentiment quickly turned once Andrew Jackson was elected President, and an era of egalitarianism and mistrust of learning ensued. These developments counteracted movements toward the professionalization of medical practices.

Between 1820 and the start of the Civil War, allopaths lost much of their status to the ever-growing numbers of conflicting medical factions. Regulars, irregulars, homeopaths, eclectics, Thomsonians, hydropaths, herbalists, and other medical sects openly competed with each other, and the public was confused. At the time, they were correct in discounting the allopaths since their effectiveness and expense did not typically compare favorably. The proliferation of ill-trained allopaths funneled through low-quality, profit-driven, private medical schools that multiplied exponentially during the period created even greater confusion.

3

Pittsburgh's first Medical Practitioners: Enter the Physician-Soldier

On 26 April 1777, George Washington wrote to his old friend Dr. James Craik, stating, "I am writing to address you on a subject which may lay some claim to your attention..." In his correspondence, Washington requested Craik consider serving as Assistant Director General of the Continental Army's Hospital Middle District. Craik readily accepted the offer at the pay of "three Dollars and six Rations per day; and two Horses plus traveling expenses found."[1] In making his proposition, Washington renewed an old friendship that had its roots many years earlier in an ill-fated expedition through the western Pennsylvania wilderness in July 1755. On this trip with General Edward Braddock to oust the French from Fort Duquesne, Craik became the earliest documented university-trained physician-soldier to ply his skills in the region. His visit was the first of a long line of transient physician-soldiers who followed over the next several decades. It would also not be Craik's last visit to the region.

Craik returned to Pittsburgh with Washington, Captain William Crawford, and others in October 1770 as part of a surveying trip to view lands Washington received in compensation for his services during the French and Indian War. The group arrived on the 17th of the month and stayed at Samuel Semple's lodge, located about 300 yards from Fort Pitt.[2] On the 18th, they dined at the lodge with Colonel George Croghan, one of the region's most noted Indian agents, and officers of the fort. While not traveling in the company of Washington and Craik, Dr. John Connolly was also in attendance. Washington reported there were approximately twenty log houses along the Monongahela River, most inhabited by "Indian traders."

Craik was a native of Scotland and product of the University of Edinburgh. He first came to this country in the service of General Braddock and marched with him, George Washington, and the British Army in 1755. He served as surgeon-in-chief on the expedition, and it was Craik and his assistants who dressed Braddock's wounds after the Battle of the Monongahela (Braddock's defeat) on 09 July 1755.

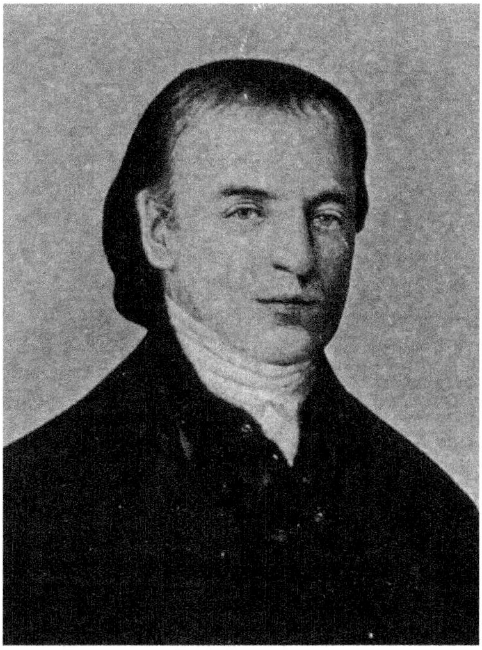

James Craik, Physician General of the United States Army. (*National Library of Medicine*)

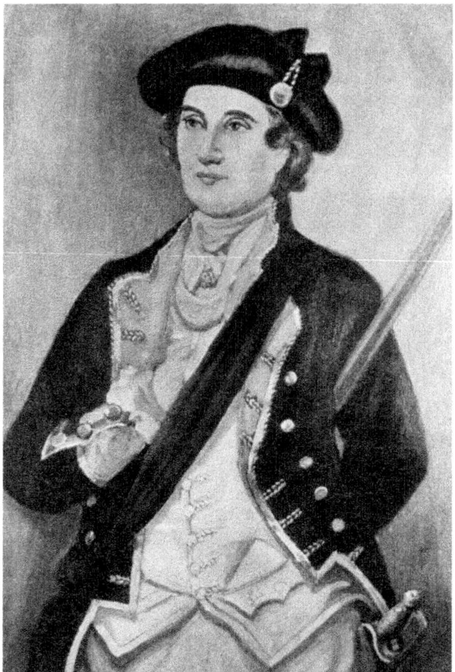

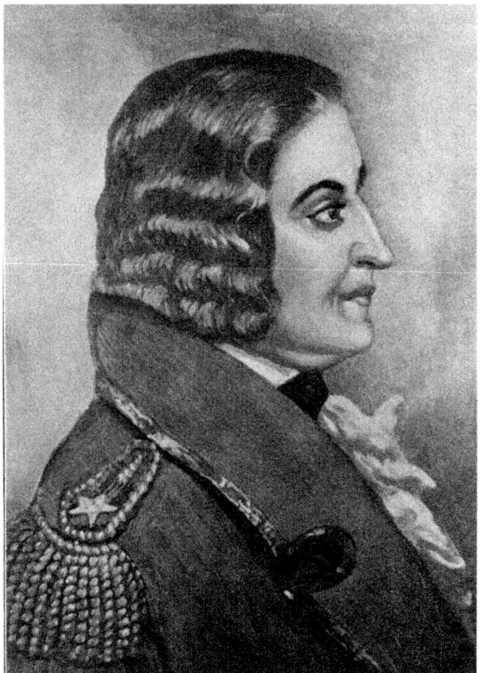

Above left: George Washington, General Braddock's *aide-de-camp*. (*Braddock Carnegie Library*)

Above right: General Braddock. (*Braddock Carnegie Library*)

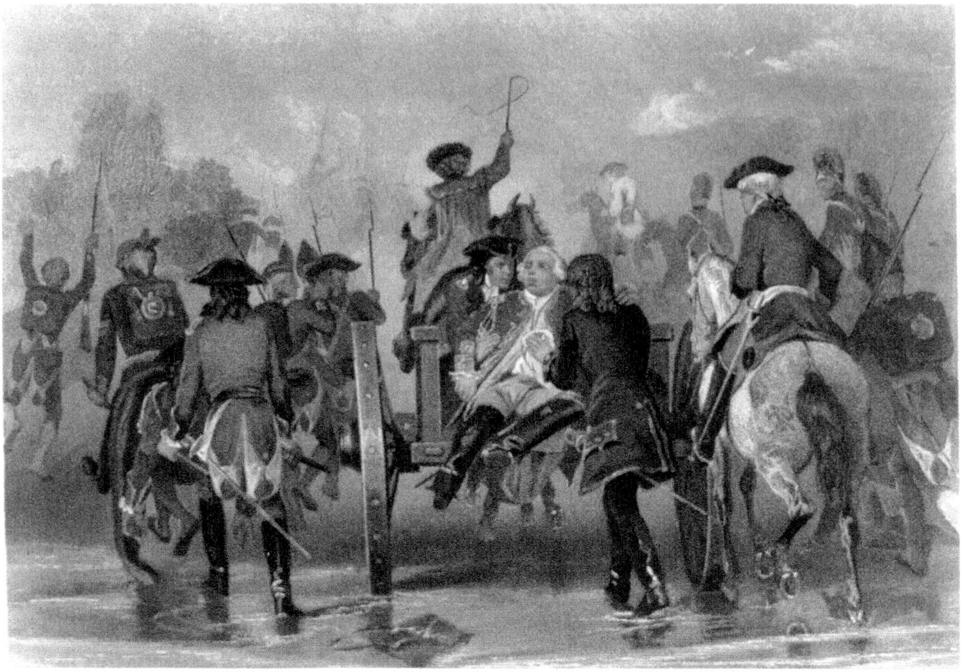

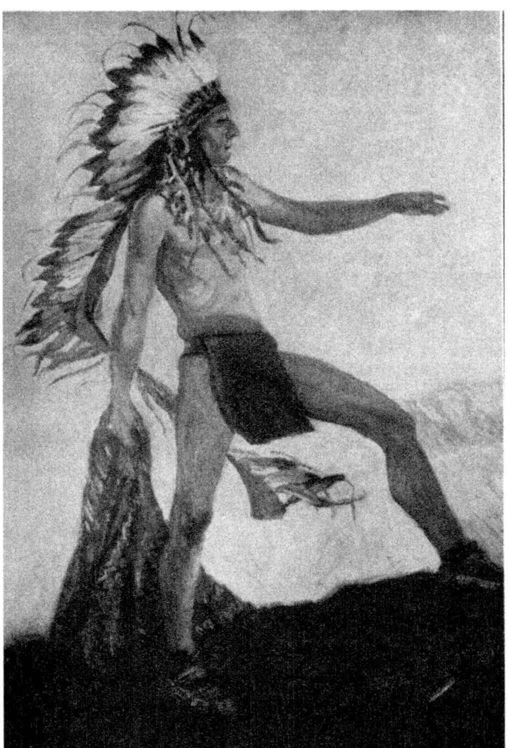

Above: General Braddock wounded and dying. (*Library of Congress*)

Left: King Shingiss, Chief of the Delawares, whose warriors aided the French in defeating General Braddock at the Battle of the Monongahela. (*Braddock Carnegie Library*)

Upon General Braddock's death, Craik attended the funeral service with Washington. Washington and Craik afterward remained steadfast friends. Craik served in numerous capacities during the Revolutionary War and subsequently became Washington's personal physician.

After Washington's death on 14 December 1799, a letter written by Dr. Craik was published in the *Times* newspaper of Alexandria, Virginia. On 13 December, he noted Washington had developed a sore throat. His treatment regimen included being bled four times, blistered twice, dosed with calomel and emetic tartar, and given a cataplasm of bran and vinegar to the throat. All were considered standard "heroic" treatments at the time. Nonetheless, Washington expired twenty-four hours later. In his will, he recognized his friendship with Craik by characterizing the doctor as "my compatriot in arms, and old and intimate friend."[3] It was a fitting tribute to Western Pennsylvania's first physician of note.

Thus began a long list of physician-soldiers arriving in Pittsburgh—some leaving a permanent mark and others of only fleeting interest. Their presence, whether transitory or permanent, laid the groundwork for a medical heritage that is uniquely Pittsburgh's.

Not long after Braddock's defeat and Craik's first visit to the area, other transient physician-soldiers followed. In 1758, several physicians, including Drs. James Young, Thomas Lloyd, John Morgan, George Armstrong, Thomas Eckerly, and Hugh Mercer, accompanied General John Forbes on a mission to remove the French from Fort Duquesne. Colonel Mercer was left in command of Fort Duquesne on November 25, 1758, and he became the first semi-permanent physician to serve in the area.

Thomas Davis wrote that on 01 March 1759, Mercer reported: "I cannot omit this opportunity of signifying to you the difficulties I am under of a surgeon to attend our sick. Mr. (Dr.) Johnston of the VA Reg. has been kind enough to attend them hitherto."[4] Mercer's stay lasted only until General Stanwix relieved him in December 1759. Like Mercer, many of the physicians who were stationed at Fort Pitt periodically reported distress over their seeming inability to provide relief for their patients. Surgeon James Miller who was based at Fort Pitt in the early 1760s was one. He is reported to have "Cut his own throat at Night in his Room with two Rayzors..."[5] in response to his inability to treat illnesses beyond his control.

At the time Mercer was relieved by General John Stanwix, there was reportedly one other physician-soldier at Fort Pitt. In his writings, Stanwix mentions a Dr. Johnston. While Drs. Mercer and Johnston are the only names recorded, there may have been others since Mercer's reports indicate that immediately before 04 April 1759, "seventeen had died and upwards of one hundred had been sick in the fort from Jan. 1st."[6]

During the Revolutionary War, upon receiving a recommendation from George Washington, Mercer was commissioned a brigadier general. He served the nation well and is recognized for his tenacity on and off the battlefield. He was present at

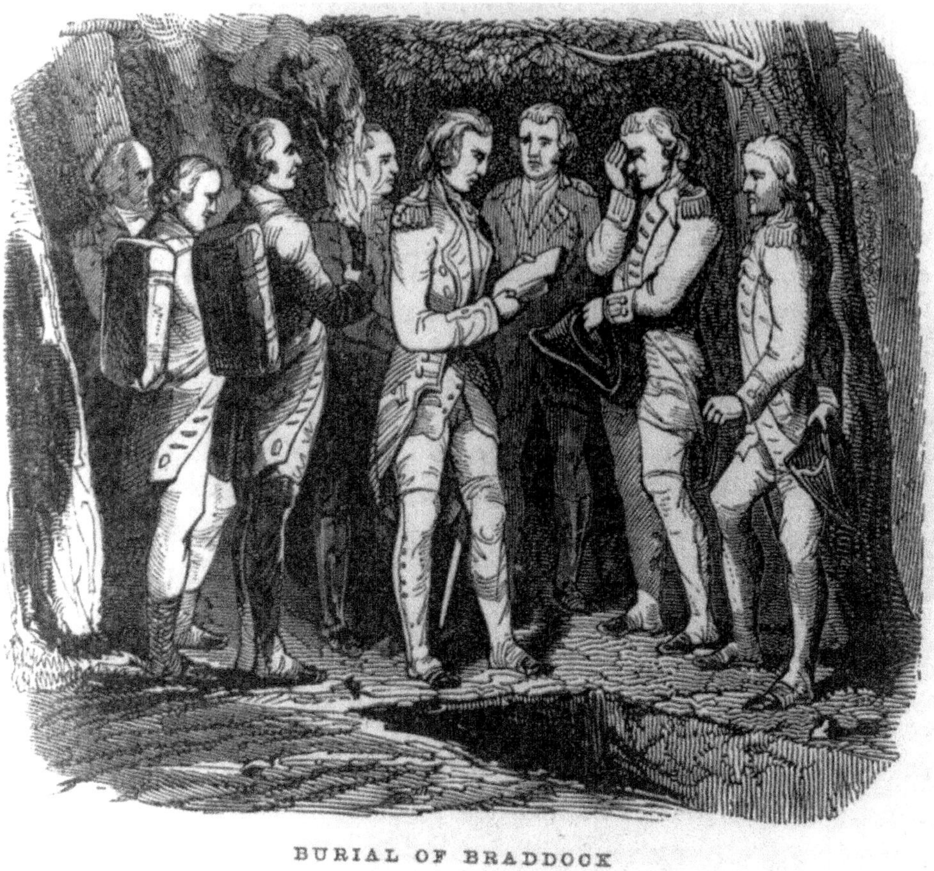

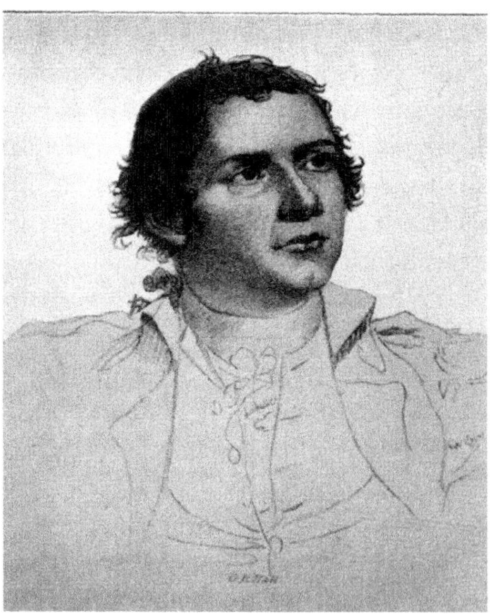

Above: George Washington reading funeral service for General Braddock by torchlight over open grave. (*Library of Congress*)

Left: Colonel Hugh Mercer. (*U.S. Army Medical Department Office of Medical History*)

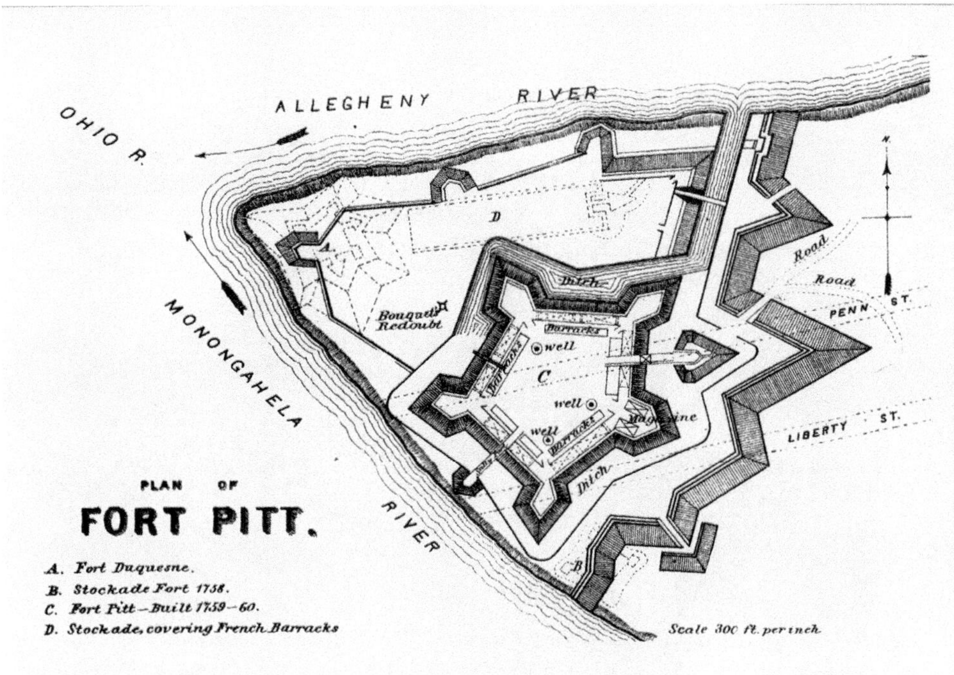

Fort Pitt, c. 1760. (*Carnegie Library of Pittsburgh. All rights reserved. Unauthorized reproduction or usage prohibited*)

the Battle of Trenton and led the charge at the Battle of Princeton, during which he was severely wounded and captured. He succumbed to his wounds on 12 January 1777.

The first temporary hospital established in Pittsburgh was a shelter at Fort Pitt in 1761. In 1763, after an epidemic of smallpox broke out, Dr. Robert Boyd, a military physician assigned to the garrison, constructed another temporary hospital shelter. Surgeon's mate Boyd was serving as the post physician at Fort Pitt when Colonel Henry Bouquet came to relieve the fort in response to Pontiac's War.[7] Under the command of Captain Ecuyer, Boyd had built another temporary hospital "under the drawbridge" in response to an outbreak of smallpox. In his reports to Bouquet, Boyd wrote: "We are so crowded in the fort that I fear disease; for, in spite of every care, I cannot keep the place as clean as I should like. Besides, the small-pox is among us; and I have therefore caused a hospital to be built under the drawbridge, out of range of musket shot."[8]

Healing the sick and wounded was a customary adjunct to the military duties of these physician-soldiers in the early years of Fort Pitt. In an odd instance of history, those responsible for healing and curing supposedly turned their medical knowledge and experience with smallpox into a weapon against the American Indians who were threatening to dispossess them of the fort and all of the lands around the forks. In

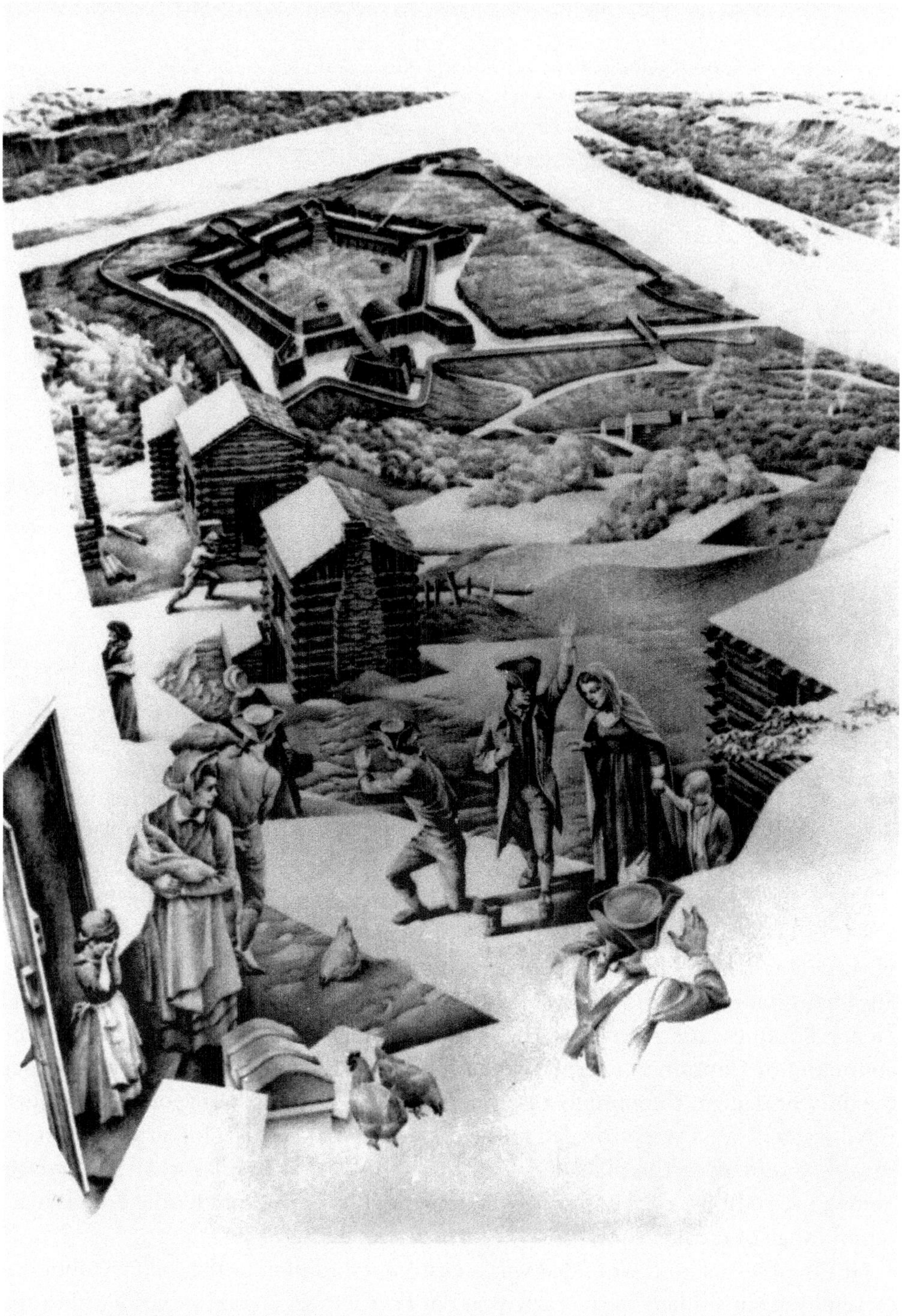

Preparing for an Indian attack. (*Carnegie Library of Pittsburgh. All rights reserved. Unauthorized reproduction or usage prohibited*)

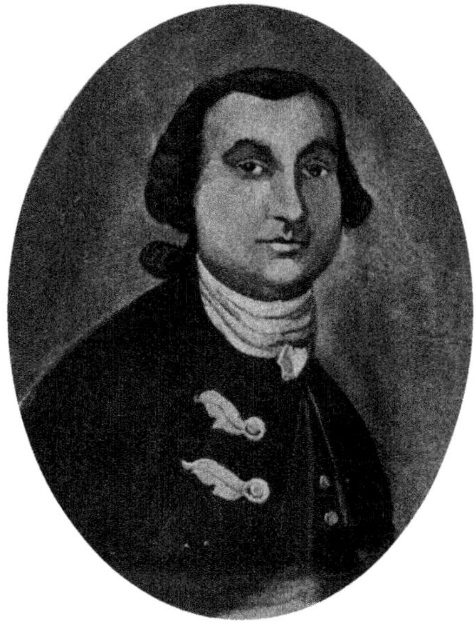

Colonel Henry Bouquet. (*Carnegie Library of Pittsburgh. All rights reserved. Unauthorized reproduction or usage prohibited*)

1763, General Jeffery Amherst, Colonel Bouquet, Captain Ecuyer, Captain William Trent, and others debated the benefit of infecting the American Indians who were threatening the fort with smallpox carried on two blankets and a handkerchief. It is from Boyd's temporary hospital the contaminated blankets and handkerchief were purportedly taken.

There is considerable debate on whether or not the plan was carried out, but sufficient evidence exists to suggest it was and it represented one of the earliest uses of biologic warfare in our country's history. At the least, epidemics of measles, smallpox, dysentery, and other diseases previously unknown to Native Americans—whether delivered through gifts or natural transmission—had a profound dilatory effect on their population.

Written between March 1765 and November 1767, an account book of a group of American Indian traders offers an interesting view of the city's population. They noted: "The little community of Fort Pitt then consisted of three blacksmiths, a minister, two brewers, a plumber for calking boats, two gunsmiths for repair of weapons, one tanner to help with furs and hides used by the community, three bakers, and five doctors."[9] The traders dealt with a wide variety of merchandise needed to satisfy both the American Indians and the military attachments assigned to the fort. Their products included furs, rum, muskets, fine linens, and "trinkets" for the Indians.

Many other recognizable names in the early history of Pittsburgh were military physicians who plied their trade in the city for a few months to many years. Dr. Arthur St. Clair served as Washington's representative on the western frontier. Dr. John Connolly served as representative of Gov. Dunmore. Dr. Edward Hand followed Hugh Mercer as Commandant of Fort Pitt and erected another temporary military hospital. Dr. William Irvine also temporarily served as Commandant of Fort Pitt.

Connolly first met Washington during his visit to Semple's tavern in 1770. At the time, he was married to the owner's daughter. Earlier, he studied medicine under Cadwallader Evans, a distinguished physician in Philadelphia. In 1773, Connolly notoriously claimed ownership of the recently abandoned Fort Pitt under the name of Lord Dunmore, the last British Governor of Virginia. He erected a stockade and took liberty in destroying much of the civic infrastructure, including dismissing and arresting local judges, discharging courts, and fostering considerable dissent among the local population as he attempted to subjugate them. Once the colonies revolted, Connolly was arrested and imprisoned until the end of the war.

In 1772, Reverend David McClure, a Presbyterian missionary to American Indians, and his associate Reverend Levi Frisbie visited Pittsburgh. Frisbie was ill, and McClure noted in his diary that Dr. Hand "attentively and gratuitously attended him during his sickness."[10] McClure's account of his visit to the city is noteworthy as it also includes a poignant description of his visit to Braddock's Field. In his diary, he wrote:

> Monday [August 31, 1772] rode to Braddock's field. This memorable spot is about 11 miles above Pittsburgh on the bank of the Monongahela. It is a gradual ascent from the bank to the top of a hill, extending about 1/4 of a mile. Up & down this Ascent the army consisting of about 1400 chosen troops were paraded, rank & file, three deep in platoons, with intervals for field pieces. They were a fatal mark for the Indians, who lay on the ground, concealed by the trees. About 1000 of the army fell; & it was not known that a single Indian was hurt. The trees in front of the army were wounded with grape shot about five feet from the ground. I got a handful of the shot from one of the trees. It was a melancholy spectacle to see the bones of men strewed over the ground, left to this day, without the solemn rite of sepulture. The fact is a disgrace to the British commanders at Fort Pitt. The bones had been gnawed by wolves, the vestiges of their teeth appearing on them. Many hundreds of skulls lay on the ground. I examined several, & found the mark of the scalping knife on all. I put one, & a jaw bone, in my portmanteau, which I afterwards presented to Mr. Stewart's Museum in Hartford. The harness of the horses remained unconsumed on the ground. A man who lives near the field of battle, & whose cornfield takes in a part of it, had humanely collected a great number of the bones & laid them in small heaps. I departed from the place with serious & solemn reflections on the vanity of life, & the deep depravity of our fallen nature, the dreadful source of fighting & war, & all the miseries that man delights to inflict on man.[11]

In the heat of battle and its aftermath, there was little that anyone could do, including physician-soldiers, to address the devastating loss of life that occurred in July 1755 when the Battle of the Monongahela was lost.

Dr. Edward Hand arrived in America as surgeon's mate of the 18th Royal Irish Regiment in 1744. He was commissioned Ensign in 1772 but subsequently resigned his commission in 1774 to practice medicine in Lancaster, Pennsylvania. At the outbreak of the Revolutionary War, Hand joined the Continental Army and was appointed colonel of the 1st Pennsylvania Regiment. Shortly afterward, he was promoted to brigadier general, and in 1777, he was given command of Fort Pitt. During Hand's stay in 1777, he developed another temporary hospital—at this point, the first federally funded hospital and the only medical institution west of the Allegheny Mountains—to confront another smallpox outbreak.

The Hand Hospital (situated in an area near the fort in what is now Crafton, Pennsylvania) was constructed by soldiers and settlers, was two stories high, and measured 30 feet by 100 feet. It contained no windows and had but two doors. The hospital served soldiers, settlers, and American Indian alike. Hand stayed at the fort for a little more than a year. Afterward, he held various higher commissions and served in the army until 1783. Between 1783 and 1784, he served as a member of the Continental Congress.

Other military physicians followed, including Drs. John Knight, George Stevenson, Andrew Richardson, and the father of Pittsburgh Medicine, Nathaniel F. Bedford. A regimental surgeon, Dr. Bedford was attached to one of the British units at Fort Pitt. He became the first university-trained physician-soldier to permanently take up residence in the city for the sole purpose of practicing medicine.

In 1781, Dr. John Rose accompanied General William Irvine as he assumed command at Fort Pitt. He had previously served as surgeon's mate in a hospital and as a surgeon in the Navy, a period of service in which he was captured but subsequently released through a prisoner exchange. Rose was appointed surgeon of the 7th Pennsylvania Regiment and served as a lieutenant and aid on General Irvine's staff. During his service with Irvine, he was assigned to accompany Colonel William Crawford on his unsuccessful "Sandusky Expedition" against the American Indians on the western front in 1782. In his official report, Irvine wrote:

> In this campaign Rose exhibited great courage in resisting the attack of the Indians and British in the disastrous battle at Sandusky. In the retreat it is said, "His cheerfulness, suavity and coolness were only equaled by his wonderful skill and intrepidity." He further added, "I must acknowledge myself ever obliged to Maj. Rose for his assistance both in the field and in the camp."[12]

William Irvine was a surgeon on a British man-of-war during the French and Indian War. Early in the Revolutionary War, he was captured in Canada and remained a prisoner from June 1776 until exchanged May 1778. He was appointed brigadier general in May 1779 and served as commandant of Fort Pitt from 1781–1783. From 1787–1788, he was a member of the Continental Congress. He returned to western Pennsylvania in 1794 as commander of the State troops during the Whiskey Rebellion.

In his *Treatise on the Prevention and Cure of Diseases*, William Buchan remarked about the special challenges of soldiers:

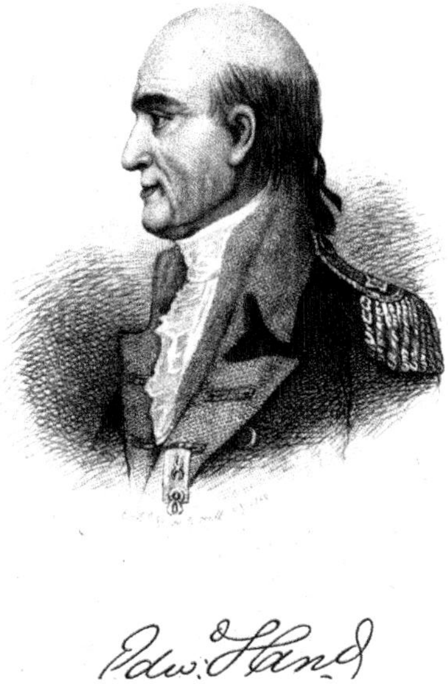

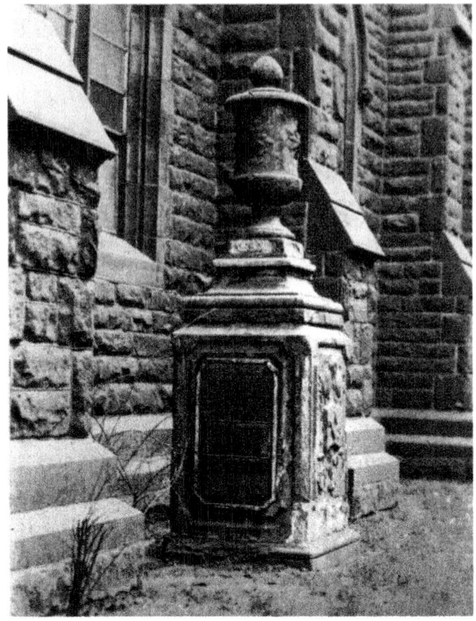

Above left: General Edward Hand. (*National Library of Medicine*)

Above right: Dr. Nathaniel Bedford monument in Trinity Cathedral Churchyard, Pittsburgh. (*Library of Congress*)

> Soldiers suffer many hardships from the inclemency of seasons, long marches, bad provisions, hunger, watching, unwholesome climates, bad water, &c. These occasion fevers, fluxes, rheumatisms, and other fatal diseases which generally do greater execution than the sword, especially when campaigns are continued too late in the season.[13]

James Gibson, in his biography of Bodo Otto, recorded many of the dire medical situations Otto observed during the Revolutionary War. He noted most wounds were caused by musket balls—round balls of about three-quarter inches in diameter. He further reported although bayonet wounds were seldom encountered, injuries from Indian clubs, knives, and hatchets were frequently seen. Gibson added:

> A soldier had ninety-eight chances out of a hundred of escaping death in battle, but the odds of his leaving a hospital alive were but seventy-five percent. The pitiful part of this greater hazard was that serious afflictions which carried men off were often contracted in the hospital where the soldiers may have gone for treatment of some simple malady.[14]

Over the previous forty years—and two devastating wars—much had been learned about the health needs of troops and citizens. Between the two groups, the military had a stronger base of medical knowledge, along with better-educated officers and physicians, and more opportunity to draw lessons from other countries and other wars than the early explorers and woodsmen of Western Pennsylvania. When the military gained knowledge, they disseminated it widely. For the astute private physician, the military offered important lessons. For example, Dr. Benjamin Rush, who served as Surgeon General of the Continental Army during the Revolution and a signer of the Declaration of Independence, published many reports on medical lessons learned during the war. His "Observations" stands out as a prime example of the lessons of war and how they could be applied to both military and public circumstances. Bodo Otto remarked on the state of affairs, and noted Rush's body of work by explaining: "Many of the patients were admitted for a 'good purging.' Dr. Benjamin Rush's observations on the sick of the Army were so full of information and suggested precautions that they were ordered published and distributed throughout the Army."[15] Some examples of his observations include:

RESULT OF OBSERVATIONS, &c.

- The army, when in tents, was always more sickly than in the open air. It was likewise more healthy when it was kept in motion, than when it lay in an encampment.
- Young men under twenty years of age were subject to the greatest number of camp diseases.
- The southern troops were more sickly than the northern or eastern troops.
- The native Americans were more sickly than the natives of Europe who served in the American army.
- Men above thirty and five and thirty years of age were the hardiest soldiers in the army.
- Those officers who wore flannel shirts or waistcoats next to their skins, in general, escaped fevers and diseases of all kinds.
- The principal diseases in the hospitals were the typhus gravior and mitior of Doctor Cullen. Men who came into the hospitals with pleurisies or rheumatisms soon lost the types of their original diseases, and suffered, or died, by the above-mentioned states of fever.
- The typhus mitior always prevailed most, and with the worst symptoms, in winter. A free air, which could only be obtained in summer, always prevented, or mitigated it.
- In all those cases, where the contagion was received, cold seldom failed to render it active. Whenever a hospital was removed in winter, one half of the patients generally sickened on the way, or soon after their arrival at the place to which they were sent.
- There were many instances of patients in this fever, who suddenly fell down dead, upon being moved, without any previous symptoms of approaching dissolution. This was more especially the case, when they arose to go to stool.
- The contagion of this fever was frequently conveyed from the hospital to the camp, by means of blankets and clothes.
- Those black soldiers who had been previously slaves died in a greater proportion by this fever, or had a much slower recovery from it, than the same number of white soldiers.

- The remedies which appeared to do most service in this disease were vomits of tartar emetic, gentle dozes of laxative salts, bark, wine, volatile salt, opium, and blisters.
- Hospitals built of coarse logs, with ground floors, with fire-places in the middle of them, and a hole in the roof, for the discharge of smoke, were found to be very conducive to the recovery of the soldiers from the hospital fever.
- In fevers and dysenteries, those soldiers recovered most certainly, and most speedily, who lay at the greatest distance from the walls of the hospitals.
- Hospitals are the sinks of human life in an army. They robbed the United States of more citizens than the sword.[16]

Like the pioneers, physician-soldiers had little initial knowledge of the illnesses and diseases encountered in the endless wilderness of the western frontier. On the frontier, often with little recourse other than individual ingenuity, they learned quickly, but it was the physician-soldiers who documented and transmitted their experiences with much greater effect. They were also quick to sense opportunity, and they seized it as they established themselves as the region's earliest permanent physicians.

The history of these pioneer physician-soldiers continues to evolve as researchers discover new sources of authoritative information. French physician-soldiers who were present in colonial Pittsburgh are not accounted for in this work as it is constructed from a predominantly British-American perspective. With that caveat noted, the story of the physician-soldiers who stayed, those who returned, and those who subsequently entered the city to establish a civilian practice with both military and medical credentials is a captivating tale.

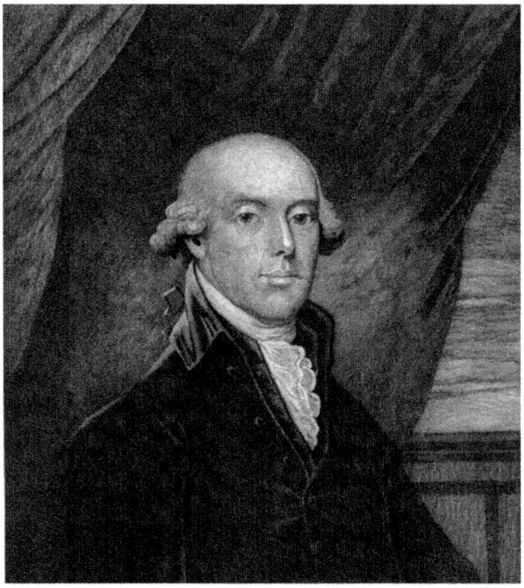

Dr. Benjamin Rush. (*Library of Congress*)

4

Pittsburgh's First Resident Physicians

As the Revolutionary War drew to a close, members of the Continental Congress wrestled with the issue of how to make good on the back pay owed to thousands of American soldiers. Once a decision was rendered to offer grants of unsettled lands on the western frontier, commerce in Pittsburgh roared back to life. Over the previous several years of war, much of the American Indian trade that had made Pittsburgh a fast-growing city was diminished, along with the number of residents who called the city home. That changed abruptly once the land grants were issued. Pittsburgh was now both a destination and a gateway. The first new residents came as traders supplying goods and materials needed by those heading west. Since the city was the last major stopover where settlers could rest and stock up on supplies before embarking on their journey, business was lucrative. Not all new residents were traders or craftsmen. Many were army veterans who had previously been stationed in the city.

Nathaniel Bedford, as previously noted, was one such military officer. He established his medical practice on Seventh Street sometime around 1765. Bedford married Jane Ormsby, the daughter of John Ormsby, a prominent local businessman. Upon his wife's death, Bedford inherited property in the Birmingham section of the city. He is recognized for developing the early design of the area and for naming "Carson Street" after an old friend. On Christmas day 1779, Bedford unsuccessfully treated Shawnee Chief Mio-Qua-Coo-Na-Caw (Red Pole) while the Chief was being detained by the military. Both the Chief and Bedford are buried, side-by-side, on the grounds of Trinity Church in downtown Pittsburgh.

Graduating with a medical degree from the University of Edinburgh, Arthur Lee visited Pittsburgh in 1784 traveling as a government emissary "to treat with the Indians." During his visit, he observed: "There are here four attorneys, two doctors and not a priest of any persuasion, nor church, nor chapel, so that they are likely to be damned without the benefit of the clergy." He added: "The place I believe

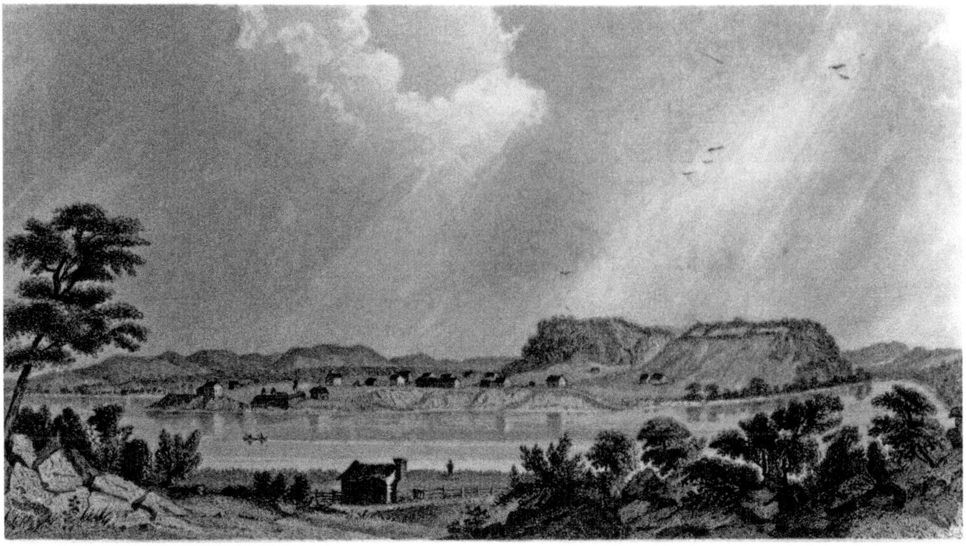

First sketch of Pittsburgh, 1790. (*Carnegie Library of Pittsburgh. All rights reserved. Unauthorized reproduction or usage prohibited*)

will never be any considerable."[1] While his prediction for the city was incorrect, his observation about the number of physicians in residence was seemingly accurate. Nathaniel Bedford was one of the physicians; the other most likely was Dr. Thomas Parker. Bedford and Parker were among the original trustees of the Pittsburgh Academy upon its founding in 1787. Today it is known as the University of Pittsburgh.

Dr. John Knight enlisted in a Virginia regiment in 1776. He was appointed surgeon of the 7th Pennsylvania Regiment in August 1778 and posted at Fort Pitt. In 1782, he joined Col. William Crawford's mission against the Indians. The Sandusky Expedition (Crawford's defeat) was launched on 25 May 1782 to end American Indian attacks on settlers on the western frontier (Pontiac's War). Crawford was defeated in a devastating battle near Sandusky, Ohio, during which Knight and others were separated from their retreating comrades. After wandering the woods for two days, the group was discovered on June 7; a number had been killed, and the rest, including Knight, were taken captive. Beatings, torture, and long marches followed their capture, but luck was with Knight, and after suffering severely, he escaped. Knight eventually made it back to Fort Pitt, arriving with much fanfare on 04 July 1782. Upon recovery, he continued his service as a surgeon at the fort until the end of the war in 1783. In 1788, Dr. McKenzie, the principal surgeon at Fort Pitt, appointed Dr. Knight as surgeon's mate.

During this period in Pittsburgh's medical history, many physicians were also apothecaries. John Russel Twiss, in his study of medical practices in colonial America, noted: "The doctor had to be his own pharmacist. He made his own pills and

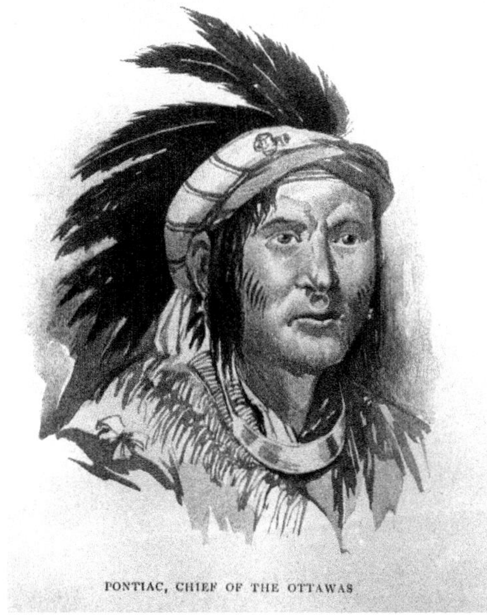

Chief Pontiac. (*Library of Congress*)

tinctures, compounded all his medicines, and generally carried all he required, as, with saddle bags across his horse, he wended his way from house to house."[2] Drs. Bedford and Richardson are recorded as selling products like "Asthmatic Elixir, Glauber's Salts, Huxham's Tincture of Bark, Mercurial Pills, and licorice juice" at their store, while other items like "Doctor Anderson's famous Scotch pills," and "Old Robert Turlington's original balsam of life" were available from other local purveyors.[3]

Bedford's legacy to medicine in Pittsburgh was Dr. Peter Mowry, the first documented physician to receive medical training in the city. Mowry began training as an apprentice under Bedford at the age of fourteen, "to be taught the science and art of medicine and surgery," and eventually established himself as the preeminent physician in the city.[4] He advised hospital experience as the best method of gaining skill as a physician at a time when there were no hospitals west of the Allegheny Mountains. He is remembered for his unwavering commitment to teaching and professing to his students that in medicine they were assuming great responsibility. In this regard, he was an outspoken critic of "irregular" medical practices, and he warned: "God help the Quacks who with little impudence rush in where conscientious men fear to enter."[5] Mowry died at the age of sixty-three, leaving two sons who both became physicians.

His nephew, Robert Bruce Mowry, studied medicine under him and subsequently graduated from Jefferson Medical College in 1836. Taking his uncle's advice, he became one of the first physicians named to the medical staff of Western Pennsylvania Hospital upon its opening in 1853. In 1882, he was one of the original incorporators of Allegheny General Hospital.

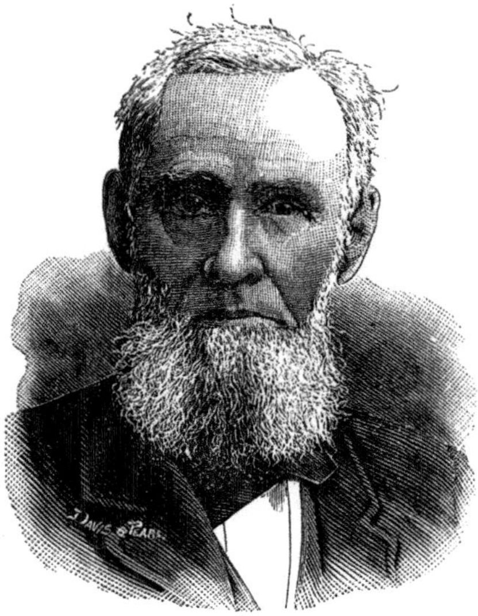

Dr. Robert Bruce Mowry. (*Cities of Pittsburgh and Allegheny and Their Resources, Souvenir of the Pittsburgh Chronicle Telegraph, 1889*)

In 1786, it was reported there were only about three-dozen homes and five small businesses in the city. In 1800, the city's population had grown to almost 1,600 residents. Between 1794 and 1797, author Thomas Davis, using ferry records to document their presence, reported two other physicians present in the city. These were Drs. Adams and Wilkins.[6] No other details about them have emerged, so their stay in the city may not have been long.

Dr. George Stevenson was another physician-soldier who served during the Revolutionary War. He saw action at the Battle of Brandywine and spent a memorable winter with Washington at Valley Forge. In 1794, he arrived in Pittsburgh with the contingent of troops sent by Washington to quell the Whiskey Rebellion. Stevenson became so enamored with the local area he resigned his commission and set up a medical practice.

In 1807, records indicate there were four physicians in the area, including Drs. Bedford, Richardson, Stevenson, and Mowry. Dr. Edward Pennington began practice in the city shortly afterward, and in 1814, a Dr. Brainard also started a practice in the area.

James Riddle published the first city directory in 1815; it lists eight physicians. Of the eight, four had served in the military or had training directly attributable to military physicians. The three most notable physicians were Drs. Joel Lewis, Peter Mowry, and George Stevenson. The other five physicians were either transient or more interested in the profitable business of compounding drugs. Drs. George Dawson, Morrell Parker, and Frederick Aigster noted their penchant for the drug business in their directory listings.

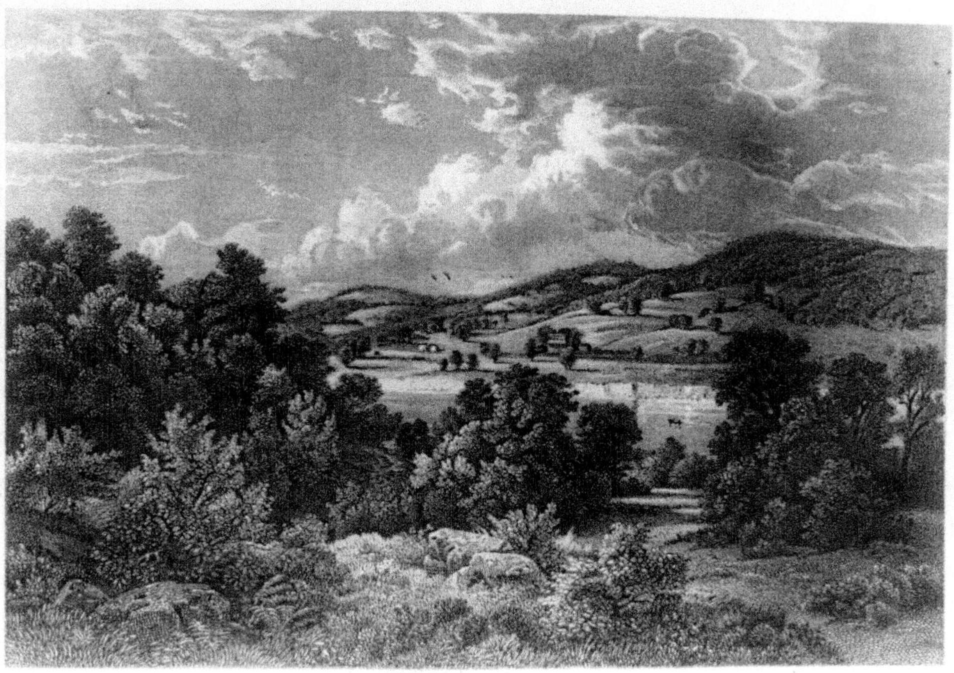

Braddock's field site and scene of meeting of the Whiskey Rebels. (*Library of Congress*)

Mowry and Stevenson's roles with the military have already been detailed. Lewis's connection to the military began around 1822 when he was named brigadier general of the Pennsylvania Militia. During the same year, he was elected president of the Pittsburgh Medical Society, which had only been founded the previous year. His death in 1824 cut short an extremely promising career.

In 1818, Drs. James Agnew and William Simpson formed a partnership to practice medicine. Shortly afterward, they opened a drug and medicinal warehouse at the corner of Wood and Third Streets. In 1819, they advertised: "...they will sell genuine drugs and medicines, wholesale and retail, also patent medicines."[7] Sometime after 1819, Dr. Agnew formed another partnership, this time with Dr. Dimitt. Dimitt is credited with being the first physician west of the Allegheny Mountains to inoculate using Edward Jenner's turn-of-the-century smallpox vaccination procedure.

The next widely available city directory arrived in 1826. Published by S. Jones, it includes entries for sixteen physicians. A little over a decade later, in 1837, Isaac Harris published the next city directory. This directory indicates there were fifty-six physicians in the city. A number of these were also connected to the military by training or service.

One retired physician, Dr. Felix Brunot, was included in the 1837 directory. He had arrived in Pittsburgh in 1797, after living in Philadelphia since the end of the Revolutionary War. Brunot, a foster brother of the Marquis de Lafayette, had

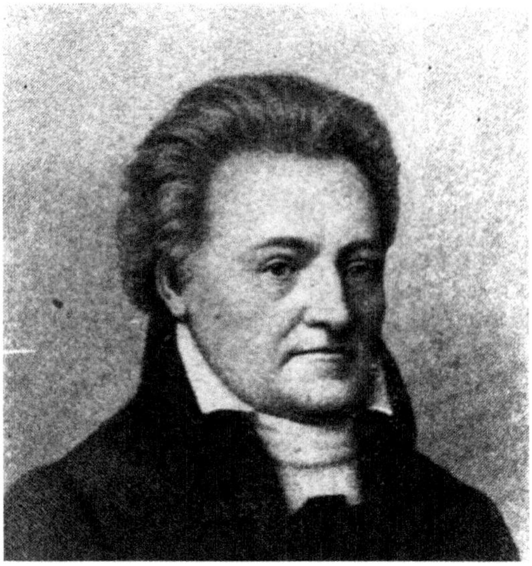

Dr. Felix Brunot, friend of La Fayette and father of Felix R. Brunot. (*Carnegie Library of Pittsburgh. All rights reserved. Unauthorized reproduction or usage prohibited*)

served as a military surgeon with our French Army allies during the war. Brunot is recognized as the first physician in the area to experiment with the therapeutic uses of electricity and is perhaps best known for the island on the Ohio River that still bears his name (Brunot Island).

The industrialization of the city, which began during the early 1800s, brought with it steady increases in the population. As the population grew, so did the city's health problems. There were some enlightened members of the community who helped form associations to endorse sanitary reform and regulation, and others who promoted the adoption of progressive medical care. Among the latter was a small group who formed one of Pittsburgh's earliest medical associations, the Pittsburgh Medical Society, in 1821.

The most prominent physicians practicing in Pittsburgh in 1837 were William Addison, George Bruce, Thomas E. Dale, Martin R. Delany, Joseph Gazzam, Sheply R. Holmes, William F. Irwin, J. H. Irwin, Robert B. Mowry, and Henry D. Sellers. Several of these physicians would subsequently play leading roles in transforming medical care in the city.

In 1842, Dr. Albert G. Walter arrived from Germany to establish a surgical practice that by many estimates was one of the most exemplary in the late 1800s. Born in 1811, Walter was orphaned at an early age and benefitted from the foresight and benevolence of a religious-minded guardian. After receiving his primary education, he studied medicine at the University of Berlin at a time when new surgical discoveries for correcting deformities were regularly advancing. A professor recommended he move to America to put the surgical techniques he had learned to use in a country with less competition and a great deal more opportunity. Before arriving in America, Walter spent a year studying at the Royal College of Surgeons in London. In Pittsburgh, he found a perfect match for his skills as the city's

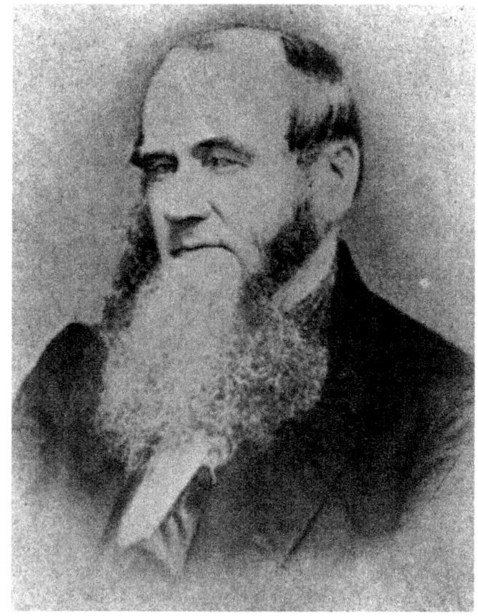

Dr. Joseph Gazzam. (*Allegheny County Medical Society*)

manufacturing plants were generating ever-growing numbers of accident victims whose injuries benefited from Walter's "corrective" surgical techniques.

In 1846, Walter married Frances Ann Butler, the daughter of Major John B. Butler, military storekeeper of the United States Arsenal in Lawrenceville, Pennsylvania. As his career in Pittsburgh matured, Walter became disillusioned with the poor state of corrective surgery available in the city. In response, he opened a proprietary hospital on Boyd's Hill near the Pittsburgh Court House. Over the years, he spent a great deal of time writing, particularly as it related to "conservative" surgery.[8] He was also known for collecting specimens of his work, from which a museum was created. The collection would ultimately reside in the Western Pennsylvania Medical College, Pittsburgh's first medical school when it opened in 1886.

Walter's progressive approach to general surgery is noteworthy. A dramatic example of his work was reported in *The Pittsburgh Medical Review* in 1890. The journal article read:

> Dr. A. G. Walter, of this city; a man whose services to the profession have never been properly recognized; among other contributions which he has made to surgery was the opening of the abdominal cavity, in a case of a ruptured bladder. In 1862, when there was no precedent for such a procedure, he boldly cut open the abdomen, washed out the peritoneal cavity, and drained the bladder by a catheter retained in the urethra. His patient recovered. This operation was not repeated until eighteen years later, but is now recognized as the proper treatment for such an injury.[9]

Walter did not have a military background; however, during and after the Civil War, he treated many soldiers. He was among the surgeons who set out from the city

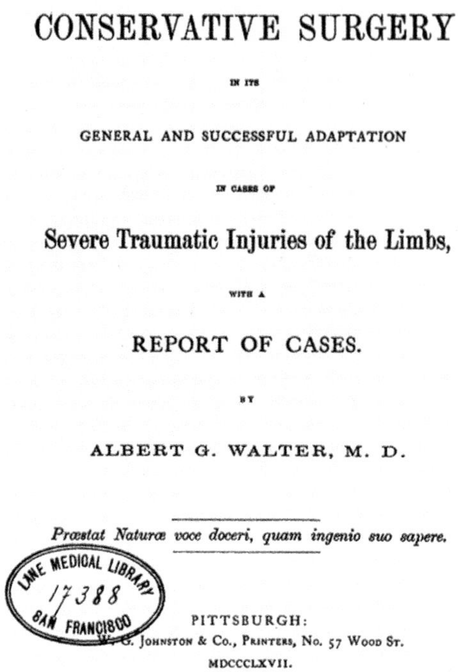

CONSERVATIVE SURGERY

IN ITS

GENERAL AND SUCCESSFUL ADAPTATION

IN CASES OF

Severe Traumatic Injuries of the Limbs,

WITH A

REPORT OF CASES.

BY

ALBERT G. WALTER, M. D.

Præstat Naturæ voce doceri, quam ingenio suo sapere.

PITTSBURGH:
W. G. JOHNSTON & CO., PRINTERS, NO. 57 WOOD ST.
MDCCCLXVII.

Title page of Albert G. Walter's 1867 *Conservative Surgery* book. (*Google Books*)

to provide care and comfort to soldiers wounded during the Battle of Gettysburg. His service to veterans was considered remarkable, his courage and work long remembered by the Grand Army of the Republic.

In the first half of the nineteenth century, citizens of Pittsburgh were impacted by the growing national distrust of professionals and learning nurtured by Andrew Jackson and his followers. In the midst of "Jacksonian democracy," the rights and status of the common man were manifest, and self-sufficiency in all things, including government, business, and medicine, were vigorously embraced. While it is true that Pittsburgh's citizens were always willing to consider the relative value of competing groups of medical practitioners—particularly when there was more than one choice available—this new wave of questioning opened the floodgates to a diverse range of medical messiahs in the city. Over a period of several decades, Pittsburgh's population gained many new choices in how their medical needs could be addressed. Thomsonians, homeopaths, eclectics, hydrotherapists, phrenologists, and many other "irregular" sects openly competed with traditional "regular" allopathic physicians. So too did the bleeders, cuppers, patent medicine purveyors, and galvanizers. Until the end of the Civil War, medical chaos reigned.

While many of the "irregulars" had success in the city—and many practitioners had a military background—it was the homeopaths that had the greatest long-term impact. In homeopathy, Pittsburgh's citizens found, many for the first time,

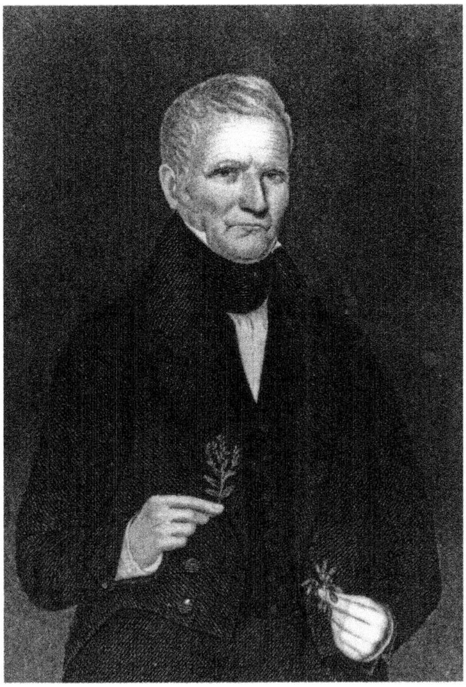

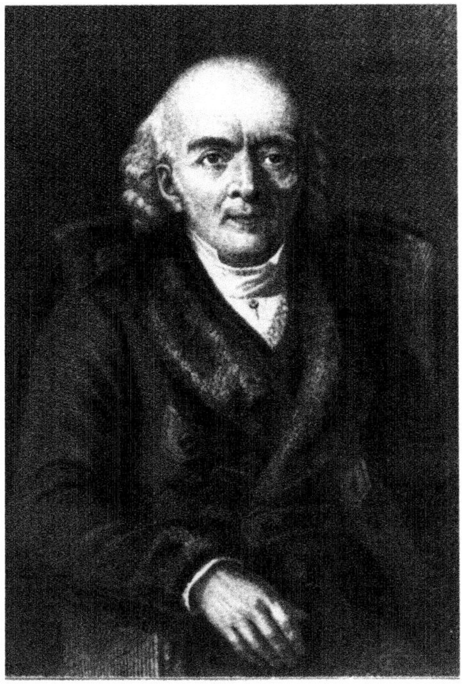

Above left: Samuel Thomson, founder of the Thomsonian system of medicine. (*National Library of Medicine*)

Above right: Samuel Hahnemann, founder of homeopathy. (*National Library of Medicine*)

practitioners "who took a holistic approach to their care by recording a lengthy patient history and detailing all their complaints and symptoms before prescribing a course of therapy."[10] They used drugs in individually calculated and highly diluted doses to produce physiologic or pathologic effects similar to those of the disease being treated. In other words, their treatment revolved around a belief that "like cures like." In contrast to the polypharmacological approach espoused by the allopaths and their "opposite suffering" mode of care, the homeopaths were typically considered less invasive, more caring, and considerably less costly.

Homeopathy first came to Pittsburgh with the arrival of Dr. Gustavus Reichhelm in October 1837. While there is no record of Reichhelm serving in the military, many of the city's other leading homeopaths were engaged in military service. Their backgrounds will be described in a subsequent chapter.

In 1864, Pittsburgh's homeopaths joined together to form the Homeopathic Medical Society of Allegheny County. With their special position in society and their livelihoods under threat, the city's allopathic physicians banded together to form the Allegheny County Medical Society four months later. At the time, Pittsburgh was served by three hospitals. All were aligned with allopathic physicians, and none

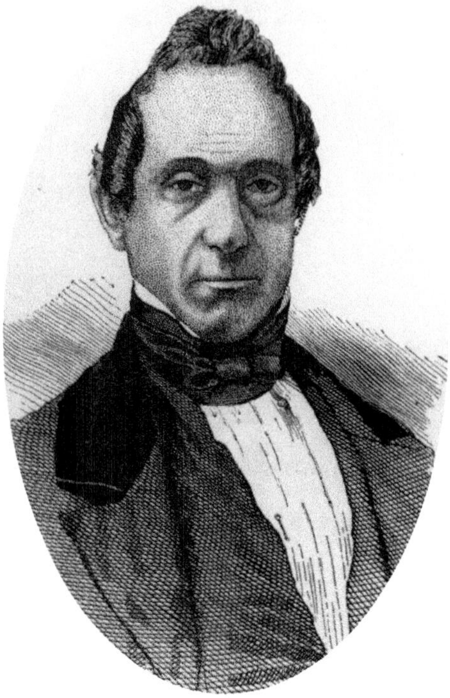

Gustavus Reichhelm, Pittsburgh's first homeopathic physician. (*Semi-Centennial Celebration of the Introduction of Homeopathy West of the Allegheny Mountains, 1887*)

would allow homeopaths to admit patients. In 1866, circumstances would change when the city's homeopaths received financial support from wealthy patrons to build a hospital of their own—the Homeopathic Medical and Surgical Hospital and Dispensary of Pittsburgh (now Shadyside Hospital).

Dr. L. Callahan arrived in the city sometime in the late 1820s. He became an outspoken champion of strict enforcement of sanitary measures in the city. In 1827, after joining the Pittsburgh Medical Society, he presented a paper on fevers. He suggested the cause stemmed from poor sanitary practices. In part, he stated:

> In the first place, I would ask the medical philosopher whether or not he has ever seen pure typhus fever prevail as an epidemic where the exciting and predisposing causes were not present on the spot, either in the surrounding atmosphere, the habitudes of the people, their regimen, or the privations to which they are exposed?[11]

In 1827, Dr. James R. Speer, a member of the homeopathic medical society, performed the earliest recorded cataract operation in the city. His patient, Frederick Albright, recovered with perfect sight, which significantly enhanced Dr. Speers' reputation. In 1835, he opened one of Pittsburgh's first temporary private hospitals, the "Eye Infirmary." The practice of physicians opening proprietary hospitals was to recur several times throughout the remainder of the nineteenth century.

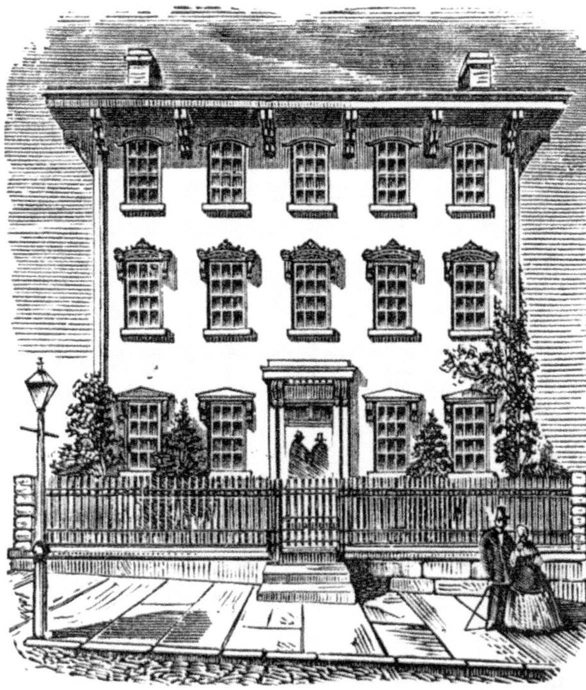

Right: Pittsburgh Homeopathic Hospital and Dispensary in 1876. (*Pittsburgh's Homeopathic Experience, 1991*)

Below left: Marcellus Cote, M.D., founder of Pittsburgh Homeopathic Hospital. (*Carnegie Library of Pittsburgh. All rights reserved. Unauthorized reproduction or usage prohibited*)

Below right: Dr. James Ramsey Speer. (*Carnegie Library of Pittsburgh. All rights reserved. Unauthorized reproduction or usage prohibited*)

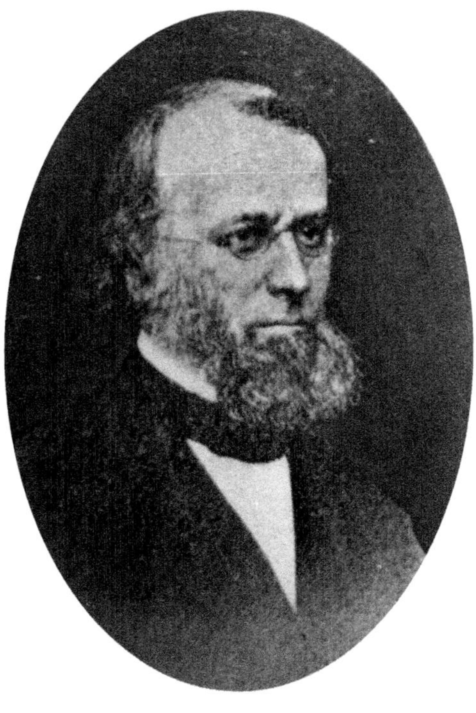

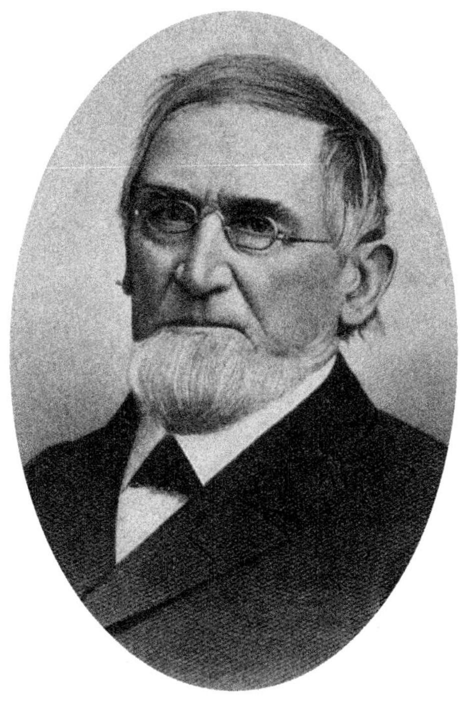

5

Civilian Health Activists and the Genesis of Professional Medical Organizations

Care of the Insane

Providing care for the insane was a major issue in early Pittsburgh. Typically, individuals suffering from mental health issues were cared for within the immediate family circle. If the family were not available to provide such care, those afflicted with mental illness often found their way into the local almshouses, poor farms, or other places that provided for the indigent. Frequently, they ended up in jail.

As hospitals began to emerge in the late 1840s, providing care for the insane challenged public notions on who should be eligible for care and how such care should be provided. The expense of delivering care was also cause for ongoing debate.

The arrival of Dorothea Lynde Dix in the city in August 1844 changed everything. At the time, Dix was recognized as one of the country's earliest crusaders for improving the care of the mentally ill. Dix was visiting cities across the country to study how the insane were cared for and under what conditions. During her stay in Pittsburgh, she visited a number of the city's public institutions. In her diary, she noted:

> Allegheny County Jail
>
> This jail combines all the faults and abuses of the worst county prisons in this state or in the United States. Hoping to find something redeeming in its earlier discipline and government, I deliberately and patiently entered upon investigation, but the nature of the revelations these inquiries brought to light, obliged me to relinquish the work to those whose more immediate duty it is to bring about a reformation. The prison was built in view of the separate imprisonment, classification, and employment of offenders; instead of which, I found transgressors of all ages, colours, sexes and degrees, promiscuously associated; little boys listening greedily to gray-headed, time and crime-hardened convicts; the youthful transgressor learning new lessons of iniquity, from those whose vices only kept pace with their crimes; here the sick were unattended, the

> ignorant untaught, the repentant (if any) unencouraged, and the insane forgotten. If it had been the deliberate purpose of the citizens of Allegheny county to establish a school for the inculcation of vice, and obliteration of every virtue, I cannot conceive that any means they could have devised, would more certainly have secured these results, than those I found in full operation in the jail last August.[1]
>
> Pittsburg: the Orphans' Asylum
> The Orphans' Asylum situated in Allegheny city, is a charity which rescues many unprotected children from early crime, and saves some from the jail. This institution, so creditable to those who support it, and to the good matron who directs it is well ordered throughout.[2]
>
> Pittsburg Poor House
> The Poor-house of Pittsburg, soon to be replaced by a more commodious establishment, is also in Allegheny city. I found it comfortably arranged, and neat. The two insane of the fifteen inmates, were kindly looked after. The entire number of epileptics, insane and idiotic in this county, was computed to be not less than seventy-five, and might be more. Allegheny County has no poor-house, but the poor in most of the townships are distributed as is customary in other counties.[3]
>
> Western Penitentiary
> Of the Western Penitentiary, I shall speak elsewhere; but I cannot refrain from saying here, that it is one of the most excellently governed prisons I have ever visited. I took sufficient time to see all the prisoners, and to learn the whole state of the institution. Here, as is universal in the state prisons, are found the insane and imbecile. Some were so when committed, and in others, the disease has been developed in prison.[4]

Her report stunned the citizens of Pittsburgh. The newspapers were rife with editorials condemning and applauding Miss Dix's assertions. The outcome of the myriad conversations and committees formed to study the situation was a public meeting called by Mayor William J. Howard on 22 November 1845. A resolution providing for the revival of the Western Pennsylvania Hospital Society and the appointment of a committee to study fundraising possibilities and a potential site for a mental hospital was approved.

Not long after her visit, Dix petitioned the Pennsylvania House of Representatives for a "state hospital for the insane." She noted in her solicitation she had traveled for months across the state visiting poor houses, jails, and prisons. In the opening paragraphs of her report, she wrote:

> Gentlemen:
> I come to represent to you the condition of a numerous and unhappy class of sufferers, who fill the cells and dungeons of the poor houses, and the prisons of your state. I refer

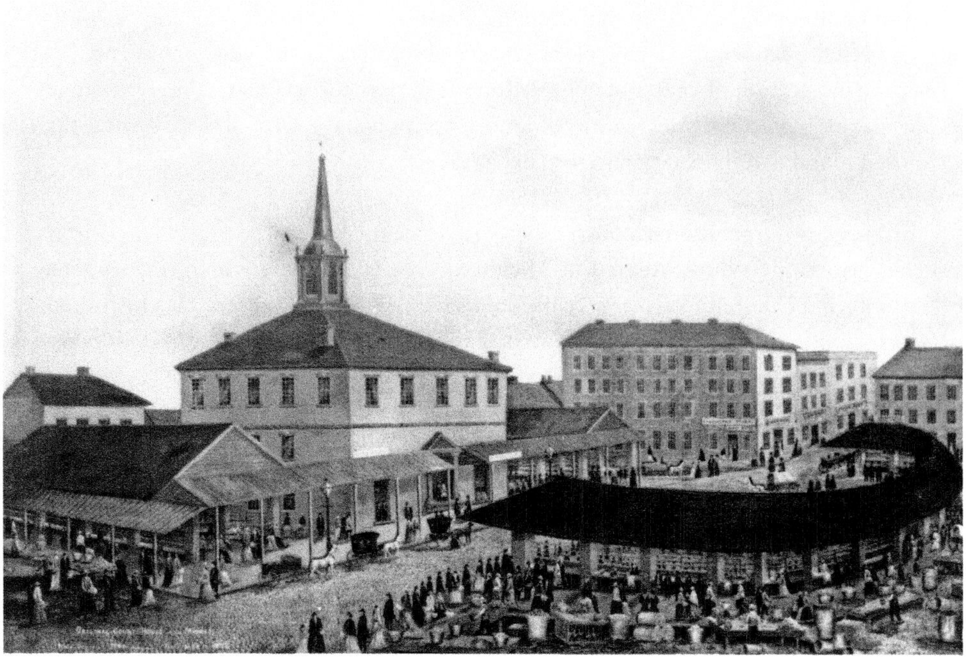

Pittsburgh's first courthouse, jail, and marketplace. (*Carnegie Library of Pittsburgh. All rights reserved. Unauthorized reproduction or usage prohibited*)

> to the pauper and indigent insane, epileptics, and idiots of Pennsylvania. I come to urge their claims upon the commonwealth for protection and support, such protection and support as is only to be found in a well conducted Lunatic Asylum.
>
> I do not solicit you to be generous; this is an occasion rather for the dispensation of justice. These most unfortunate beings have claims, those claims which bitter misery and adversity creates, and which it is your solemn obligation as citizens and legislators to cancel. To this end, as the advocate of those who are disqualified by a terrible malady, from pleading their own cause, I ask you to provide for the immediate establishment of a State Hospital for the Insane.[5]

As noted, the immediate result of her report was the revival of the Western Pennsylvania Hospital Society, which tasked itself with addressing the city's mental health situation. The outcome of the Society's work concluded with the incorporation of the Western Pennsylvania Hospital in 1848, and later in 1861, the creation of Dixmont Hospital for the Insane.

Dix subsequently met periodically with members of the Western Pennsylvania Hospital board of managers as they struggled to provide adequate care for the city's insane. She supported their efforts by providing counsel on best practices and corresponded frequently with the board's officers about levels and settings of care. She was also a determined fundraiser, and her solicitation efforts with the Pennsylvania State Legislature routinely proved critical to the hospital's ongoing financial viability. A newspaper account of one of her visits in 1857, stated:

> Miss Dix, the philanthropist, who has devoted her talents and her energies, for many years past, to the amelioration of the condition of insane persons in hospitals, prisoners in jails and paupers in poor houses, is now in our city, the guest of Mr. Langdon, at the Western Pennsylvania Hospital. On Friday [10 July 1857], she visited the City Poor Farm and inspected the recent purchase of the Trustees of the Hospital from an Insane Asylum. She will remain in the city for a portion of the present week. This lady has by her personal exertions and influence, procured grants in aid of insane institutions and hospitals, from Legislatures of several States, and influenced large private subscriptions towards the same noble charities.[6]

Dix would eventually receive credit for motivating Pittsburgh's citizens to create her namesake hospital in the city: Dixmont Hospital for the Insane. Her work inspired action and her visits and consultations with the board of managers of the Western Pennsylvania Hospital determined its physical location.

Stimulating action in support of the insane—in Pittsburgh and other cities in the State and across the county—was not her only act of leadership. During the Civil War, Dix is credited with almost singlehandedly changing nursing care from a secondary thought to a necessary and crucial ingredient for recovery of sick and wounded soldiers on the battlefields and in military hospitals.

Secretary of War Simon Cameron and Acting Surgeon General D. C. Wood named Dix Superintendent of Women Nurses on 10 June 1861. Her appointment, however, did not negatively affect the ongoing use of Catholic nuns. They were already highly valued in military circles since they worked virtually for free, they were quiet, and they were obedient. Their numbers, however, were not sufficient to meet the growing need of the military, particularly early in the war, that was producing sick and wounded soldiers at an alarming rate.

Along with the title came an immense challenge, as Dix was then responsible for recruiting, selecting, and assigning women nurses to virtually all of the Union's military hospitals. By nature, Dix was strong spirited and determined to elevate the skills, stature, and purview of nurses, often to the chagrin of military officials. Due principally to the friction between Dix, military officers, and hospital physicians, her tenure as superintendent lasted only until the fall of 1863. The War Department issued General Order No. 351 giving Surgeon General Joseph K. Barnes the same authority as Dix, effectively relieving her of operational responsibilities. Nonetheless, over the two-year period, she was able to recruit, train, and place approximately 3,000 nurses. From that point forward, the hiring of qualified nurses became the rule rather than the exception in hospitals—both military and civilian—across the country.

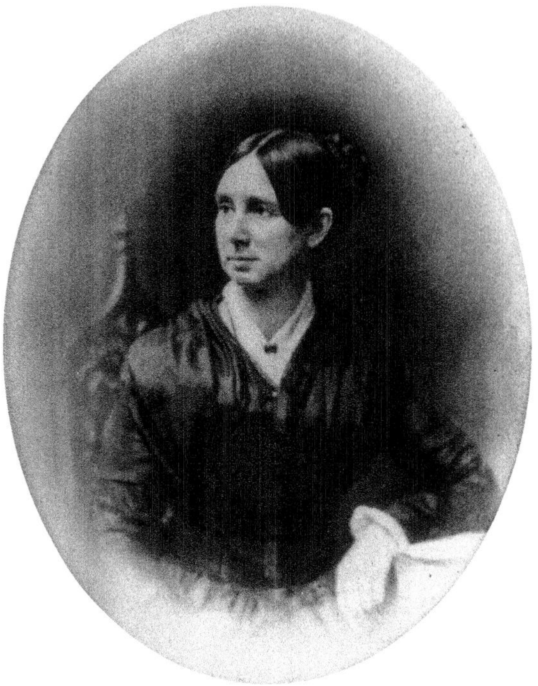

Dorothea L. Dix. (*National Library of Medicine*)

The Genesis of Pittsburgh's Professional Medical Organizations

In the first half of the 1800s, Pittsburgh's physicians remained an eclectic group. Many had been trained through apprenticeship, and some had attended medical school in Europe. Fewer still attended one of the few university-based medical schools that had developed in the eastern United States. With no medical school in Pittsburgh until 1886, another way early nineteenth-century physicians became informed on the latest medicines, treatments, and procedures was through membership in professional medical societies. As these groups emerged intermittently between 1814 and the end of the Civil War, the names of physicians with direct or indirect military experience are always found among the originators and earliest members.

One of the first to form was the Western Medical Society in 1814.[7] Little is known about the organization except that it was short-lived. Another professional organization operating in the city at the time was the Pittsburgh Chemical and Physiological Society. While not focused on medicine, members of the medical profession participated in its meetings—if not as members, then as lecturers.[8]

The next to form was the Pittsburgh Medical Society in 1821. This society survived a bit longer as it was last mentioned in 1829.[9] Members of this society were a close-knit group and represented most, if not all of the physicians practicing in the city at the time. Little is known of their work except they united together in

May 1822 to petition the city to purchase "an apparatus for the resuscitation of persons who had been partially drowned."[10] The years between 1829 and 1848 are devoid of any references to professional medical societies.

Another society was born in August 1848, repeating the pattern. The new society was named the Allegheny Medical Society, but it too would not last long. Its membership of thirty-nine in 1854, however, indicates there were more than twice as many physicians now resident in the city than there were in 1826. After 1854, there is no discernable evidence of any medical societies operating in the city until late in the Civil War.

One explanation for the disappearance of medical societies may be that the prospects of war in the early 1860s preoccupied everyone's attention. There were other pressing civic matters that required the attention of physicians and layman.

The first societies to emerge near war's end were the Pittsburgh Homeopathic Medical Society and the Nathaniel Bedford Society. The Homeopathic Society was formed on 09 December 1864. As the name implies, the group was devoted to advancing the cause and practice of homeopathy. Two years after forming the society, its members were among the founders of the Pittsburgh Homeopathic Medical and Surgical Hospital (which later became Shadyside Hospital).

The Nathaniel Bedford Society was also initiated in 1864. Its purpose was principally to provide professional enrichment and social interaction. Neither its design nor its aspirations allowed it to grow substantially over the years. Among its leaders, however, were Drs. Robert B. Mowry and David N. Rankin, both of whom were leading advocates for the creation of a medical school in Pittsburgh. It would take almost twenty years for their efforts to be effective, as Western Pennsylvania Medical College would be chartered in June 1883, with the school's doors opening in 1886. Around the time the medical school opened, the Bedford Society ceased operating with its members forming the nucleus of the Pittsburgh Academy of Medicine upon its formation in 1888.

Pittsburgh's mainstream physicians, many of whom had recently returned from war service, did not take long to act in creating a new medical society once the war ended. In less than two weeks after Lee's surrender, the city's allopathic physicians came together to create the Allegheny County Medical Society. As demonstrated by its continued existence today, the outcome was different this time.

The driving force in organizing the new society was Dr. H. T. Coffee. Shortly after he called a planning meeting to order at the Pittsburgh Board of Trade Rooms, on 20 April 1865, the society was formed, its officer's elected, and formal plans for the organization initiated. Founding members included many of the leading physicians in the city at the time, including a significant number who served in the war as regular or volunteer surgeons, or as members of volunteer medical teams that treated sick and wounded soldiers on both the battlefront and in the city. The inaugural group of members included A. H. Gross; D. W. Lewis; A. J. Davis; H. Neal; J. H. Grouard; M. R. Trevor; R. B. Mowry; George M. Maclean; A. Fleming; George L. McCook;

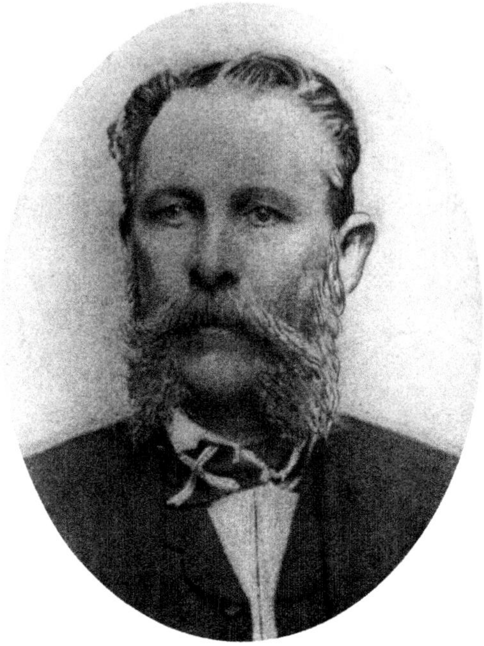

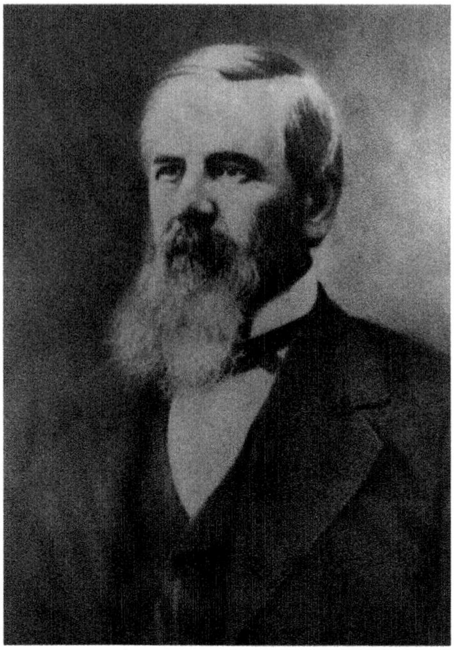

Above left: A. H. Gross, M.D., first president of the Allegheny County Medical Society. (*Carnegie Library of Pittsburgh. All rights reserved. Unauthorized reproduction or usage prohibited*)

Above right: James King, M.D. (*Allegheny County Medical Society*)

N. McDonald; A. H. Achenbach; Thos. J. Gallaher; B. C. Jillson; S. N. Benham; H. T. Coffee; M. O. Jones; James King; and William F. Knox.

At this point, with the war settled, the nation began the process of reconstruction and healing, both metaphorically and physically. The physicians, nurses, and volunteer medical support teams that returned to the Pittsburgh represented a cathartic harbinger of change. Medical care delivery in the city would never be the same.

Patriotism and Volunteer Support during the Civil War Period

Three days after the Confederates fired on Fort Sumter, President Lincoln called for the formation of a 75,000-man militia to serve for three months. Believing the war could be suppressed in short order, his call was quickly answered in Pittsburgh, as were subsequent calls for the "second requisition" of 03 May 1861, and "third requisition" of 02 July 1862. On 15 April 1861, the day of Lincoln's initial call to arms, a mass meeting of the citizens of Pittsburgh was organized. The meeting was held at City Hall, where a range of patriotic resolutions supporting the Union was adopted, including the creation of a Committee of Public Safety "to see that

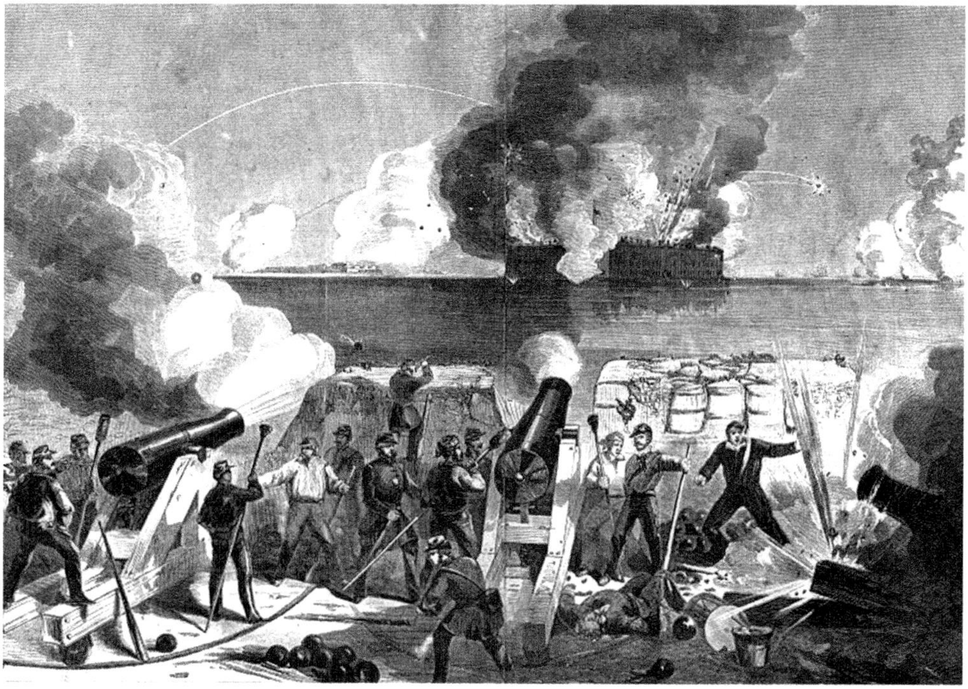

Above: Bombardment of Fort Sumter by the batteries of the Confederate states April 13, 1861. (*Library of Congress*)

Right: Abraham Lincoln, President of the United States. (*Library of Congress*)

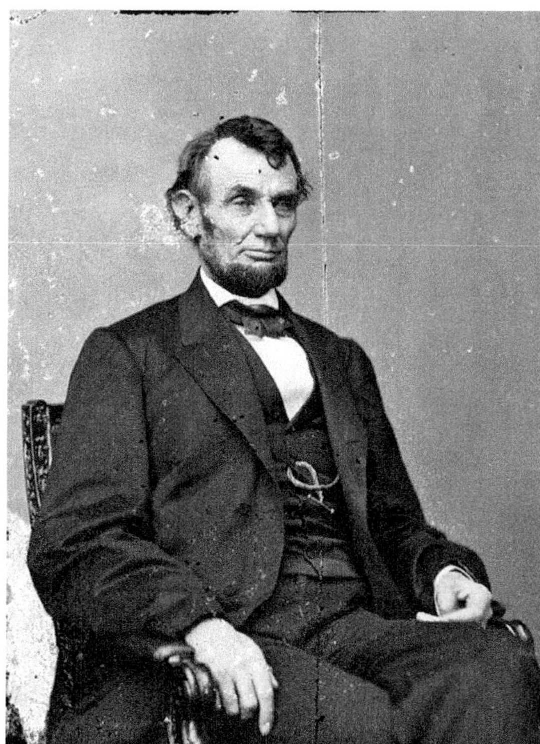

the patriot cause receives no detriment in this region, and to convene the people whenever in their judgment such a step is necessary."[11]

On 18 April 1861, the first organized meeting of the Committee of Public Safety took place, during which three subcommittees were formed. They included the Executive, Finance, and Home Defense committees. Initially, the three subcommittees worked clandestinely to reduce the possibility of their work informing southern sympathizers then working in the city to support the Confederacy through intelligence gathering and transmission of contraband materials.

One of the very first efforts of the subcommittees was the creation of the "Home Guards," to serve as a foundation for volunteer military recruitment in the city. Two days after the first meeting at City Hall, recruitment began. In less than two weeks, twenty-six companies had been formed with many already on their way to the front. By 02 May, sixty-four volunteer companies of approximately seventy men each were assembled, equipped, and armed.

As the volunteer units formed, the Committee of Safety had other important issues to consider. The powder and munitions held at Allegheny Arsenal were thought to be in jeopardy. Three months before the firing on Fort Sumter, Pittsburgh's citizens had expressed concern about potential shipments of munitions and armaments to southern states and sympathizers. At the time, credit was given to Pittsburgh physician Dr. J. S. Speer for interceding with his cousin, President James Buchanan, to stop shipments of armaments already clandestinely moving to the docks to be loaded aboard the steamer *Silver Wave*.[12]

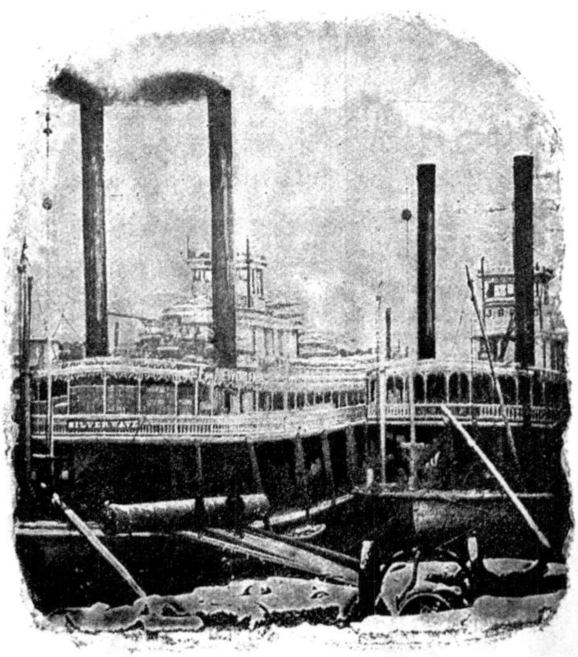

Steamboat *Silver Wave*. (*The 28th National Encampment of the Grand Army of the Republic, Official Program 1894*)

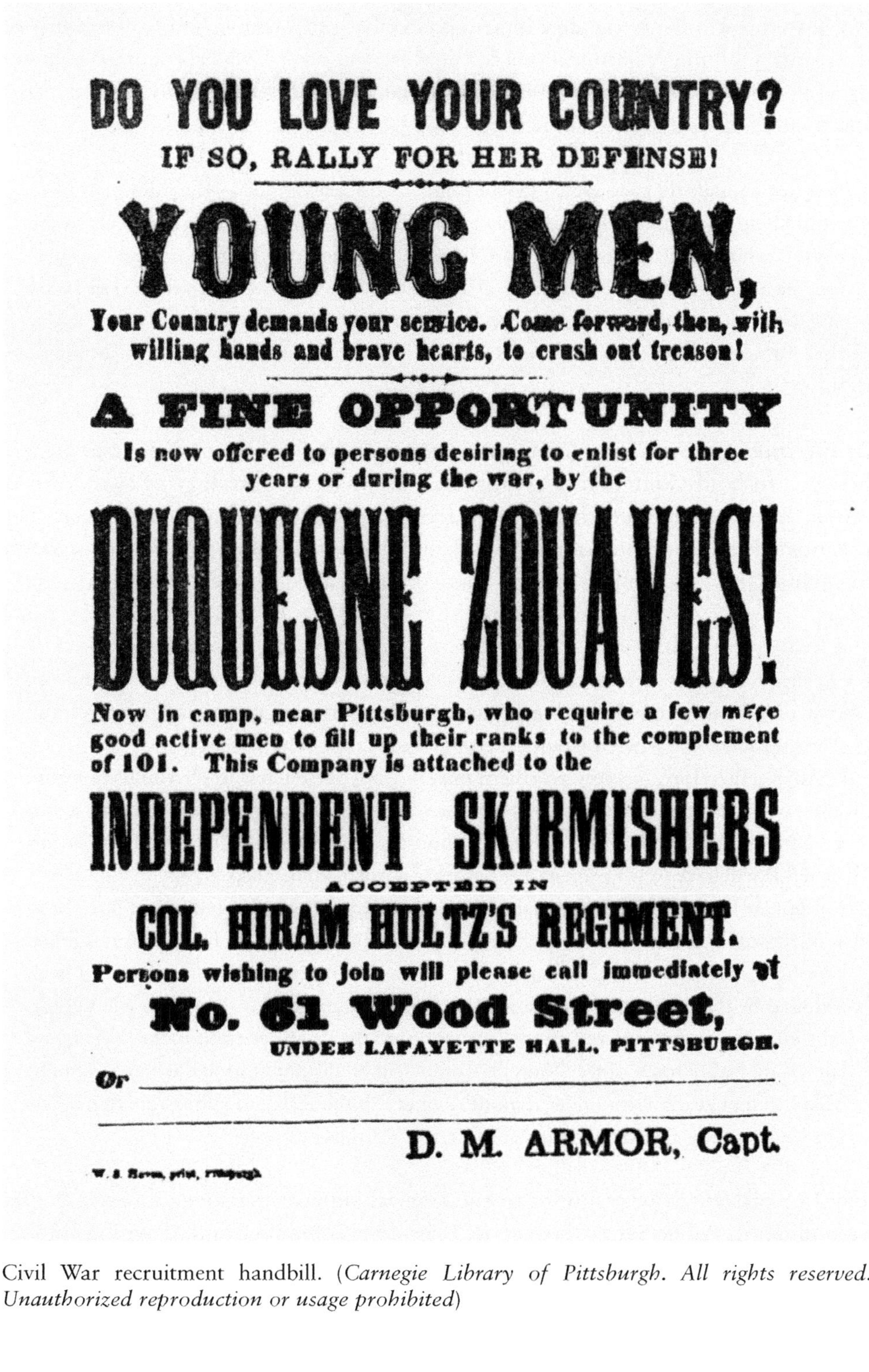

Civil War recruitment handbill. (*Carnegie Library of Pittsburgh. All rights reserved. Unauthorized reproduction or usage prohibited*)

Located just outside the city in Lawrenceville, the Arsenal had become one of the primary suppliers of munitions to the west, but now it was recognized some of its equipment and products were being shipped down river allegedly for illicit use. Local newspapers expressed concern:

> Is it not enough that we are to be sold out to the secessionists—the administration would bind us hand and foot, deprive us of arms, and deliver us neck and heels to the traitors who would destroy the Union! It has already ordered one hundred and twenty-four heavy guns from our Allegheny arsenal to the far South,—not to defend the stars and stripes, for which our skillful mechanics made them, but to batter it down under the pirate flag of some Lone Star or Rattlesnake government. Will our people submit to this?[13]

At the time, Colonel John Symington, commanding officer of the Arsenal, was believed to hold Confederate sympathies, as was U.S. Secretary of War John B. Floyd. Rumor suggested they were actively diverting war materials south. The potential diversion of munitions caused justifiable panic among Committee of Safety members. On 27 December, a newspaper editorial called for local citizens to arm:

> Let the People Arm.
> We give this advice reluctantly. We have been last to believe it necessary. But events are crowding on us so rapidly and rendering it so necessary, that we can no longer refrain. The time has come when it would be criminal to withhold it.
>
> Advice, therefore, to every Northern man is arm yourself at once. If you have a gun, get it ready for instant use; if you do not own one, get one as soon as possible. For it will take time to get one. The north is, today, almost bare of arms, and he who orders one to be made will have to wait some time before his order can be filled.
>
> Look at the facts. The northern Arsenals belonging to the United States have been eroded, within the last 3 months, every available arm within them having been shipped South. The state Arsenals are empty. The rifle and pistol manufacturers have all been emptied by the Southern demand, and have orders far ahead of their ability to supply. The government has ordered all the U.S. troops to the Pacific coast, out of the way; and all the available force of the Navy has been sent to distant stations, where orders to recall cannot reach them under a month's time. All these facts demonstrate that while the south is fully armed and ready for war, the North is defenseless.[14]

On 25 April 1861, in response to the general state of perceived emergency, the Committee of Public Safety through its Executive Committee and Munitions of War subcommittee passed several resolutions seeking to limit the movement of contraband leaving Pittsburgh. Two of Pittsburgh's other prominent physicians, Drs. Edward D. Gazzam and George L. McCook, played a leading role in drafting resolutions designed to take control of the situation. As enacted, the resolutions stated:

> Resolved, That all goods arriving in Pittsburg, and destined for the Southern States, be stopped for the present, stored and insured.
>
> Resolved, That no packages whatever shall be allowed to go forward to Southern States till they have been opened and examined by the Committee.
>
> Resolved, That one or more packers be employed to attend to the opening of the boxes and other packages and repacking the same.

With the support of Dr. McCook and others on the executive committee's "Committee on Munitions of War," Dr. Gazzam, serving as chairman of the committee, promptly communicated the city's concerns to Washington. In response to his telegraph, Gazzam received the following reply:

> Ordnance Office, Washington, D.C.,
> May 3, 1861.
>
> E. D. Gazzam, Chairman, Pittsburg, Pa.:
>
> Sir: Your telegram of May 1 to the Secretary of War about powder now held by the Committee is received and sent to this office. If any of the powder is needed by the commanding officer of Allegheny Arsenal, and is in his judgment of suitable quality for the United States service, it may be delivered to him. The Committee must use their discretion about the residue, throwing every proper guard around the disposition to be made of it.
>
> Respectfully, Your Obedient Servant,
> James W. Ripley, Lt.-Col. U.S.A.
>
> "The powder referred to was seized by the Committee of Safety when about to be shipped south, from which the importance of the step taken can readily be discerned."[15]

Within a few weeks, most of the illicit transport of contraband was stopped, and joint federal and state authority took control of the Arsenal's munitions. The Committee of Public Safety through the Committee on Munitions of War and the Committee on Transit of Contraband Goods, now effectively controlled the distribution of all products manufactured in Pittsburgh, as well as those arriving from other regions for transit through the city.[16]

Through the actions of Pittsburgh's leading citizens and three of its most prominent physicians, a crisis was averted, and the importance of their attentiveness was soon understood. Exactly one month after the Ripley telegram, it was reported that on 03 June 1861, the Union Army won the Battle of Philippi, and "the first Union victory was won with ammunition furnished from Pittsburgh."[17] Thus, the ammunition used at Philippi by a regiment of mostly West Virginia troops may not

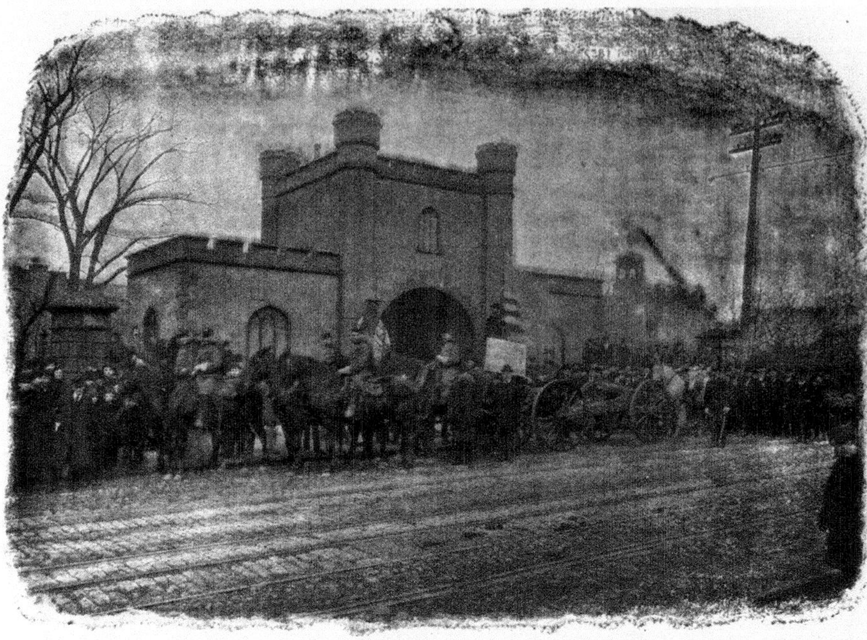

THE HISTORIC GUN.

Allegheny Arsenal parade. (*Grand Army of the Republic 28th National Encampment program, Pittsburgh, 1894*)

have arrived to fuel the muskets provided by Governor Andrews of Massachusetts if it were not for the actions of Drs. Speer, Gazzam, and McCook. From then on, "Pittsburgh began a point of military prominence."[18]

By the end of the Civil War, it was estimated that "twenty thousand of Pittsburgh's young men carried a musket or the sword in all the prominent battles of the war."[19] The citizens of Pittsburgh who volunteered their services to the war effort were not limited to military duty. Thousands of others supported the cause by contributing material goods, medical care, and supportive services to not only Pittsburgh's volunteers but to all Union and Confederate soldiers who were transported through the city.

Almost every one of the city's businesses, hospitals, churches, public agencies, and civic groups made some contribution. In many cases, they acted individually, in others, they merged resources and supported newly organized agencies developed to address matters of particular interest. The most prominent included:

The Pittsburgh Subsistence Committee

In Pittsburgh, early in the war, no camps had yet been formed to accommodate the regiments being established. Men were temporarily billeted in homes, or a local "house of entertainment," and no plan had yet been developed for their provisioning.

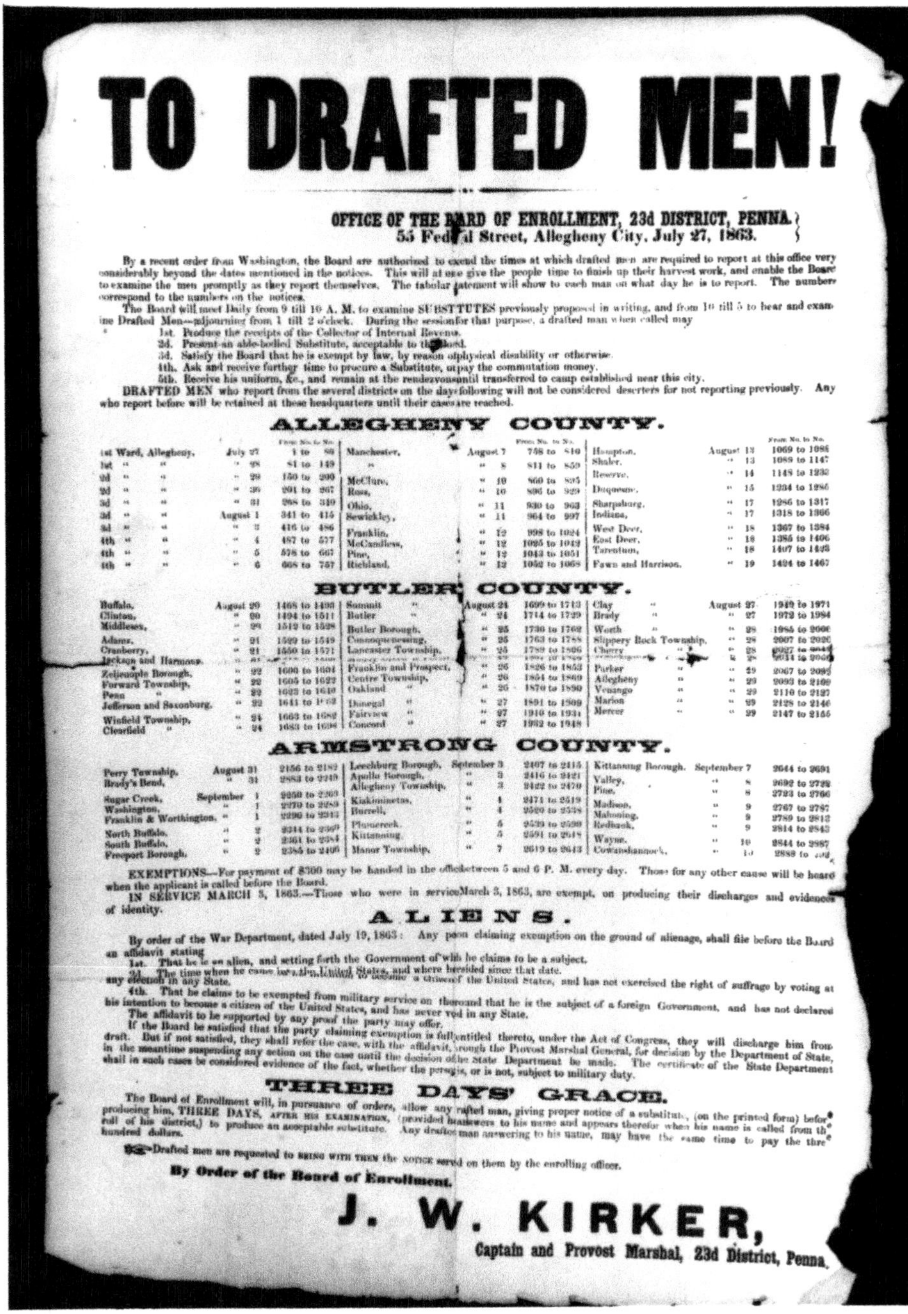

TO DRAFTED MEN!

OFFICE OF THE BOARD OF ENROLLMENT, 23d DISTRICT, PENNA.
55 Federal Street, Allegheny City, July 27, 1863.

By a recent order from Washington, the Board are authorized to exend the times at which drafted men are required to report at this office very considerably beyond the dates mentioned in the notices. This will at one give the people time to finish up their harvest work, and enable the Board to examine the men promptly as they report themselves. The tabular statement will show to each man on what day he is to report. The numbers correspond to the numbers on the notices.

The Board will meet Daily from 9 till 10 A. M. to examine SUBSTITUTES previously proposed in writing, and from 10 till 5 to hear and examine Drafted Men—adjourning from 1 till 2 o'clock. During the session for that purpose, a drafted man when called may

1st. Produce the receipts of the Collector of Internal Revenue.
2d. Present an able-bodied Substitute, acceptable to the Board.
3d. Satisfy the Board that he is exempt by law, by reason of physical disability or otherwise.
4th. Ask and receive further time to procure a Substitute, or pay the commutation money.
5th. Receive his uniform, &c., and remain at the rendezvous until transferred to camp established near this city.

DRAFTED MEN who report from the several districts on the days following will not be considered deserters for not reporting previously. Any who report before will be retained at these headquarters until their cases are reached.

ALLEGHENY COUNTY.

		From No. to No.			From No. to No.			From No. to No.
1st Ward, Allegheny,	July 27	1 to 80	Manchester,	August 7	758 to 810	Hampton,	August 13	1069 to 1088
1st " "	" 28	81 to 149	"	" 8	811 to 859	Shaler,	" 13	1089 to 1147
2d " "	" 29	150 to 200	McClure,	" 10	860 to 895	Reserve,	" 14	1148 to 1233
2d " "	" 30	201 to 267	Ross,	" 10	896 to 929	Duquesne,	" 15	1234 to 1285
3d " "	" 31	268 to 340	Ohio,	" 11	930 to 963	Sharpsburg,	" 17	1286 to 1317
3d " "	August 1	341 to 415	Sewickley,	" 11	964 to 997	Indiana,	" 17	1318 to 1366
3d " "	" 3	416 to 486	Franklin,	" 12	998 to 1024	West Deer,	" 18	1367 to 1384
4th " "	" 4	487 to 577	McCandless,	" 12	1025 to 1042	East Deer,	" 18	1385 to 1406
4th " "	" 5	578 to 667	Pine,	" 12	1043 to 1051	Tarentum,	" 18	1407 to 1423
4th " "	" 6	668 to 757	Richland,	" 12	1052 to 1068	Fawn and Harrison,	" 19	1424 to 1467

BUTLER COUNTY.

Buffalo,	August 20	1468 to 1493	Summit "	August 24	1699 to 1713	Clay "	August 27	1949 to 1971
Clinton,	" 20	1494 to 1511	Butler "	" 24	1714 to 1729	Brady "	" 27	1972 to 1984
Middlesex,	" 20	1512 to 1528	Butler Borough,	" 25	1730 to 1762	Worth "	" 28	1985 to 2006
Adams,	" 21	1529 to 1549	Connoquenessing,	" 25	1763 to 1788	Slippery Rock Township,	" 28	2007 to 2026
Cranberry,	" 21	1550 to 1571	Lancaster Township,	" 25	1789 to 1806	Cherry "	" 28	2027 to [illegible]
Jackson and Harmony,	[illegible]	[illegible]	[illegible]	[illegible]	[illegible]	[illegible]	[illegible]	2044 to 2066
Zelienople Borough,	" 22	1600 to 1604	Franklin and Prospect,	" 26	1826 to 1853	Parker "	" 29	2067 to 2092
Forward Township,	" 22	1605 to 1622	Centre Township,	" 26	1854 to 1869	Allegheny "	" 29	2093 to 2109
Penn "	" 22	1623 to 1640	Oakland "	" 26	1870 to 1890	Venango "	" 29	2110 to 2127
Jefferson and Saxonburg,	" 22	1641 to 1662	Donegal "	" 27	1891 to 1909	Marion "	" 29	2128 to 2146
Winfield Township,	" 24	1663 to 1682	Fairview "	" 27	1910 to 1931	Mercer "	" 29	2147 to 2155
Clearfield "	" 24	1683 to 1698	Concord "	" 27	1932 to 1948			

ARMSTRONG COUNTY.

Perry Township,	August 31	2156 to 2182	Leechburg Borough,	September 3	2407 to 2415	Kittanning Borough,	September 7	2644 to 2691
Brady's Bend,	" 31	2183 to 2249	Apollo Borough,	" 3	2416 to 2421	Valley,	" 8	2692 to 2722
			Allegheny Township,	" 3	2422 to 2470	Pine,	" 8	2723 to 2766
Sugar Creek,	September 1	2250 to 2269	Kiskiminetas,	" 4	2471 to 2519	Madison,	" 9	2767 to 2787
Washington,	" 1	2270 to 2289	Burrell,	" 4	2520 to 2538	Mahoning,	" 9	2789 to 2813
Franklin & Worthington,	" 1	2290 to 2313	Plumcreek,	" 5	2539 to 2590	Redbank,	" 9	2814 to 2843
North Buffalo,	" 2	2314 to 2360	Kittanning,	" 5	2591 to 2618	Wayne,	" 10	2844 to 2887
South Buffalo,	" 2	2361 to 2384						
Freeport Borough,	" 2	2385 to 2406	Manor Township,	" 7	2619 to 2643	Cowanshannock,	" 10	2888 to [illegible]

EXEMPTIONS.—For payment of $300 may be handed in the office between 5 and 6 P. M. every day. Those for any other cause will be heard when the applicant is called before the Board.

IN SERVICE MARCH 3, 1863.—Those who were in service March 3, 1863, are exempt, on producing their discharges and evidences of identity.

ALIENS.

By order of the War Department, dated July 19, 1863: Any person claiming exemption on the ground of alienage, shall file before the Board an affidavit stating

1st. That he is an alien, and setting forth the Government of which he claims to be a subject.
2d. The time when he came into the United States, and where he resided since that date.
[illegible] intention to become a citizen of the United States, and has not exercised the right of suffrage by voting at any election in any State.
4th. That he claims to be exempted from military service on the ground that he is the subject of a foreign Government, and has not declared his intention to become a citizen of the United States, and has never voted in any State.

The affidavit to be supported by any proof the party may offer.

If the Board be satisfied that the party claiming exemption is fully entitled thereto, under the Act of Congress, they will discharge him from draft. But if not satisfied, they shall refer the case, with the affidavit, through the Provost Marshal General, for decision by the Department of State, in the meantime suspending any action on the case until the decision of the State Department be made. The certificate of the State Department shall in such cases be considered evidence of the fact, whether the person is, or is not, subject to military duty.

THREE DAYS' GRACE.

The Board of Enrollment will, in pursuance of orders, allow any drafted man, giving proper notice of a substitute, (on the printed form) before producing him, THREE DAYS, AFTER HIS EXAMINATION, (provided he answers to his name and appears therefor when his name is called from the roll of his district,) to produce an acceptable substitute. Any drafted man answering to his name, may have the same time to pay the three hundred dollars.

☞ Drafted men are requested to BRING WITH THEM the NOTICE served on them by the enrolling officer.

By Order of the Board of Enrollment.

J. W. KIRKER,
Captain and Provost Marshal, 23d District, Penna.

Civil War draft notice 1863. (*Carnegie Library of Pittsburgh. All rights reserved. Unauthorized reproduction or usage prohibited*)

Initiated in concept by businessman Benjamin Franklin Jones (of Jones & Laughlin Steel fame) in July 1861, a group of leading citizens came together to help feed and provide comfort for these "three months' service" volunteers as they arrived and left the city.

Wishing to take control of the situation, a volunteer citizen's group led by James Park, Jr., Hon. Thomas M. Howe, and other leading businessmen joined Jones in creating the Pittsburgh Subsistence Committee on 03 August 1861. By design, its sole purpose was to provide sustenance for soldiers in the various stages of recruitment before being mustered into the army and for the provision of transient soldiers passing through the city. An executive branch composed of four of the city's most patriotic citizens, including Dr. Andrew Fleming, served as the organization's executive committee. An October 1862 report of the committee's work described its initial efforts as follows:

> The duty of the Committee was to attend to the subsisting of such companies as were forming, until they were regularly mustered into the U.S. service. After subsisting Col. Black's Regiment for some ten days, until they left for Washington City, the attention of the Committee was directed to the wants of the regiments and companies passing through our city. On the 28th of July, 1861, the first Regiment, the 24th Ohio, was fed by the Committee. This Regiment was ordered to report at Washington city, and passed through our city Saturday evening, July 27th. They had gone but a few miles when they were ordered back to Western Virginia. They were quartered Saturday night at City Hall, and on Sunday morning a breakfast was given to them by the Committee. As no rooms had been as yet fitted up, the meal was given to them standing in the street. The

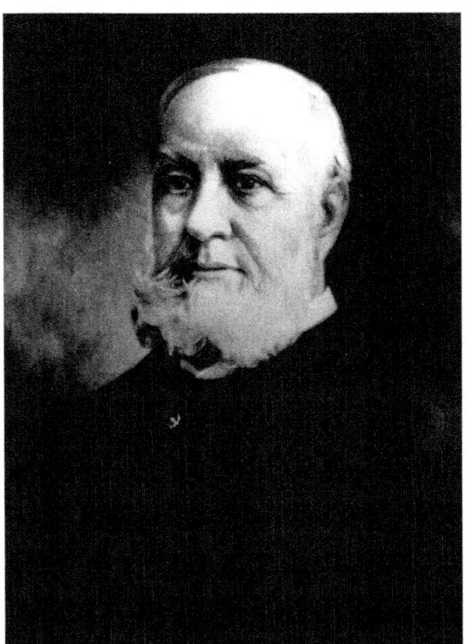

B. F. Jones, Pittsburgh industrialist. (*Carnegie Library of Pittsburgh. All rights reserved. Unauthorized reproduction or usage prohibited*)

> following week, the Committee had the "Old Leech Warehouse," corner of Penn and Wayne streets, fixed with tables, &c., for accommodating a regiment at one time. On Sunday morning. August 3d, 1861, the first regiment, the 20th Indiana, Col. Brown, was furnished with a substantial meal of bread and butter, ham and coffee. A number of young ladies and gentlemen was appointed by the committee to take charge of this part of the work—the giving of a meal to regiments and companies on their way to the seat of war, and on the 17th of August, 1861, the Committee resigned into the hands of these ladies and gentlemen the whole management of its operations.[20]

In addition to meals, accommodations were also made by the committee to provide assistance to sick or wounded soldiers. Dr. Fleming took charge of the "medical department" and set up a small hospital in a room adjoining the dining hall for the accommodation of the sick and wounded. The room contained beds, medicines, and "little delicacies which often do more good than medicines."[21]

Building upon their initial success, the Committee, in October 1862, moved into more spacious quarters by utilizing City Hall for its dining hall. At the time, the building was one of the largest in the city. The new dining area afforded facilities for feeding 1,200 soldiers, seated at ten long tables, at one time. This was almost double the capacity of the old hall: "Coffee, meat, and bread for as many as five thousand men in a night was not unusual..."[22] In a report issued in the same month, it was noted that since the committee's organization, more than 76,000 soldiers were been fed and an additional 5,768 sick and wounded had been cared for through the medical department.[23]

When it was determined some soldiers could not take advantage of the hospitality of the new quarters because of the distance from the train station and limited amount of time available between transit, yet another, albeit smaller, accommodation was found in a converted warehouse at 347 Liberty Street. This satellite rest area was officially designated the "Soldiers' Home." Upon opening this new facility, the Committee prepared special handbills offering assistance, food, respite, and medical care, which were distributed to soldiers on all trains entering the city.

It was not long before the committee was faced with a new, but familiar challenge. There were growing numbers of soldiers requiring attention at the Soldiers' Home, and additional space was needed. At first, the committee expanded into another area on the first floor; they then added a second floor; and finally, a third floor. Even with all the expansions there still was not enough space: "... only fifty soldiers could be accommodated at one time, while frequently from one to three hundred would require care and attention."[24]

In addition to providing meals and medical attention, the Subsistence Committee began collecting and distributing supplies, including bandages, shirts, drawers, pillows, canned fruit, and other materials to hospitals. These "hospital" items were distributed through the U.S. Christian Committee's Army Committee. Between 15 January and 06 April 1863, more than $60,000 in goods had been received and

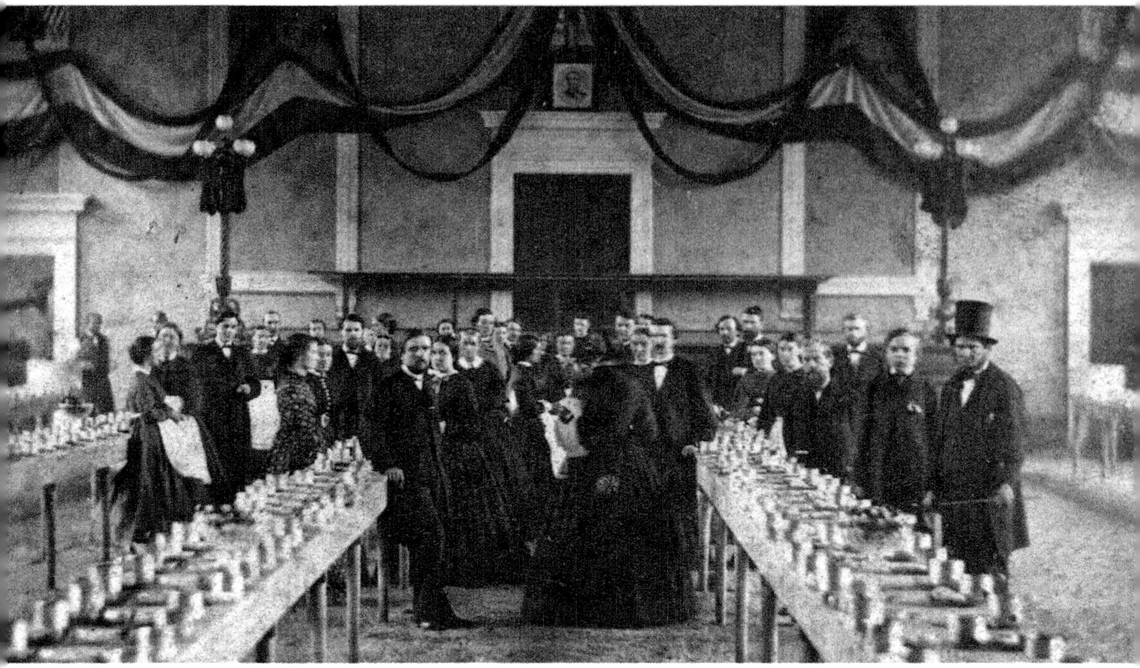

Above: Subsistence Committee members awaiting guests at City Hall, 1861. (*Heinz History Center*)

Below left: Soldiers' Home handbill. (*The 28th National Encampment of the Grand Army of the Republic, Official Program 1894*)

Below right: : Pittsburgh Subsistence Committee advertisement 1864. (*Library of Congress*)

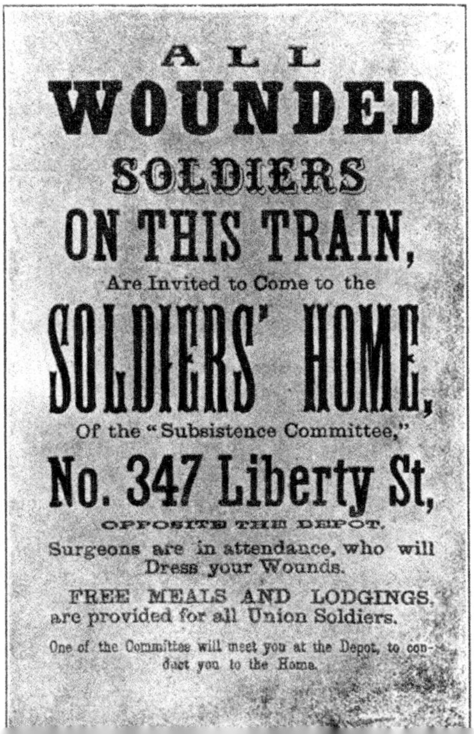

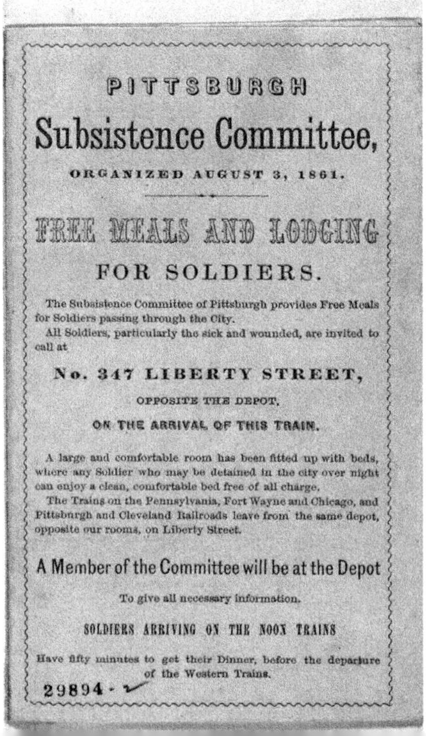

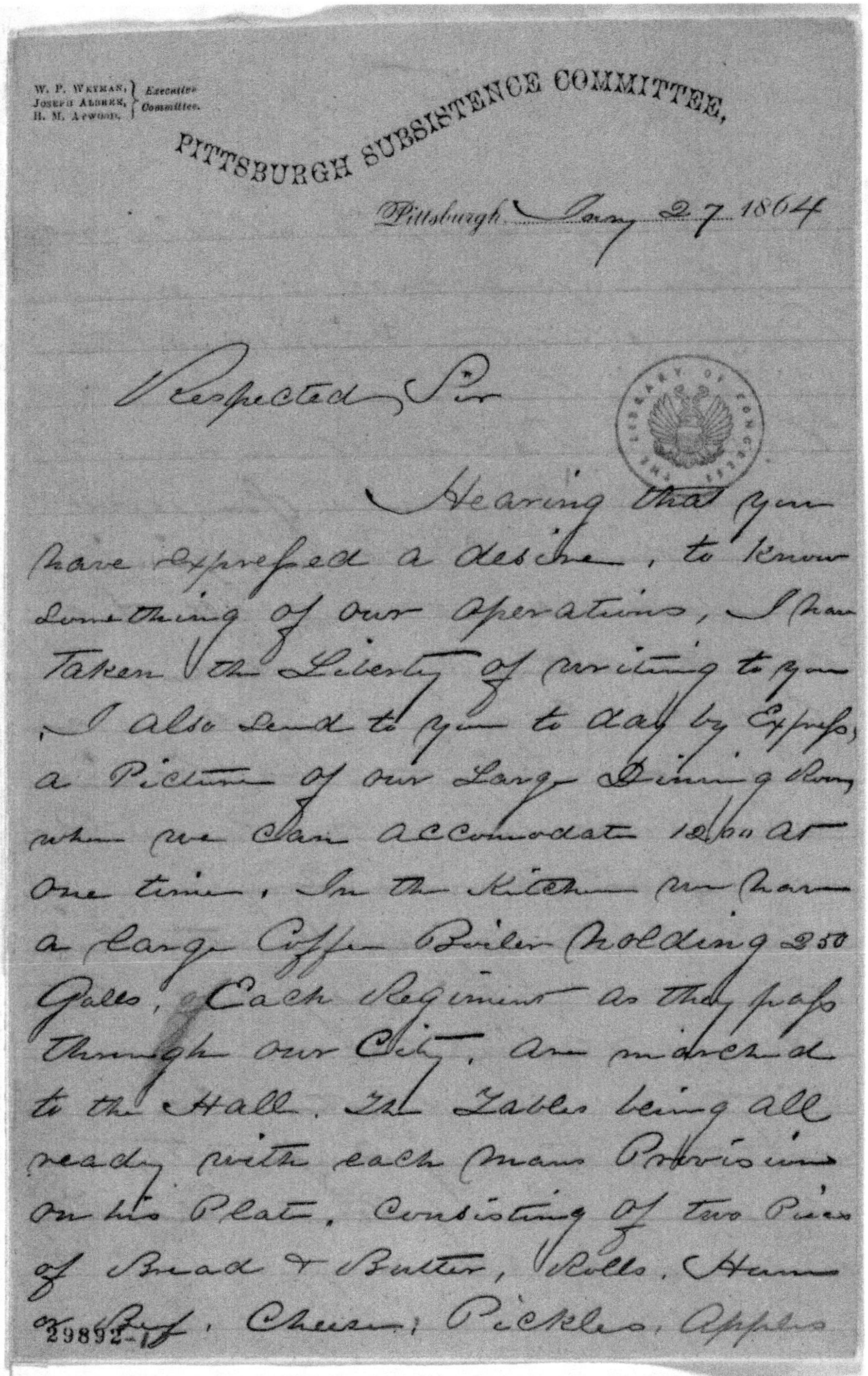

W. P. Weyman, Joseph Albree, R. M. Atwood, } Executive Committee.

PITTSBURGH SUBSISTENCE COMMITTEE,

Pittsburgh Jany 27 1864

Respected Sir

Hearing that you have expressed a desire, to know something of our operations, I have taken the Liberty of writing to you, I also send to you to day by Express, a Picture of our Large Dining Room where we can accommodate 1200 at one time, In the Kitchen we have a Large Coffee Boiler holding 250 Galls, Each Regiment as they pass through our City, are marched to the Hall. The Tables being all ready with each mans Provision on his Plate, consisting of two Pieces of Bread & Butter, Rolls, Ham or Beef, Cheese, Pickles, Apples

Pittsburgh Subsistence Committee letter from W. P. Weyman to President Lincoln 1864. (*Library of Congress*)

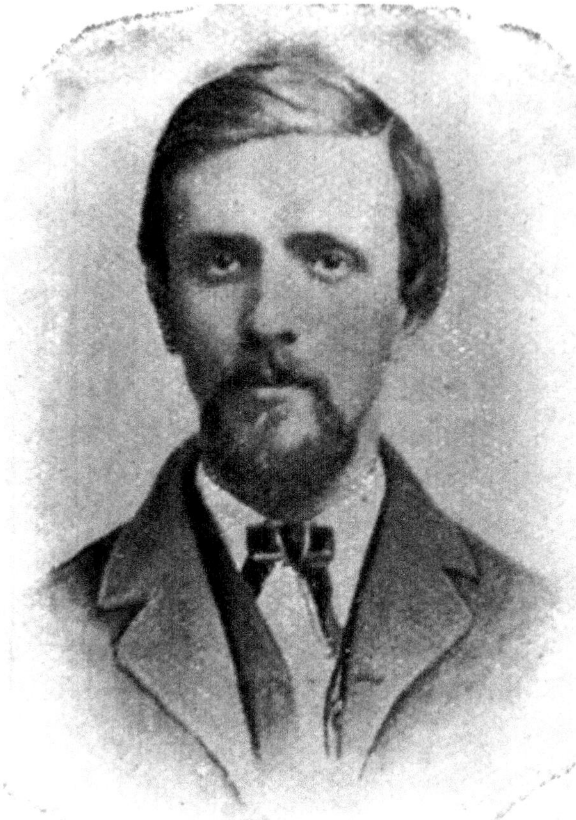

Left: W. P. Weyman, Chairman of the Pittsburgh Subsistence Committee. (*The 28th National Encampment of the Grand Army of the Republic, Official Program 1894*)

Below: Soldiers' Dining Room. (*Annals of the United States Christian Committee, 1868*)

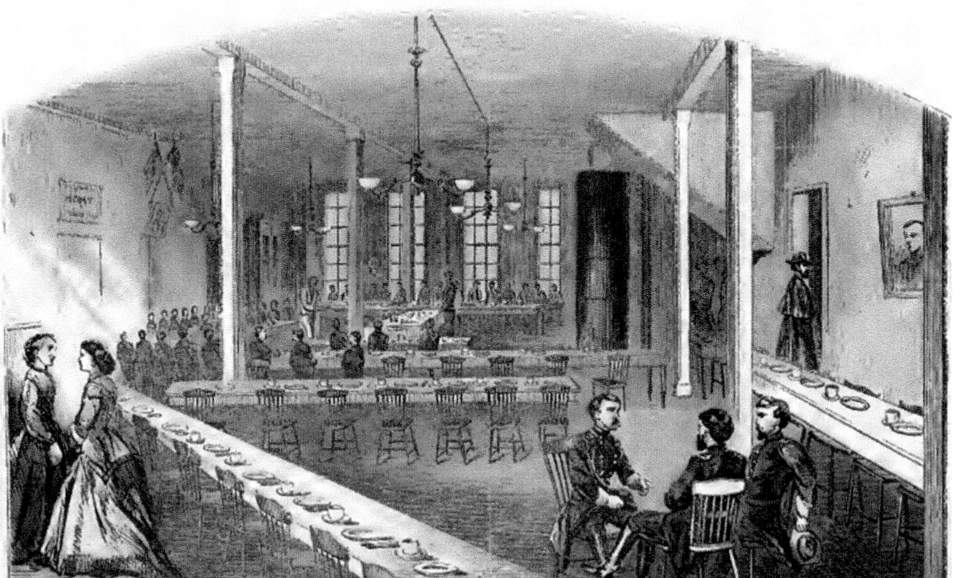

distributed. The Subsistence Committee also collected and distributed more than 246,000 religious books and papers to soldiers.

When the Subsistence Committee was disbanded in January 1866, it was determined it had fed 409,745 soldiers during their short existence. The Soldier's Home had cared for another 79,460 soldiers bringing the combined total to 489,205.

The U.S. Christian Committee

The Western Pennsylvania branch of the U.S. Christian Commission was organized on 06 April 1863, with its first public meeting held on 16 April. The commission's original goal was ministering to the spiritual needs of soldiers rather than the physical needs. However, they quickly realized "That man's soul could most easily be reached through his stomach, and the activities of the Christian Commission gradually embraced not only the distribution of religious tracts, but also the distribution of delicacies to the soldiers."[25] Upon its organization, the commission effectively relieved the Pittsburgh Subsistence Committee of its duties, except for the provision of food, refreshments, and medical care.

The commission's agents covered a territory that included Western Pennsylvania, eastern Ohio, and West Virginia. Besides its main goal of providing ministerial support, the Pittsburgh branch had seven specific responsibilities:

1) Gathering such funds and supplies as may be necessary.
2) Supplying nurses for the sick or wounded when and as far as practicable.
3) Bringing home such sick and wounded soldiers as may be proper.
4) Purchasing clothing, provisions, and matters of comfort, which rations and camp allowances may not provide, and which would contribute to the soldiers' happiness.
5) Placing in camp such Bibles, books and papers as would instruct and amuse their days of rest and quiet and keep them informed of passing events.
6) Gathering the dates and making a record of the name and history of each soldier and his services.
7) Holding constant communication with paymasters or other officers of our regiments, that friends may interchange letters and packages.[26]

By the end of the war, total cash receipts of the commission were $158,334.37, and the total dollar value of materials and stores was $679,664.89. The combined cash value of all receipts equaled $837,999.26, which was more than any other branch of the commission had collected and only slightly less than the central office. All of these supplies were transported and delivered to the needy soldiers for only $3,787.35 indicating an enormous amount of gratuitous effort went into the endeavor.[27]

Four members of the Pittsburgh branch of the Christian Commission deserve note. Of the four, three were brothers, all physicians, who left their practice in Pittsburgh to serve as volunteer surgeons under the auspices of the Commission. Thomas, John, and Joseph Dickson all served the Army of the Potomac with distinction. Thomas gave the greatest gift, his life, after contracting typhoid fever during one of the first battles of the war. John and Joseph continued their service until the end of the war.

The fourth notable member of the Pittsburgh Branch of the U.S. Christian Commission was Felix R. Brunot. He was the son of a physician, Dr. Felix Brunot, the foster brother of the Marquis de Lafayette. Felix R. was born at the United States arsenal in Newport, Kentucky. Thus, he was exposed to both medicine and the military at an early age.

Though not a physician, Brunot had a considerable influence on medical care during the war. Even though Brunot was past the age of military service when the war broke out, he was offered both rank and military command as a reflection of his high standing in the community. He declined and instead chose to work as a volunteer of the U.S. Christian Committee. He began his work immediately after the Battle of Pittsburg Landing (Battle of Shiloh) in early April 1862, by leading a contingent of volunteer doctors and nurses to the battlefield.

A list of those who volunteered was documented in a newspaper on 04 March 1862. The group included thirteen physicians and twenty-eight nurses who were chosen from among the volunteers to make the trip to the war front.[28] They traveled as part of the "Pittsburgh Sanitary Committee," which had not yet been officially connected to the United States Sanitary Commission. The commission had been formed during June of the previous year to supplement the Union Army's medical and relief efforts.[29]

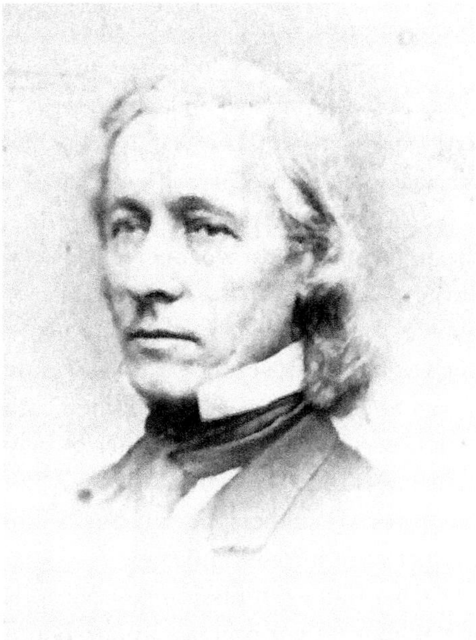

Felix Reville Brunot. (*Heinz History Center*)

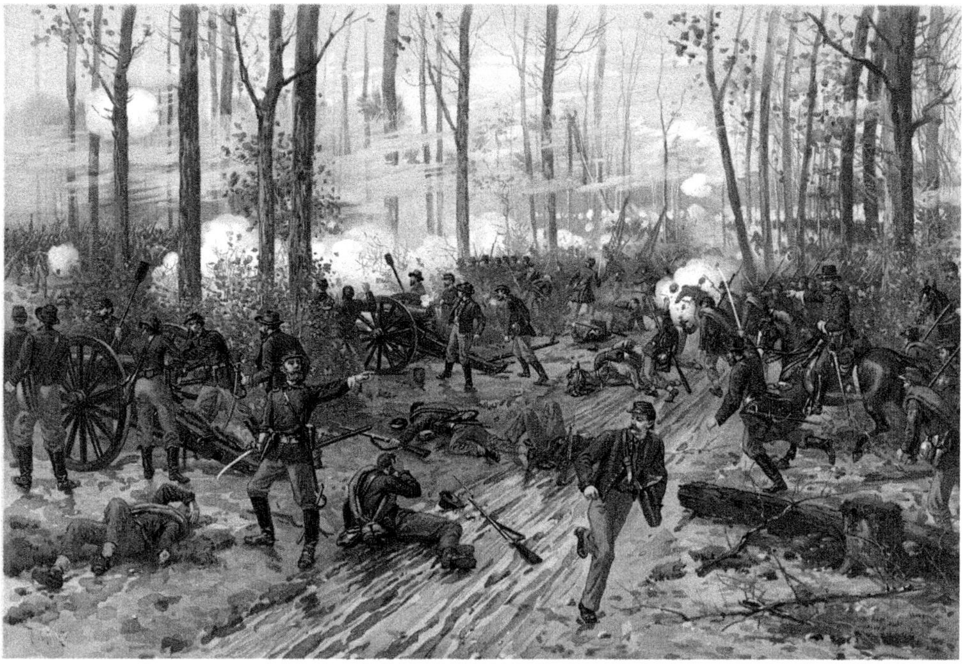

Battle of Shiloh. (*Library of Congress*)

On 12 April 1862, a newspaper described the plans for the relief expedition (referred to subsequently as the "Expedition to the Tennessee River"), including the final list of physicians and nurses who were selected to make the trip:

> The Expedition To The Tennessee River—Two Steamers To Be Sent—Volunteer Surgeons and Nurses.[30]
>
> The committee to make arrangements for fitting out an expedition to the Tennessee River for the purpose of sending Aid and assistance to the wounded soldiers, met this morning at the Board of Trade rooms, and agreed to fit out two steamers, "the *J. W. Hailman*" and "*Marengo*," one of which will be chartered by the Government, and the other by the citizens—both being furnished with surgeons, nurses, supplies, etc. at the expense of the citizens.
>
> F. R. Brunot and Rev. W. D. Howard were instructed to go in advance and make the necessary arrangements for the reception of the boats at their destinations, and the conveyance of the wounded to this city. These gentlemen left by railroad at one o'clock this afternoon.
>
> Messrs. F. R. Brunot, James I. Bennett, and Joseph R. Hunter, Committee, authorize the publication of the following notice:
>
> Any of the citizens or ladies who have hospital stores or comforts for the sick, as named below, are requested to send them at once to the warehouse of Graff, Bennett

& Company, Water street, near Market, for the use of the boat expedition about being started for Pittsburgh Landing, on the Tennessee river, and for the use of the wounded when brought to this city:

Bandages of old linen or cotton, (white); sheets, pillows or pillow slips; comforts, slippers, night shirts and drawers; dressing gowns, battling, fruits, etc.

Dr. George McCook was directed to make a list of medical supplies to be furnished by Joseph Abel and Simon Johnston, Druggists, with the understanding that such supplies as are not used shall be returned at the invoice prices.

Dr. W. D. Howard and Dr. J. F. McLaren having volunteered their services, will act as Chaplains of the expedition.

Messrs. George L. McCook, Wm. Bagaley and J. F. McLaren, the Committee appointed at the citizens meeting to procure physicians and nurses, made the following report to the General Committee, which was adopted:

The Committee, appointed to name the physicians and nurses for the expedition to the Tennessee river, have appointed the following named persons to act in that capacity:

Physicians
Dr. Geo. McCook
Dr. Patterson
Dr. Duncan
Dr. Fisher
Dr. Fundenburgh
Dr. Perchment
Dr. Metzger

Nurses

Males,
F. B. Goddard
C. D. Huston
R. B. Farrar
J. D. Johnston
J. W. Wells
Josiah Copley
Rev. B. Single
R. Allingham
George F. Irwin
Wm. McCreery
Thomas G. Smythe
W. W. McGreggor
James S. Thorn

Females,
Miss Mary M. Robinson
Mrs. Jas. Little
Mrs. Pollard
Mrs. Bese
Miss Emma Davis
Mrs. Christian Ernest
Miss Sarah Shepler
Mrs. Mary Miller
Mrs. Mary McDermot
Miss Lizzie H. Wright
Mrs. Eliza A. Lloyd
Mrs. Hawdon
Miss Anne Johnston
Mrs. Sarah J. Ammond
Mrs. Wm. McCreery

The Second Medical Corps was organized as follows:
Dr. John Dickson
Dr. Dickie Kearns
Dr. Wm. Hamilton
Dr. J. H. Dickson
Dr. J. B. Herron
Dr. W. C. Reiter

Upon arriving at the battlefield, they found most of the 13,000 Union troops who were wounded had already been evacuated. The Pittsburgh Sanitary Committee's first report in 1863 stated: "When the expedition arrived at Pittsburgh Landing, it was too late to aid the wounded, most of whom had been already removed."[31]

While the battlefield was cleared, the group was successful in loading between 400 and 500 sick and wounded on board the steamers. In a short time, they returned a majority of them to cities, like Paducah, Evansville, Louisville, Cincinnati, and others along their return trip to Pittsburgh. Ten died on the return trip—six on the *Marengo* and four on the *Hailman*. Sixty-eight were returned to Pittsburgh, including several who were suffering from "typhoid fever and diarrhea." The majority of the sick and wounded were left at the Marine Hospital and the remainder at Passavant Infirmary. Those who were brought to the city included soldiers from Illinois, Michigan, Missouri, Indiana, Ohio, and Vermont. Two Rebel soldiers were included in the group, one from Mississippi and the other from Alabama.[32]

During his return to Pittsburgh, Brunot became ill from blood poisoning, which caused him to remain in the city for several weeks. Once recuperated, he subsequently served on the Virginia Peninsula during the Seven Days Battles, including the Battles

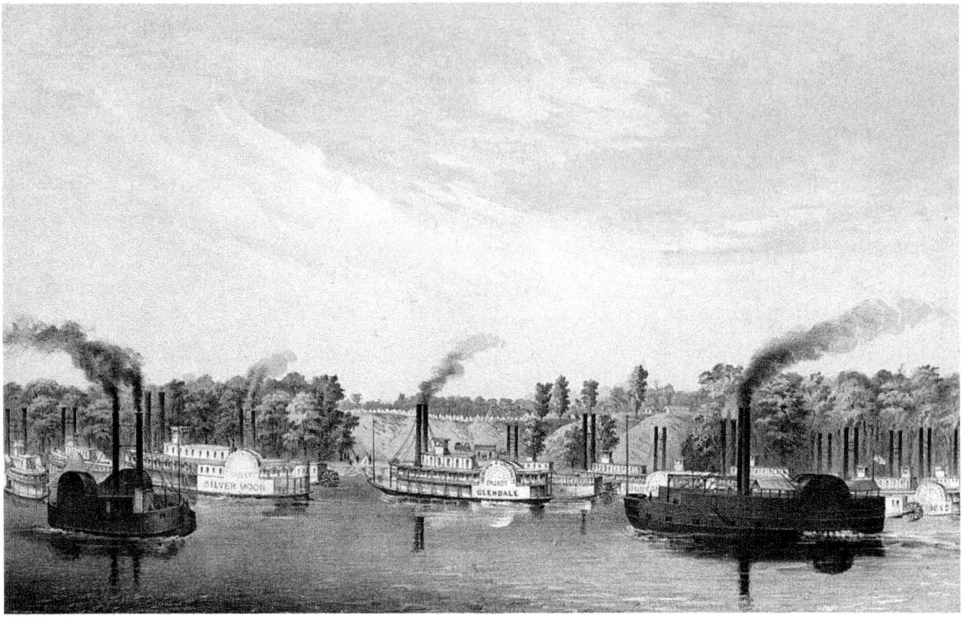

Boats arriving at Pittsburg Landing, Tennessee, May 1862. (*Library of Congress*)

of Gaines' Mills (27 June 1862; also known as the First Battle of Cold Harbor) and Savage Station (29 June 1862).

During McClellan's retreat, the Confederates captured many thousands, including the sick and wounded in field hospitals. Surgeons, nurses, attendants, and members of the Christian Committee were among those captured. Brunot was among twelve members of the Pittsburgh relief contingent who had elected to stay behind to care for the wounded. He was sent to the notorious Libby prison due to the failure of the Confederates to recognize him as a non-combatant. Brunot was subsequently invited by the Confederate authorities to visit Secretary of War Stanton in Washington to secure a modification of existing orders regarding the ban on sending medical supplies into any part of the Confederacy.

The Confederate army was ill-prepared to care for their own sick and wounded without the additional burden of maintaining the vast number of Union casualties. Stanton declined Brunot's request. It was suggested he forego returning to Libby prison and disregard his oath of parole to the Confederate authorities guaranteeing his return. Discounting the suggestion, he returned to Richmond and delivered Stanton's reply much to the chagrin of the Confederates. Frustrated, Confederate authorities paroled all of the sick and wounded. On 04 August 1962, the *Pittsburgh Daily Gazette* reported the *New York Herald* received a dispatch from Washington indicating:

> Dr. Brunot, of Pittsburgh, who was captured at the hospital at Savage's Station, and granted a limited parole to procure an exchange, left here today, en route for Richmond,

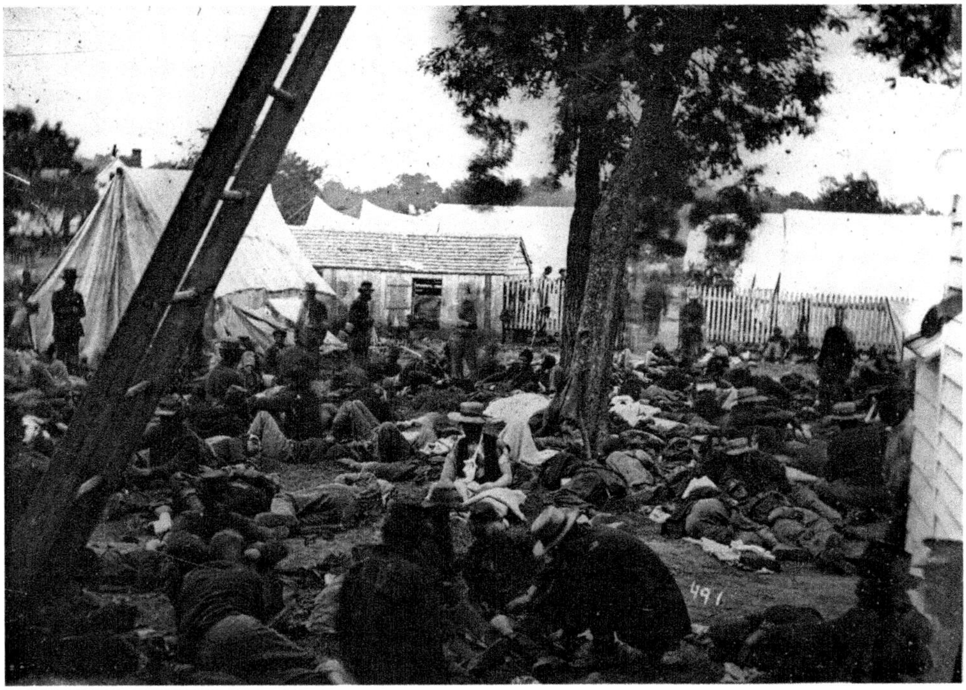

Savage Station field hospital after the battle of June 27, 1862. (*Library of Congress*)

> to redeem his pledge. He will probably find, in communicating with the rebel officers in charge of the exchange of prisoners, that he has been included in the agreement for a general exchange.[33]

Brunot was, indeed, among those released, and he quickly resumed his duties with the commission. He continued his volunteer efforts until he found himself suffering from the lingering effects of malaria. His illness caused him to retire before the end of the war. He subsequently left the city for an extended trip to recover in Europe, returning in better health during the fall of 1865. In 1868, President Grant called upon him to serve on a newly formed Indian Commission and work among the Indian tribes in the northeastern United States. In addition to his work among the American Indians, he served on the board of directors of both Western Pennsylvania and Allegheny General hospitals.

United States Sanitary Commission

Appointed by Secretary of War Simon Cameron on 09 June 1861, the Sanitary Commission (sanitary meaning relating to the preservation of health) was established as a volunteer organization committed to cooperation with the army medical staff, but independent of it. Its headquarters were in the Treasury Building

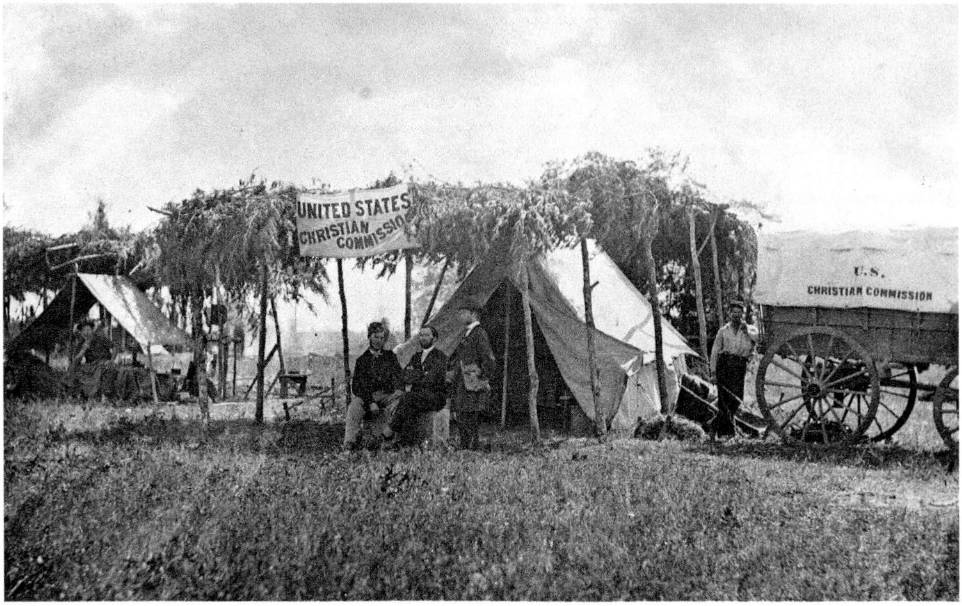

Headquarters of the U.S. Christian Commission at Germantown, Virginia, 1863. (*Library of Congress*)

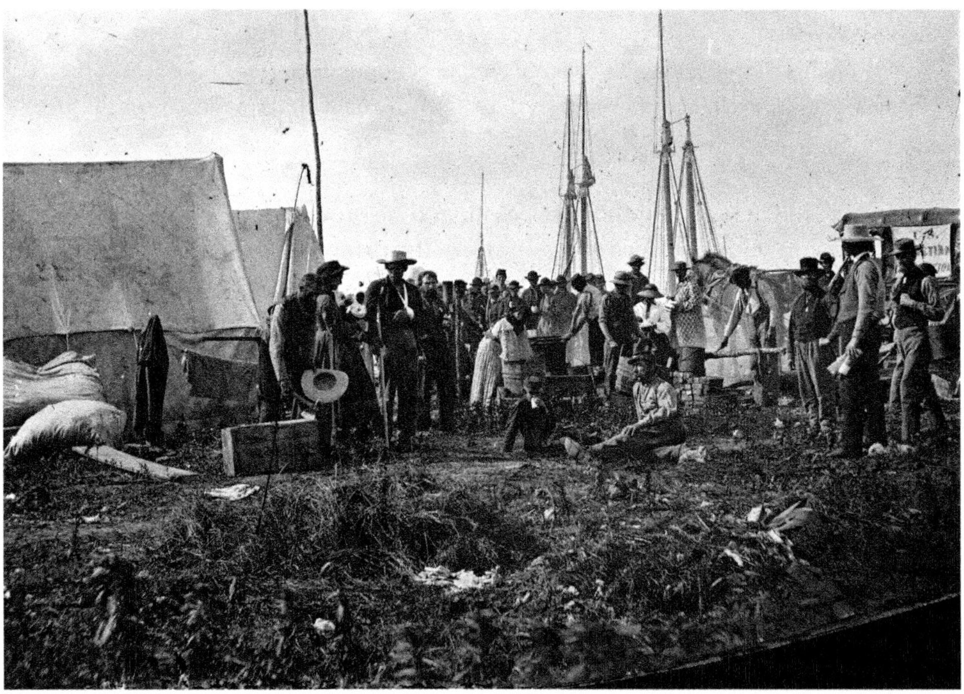

Headquarters of the U.S. Christian Commission at White House Landing, Virginia, 1864. (*Library of Congress*)

in Washington, D.C. However, local chapters throughout the many big cities of the North and Midwest provided the largest amount of services. Its mission:

> ... to enquire into the principles and practices connected with the inspection of recruits and enlisted men; the sanitary condition of the volunteers; to the means of preserving and restoring the health, and of securing the general comfort and efficiency of troops; to the proper provision of cooks, nurses, and hospitals; and to other subjects of like nature.[34]

Pittsburgh did not have a formal affiliation with the Sanitary Commission until later in the war. It was not until early 1863 that the Pittsburgh branch of the Sanitary Commission was formally launched. All of its founding officers were leading citizens and businessmen; two were intimately connected with medical care in the city. Thomas Bakewell was elected president of the Pittsburgh branch. Among his many business and civic offices, he served as president of the board of managers of Western Pennsylvania Hospital from its incorporation in 1848 until his death in 1865. Felix R. Brunot was named vice president.

The first report of Pittsburgh's newly formed alliance with the Sanitary Commission contained an account of their work:

> The main efforts of the Sanitary Commission are directed—
>
> 1. To maintain constant inspection of all the camps and hospitals by eminent medical men, for the prevention of sickness, the correction of evils, and the removal, as far as possible, of the radical sources of suffering.

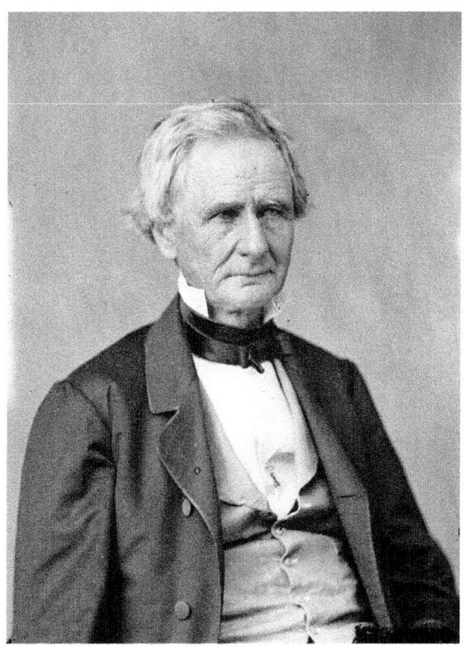

Simon Cameron, Secretary of War. (*Library of Congress*)

2. To prepare and widely distribute short but thorough Medical and Sanitary Papers for the guidance of medical and other officers.
3. To afford Special Relief at the various "Soldiers' Homes" for the sick and wounded who are in transit from camps and hospitals, and to aid discharged men to get their pay and to return to their families.
4. To maintain, for the benefit of all, Hospital Directories, from which can be learned many particulars regarding any soldier in the General Hospitals.
5. To collect and distribute the Supplies furnished by the homes of the land, among the sick and wounded in the hospitals and on the battle fields, where the need is greatest—a business requiring great labor and expense, and thorough system and organization.
6. To make the general wants and condition of sick and wounded men a constant study, and strive, by influences on Government, on Congress, and the public, to secure such new laws, or general orders, or to make such a public opinion as will induce constant improvement in their condition.[35]

Throughout the Civil War, the "Medical and Sanitary Papers" the national office of the Sanitary Commission prepared and distributed were often the only guidance available for military medical personnel. Examples of the monographs include: Report on Military Hygiene and Therapeutics; Directions to Army Surgeons on the Battlefield; Rules for Preserving the Health of the Soldier; Report on the use of Quinine as a Prophylactic against Malarious Diseases; Report on the Value of

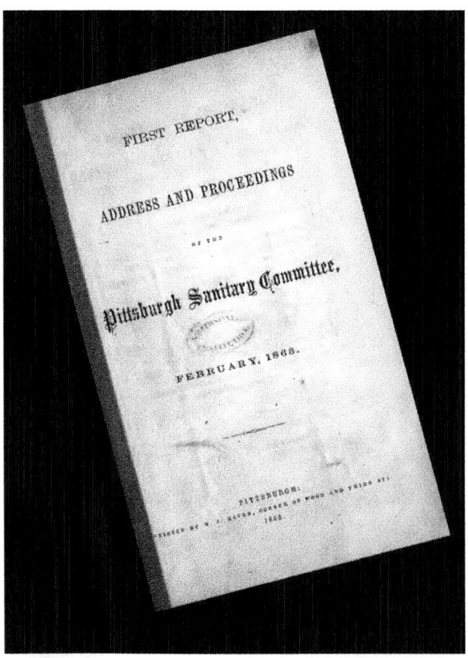

Title page of the First Report Pittsburgh Sanitary Committee, 1863. (*Internet Archive*)

Vaccination; Report on Amputations; Report on Venereal Diseases; Report on Dysentery; Report on Scurvy; Report on the Nature and Treatment of Miasmatic Fevers; Report on the Nature and Treatment of Yellow Fever; and Report on the Treatment of Infectious Diseases.[36]

In the Sanitary Commission's report to the Secretary of War in 1861, it was stated:

> The Commission has distributed gratuitously to the surgeons and officers of the volunteers, three thousand each, on an average, of five concise treatises on the best means of preserving health in camps, and on the treatment of the sick and wounded in camp and the battle field. As the surgeons of the volunteer army are almost altogether drawn from civil practice, and as no books, or even circulars of instruction in regard to their novel responsibilities, have yet been supplied them by Government, these modest works have been found of considerable value.[37]

In April 1864, a local newspaper took the opportunity to describe the manner in which supplies collected in Pittsburgh were distributed to battlefields and hospitals:

> How Sanitary Stores are distributed in the Army of the Cumberland
> They are placed in store rooms as convenient as possible to the hospitals and camps, in the exclusive charge of a confident storekeeper, and are given out by him, first and principally on the written request of the surgeon in charge, who in his request states the number for whom he desires to procure stores, and the special wants.

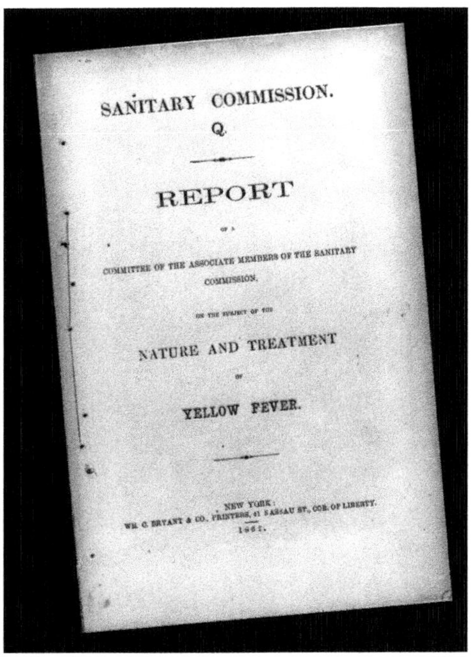

U.S. Sanitary Commission Medical and Sanitary monograph on Yellow Fever, 1862.

> Secondly, the store-keeper issues stores on the application of ladies in charge of what is called the "light diet kitchen" in hospitals. Those drawn by the surgeons are, as a general rule, placed in charge of those ladies, when the hospitals are so fortunate as to have such help. These ladies cook and distribute them to the sick.
>
> Thirdly, The Stores are given to "Hospital Visitors,"—agents who go to hospitals and camps, seeking out from every possible source any special cases of want, and supplying them. Such visits are made as often as possible.
>
> Fourthly. The storekeepers fill all orders given by State agents for any soldier they may find to be needy, or who apply to them for relief. They also furnish to individual soldiers, who may apply to any of the agents for relieve, as soon as it can be ascertained they are really needy. Under a general order from the Secretary of the Departments, they extend to the agents of the Christian Commission the same privileges as are enjoyed by the Sanitary agents, distributing to them to supply any individual cases of neglect or suffering which they may discover.
>
> Fifthly. They furnish goods to the "Soldiers' Homes" and to the "Hospital Trains." When application is made by the surgeons or the soldiers for such articles as a government has for distribution, effort is made by the agents of the Commission to have them supplied from Government stores.[38]

The work of the United States Sanitary Commission was groundbreaking. Without its efforts, countless lives would surely have been lost. The war might have had an entirely different outcome if Lincoln had elected not to accept the commission's assistance. The commission's work not only changed the outcome of the war, but it also established a template for how relief organizations would organize in the future.

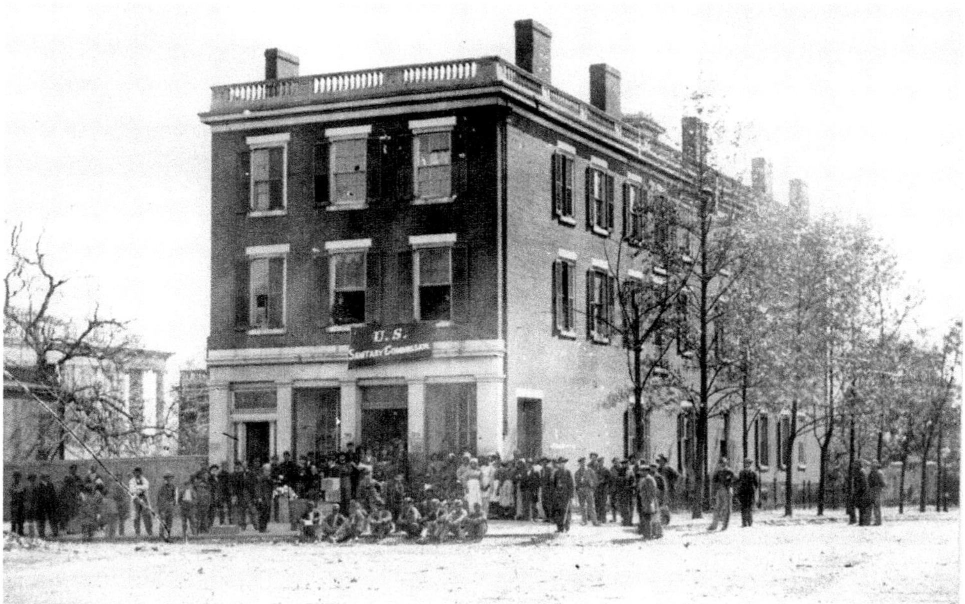

United States Sanitary Commission headquarters Richmond, Virginia, April 1865. (*Library of Congress*)

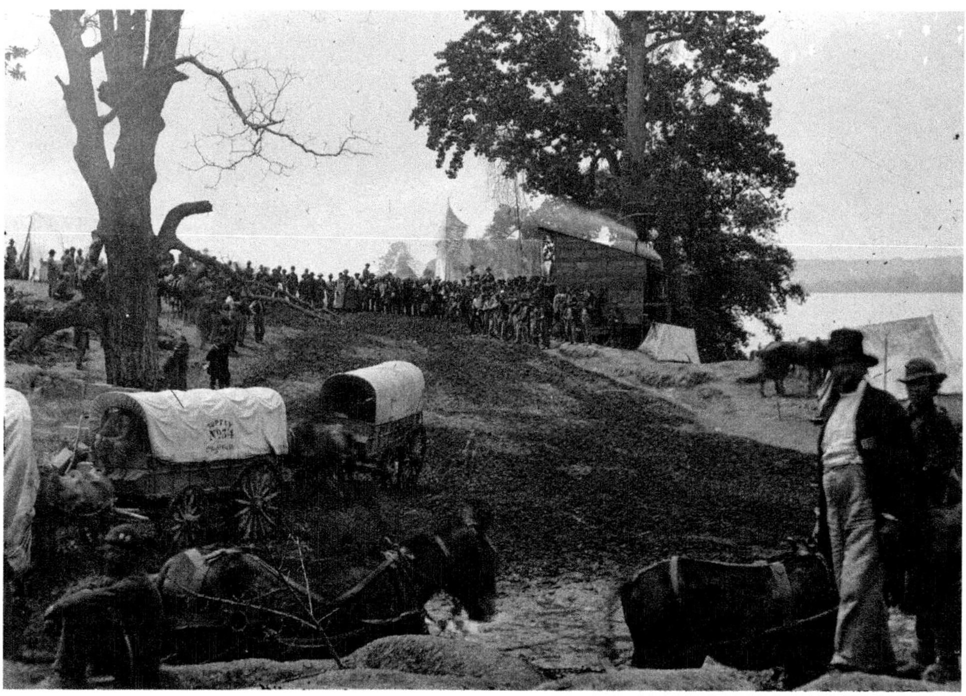

Supply wagons of United States Sanitary Commission at Belle Plain Landing, Virginia, May 1864. (*Library of Congress*)

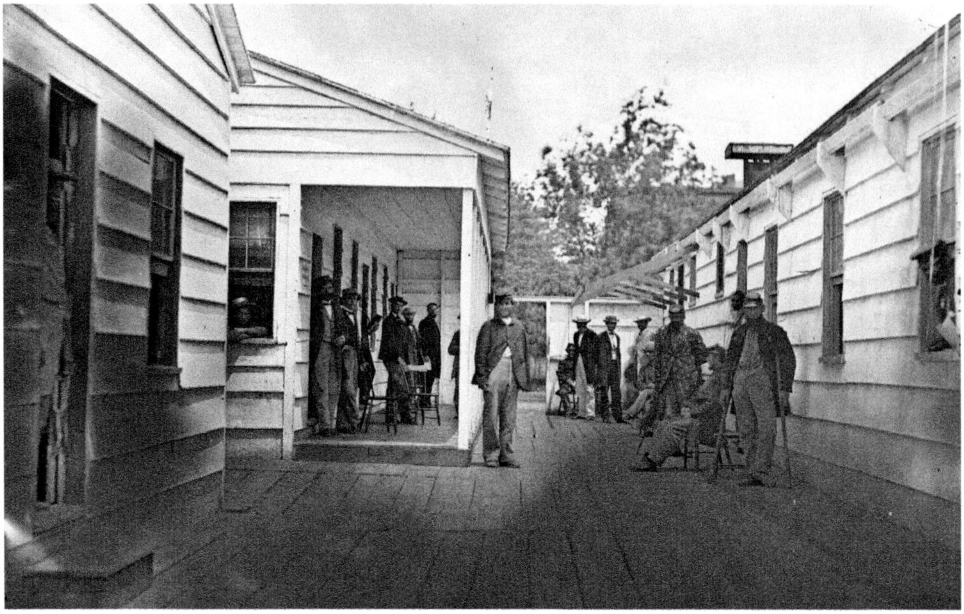

Convalescent soldiers outside quarters of the United States Sanitary Commission Home Lodge, Washington, D.C., 1865. (*Library of Congress*)

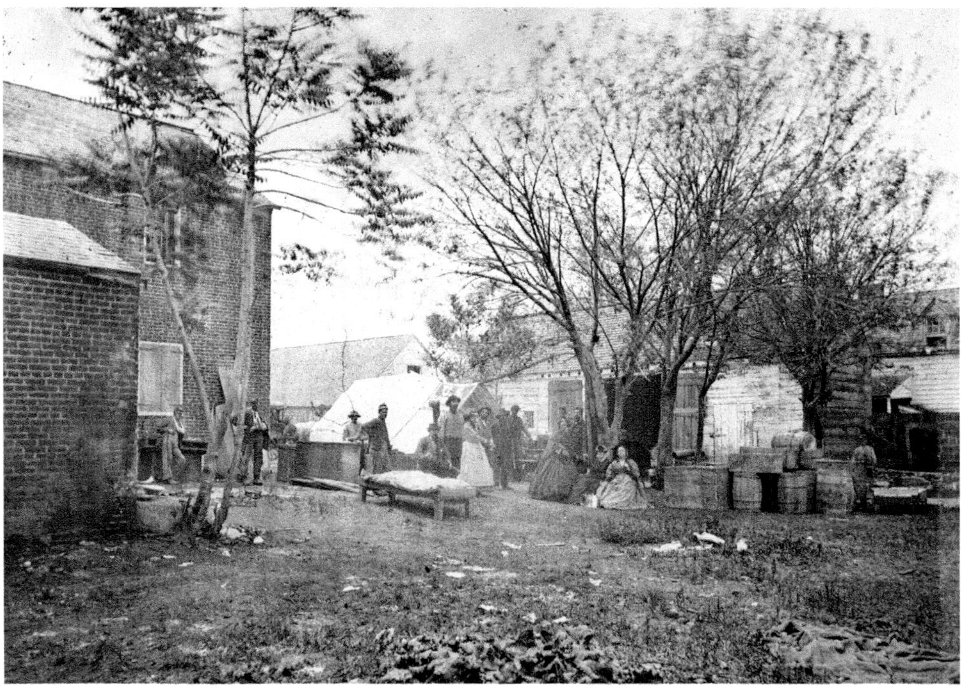

United States Sanitary Commission cooking tent, Fredericksburg, Virginia, 1864. (*Library of Congress*)

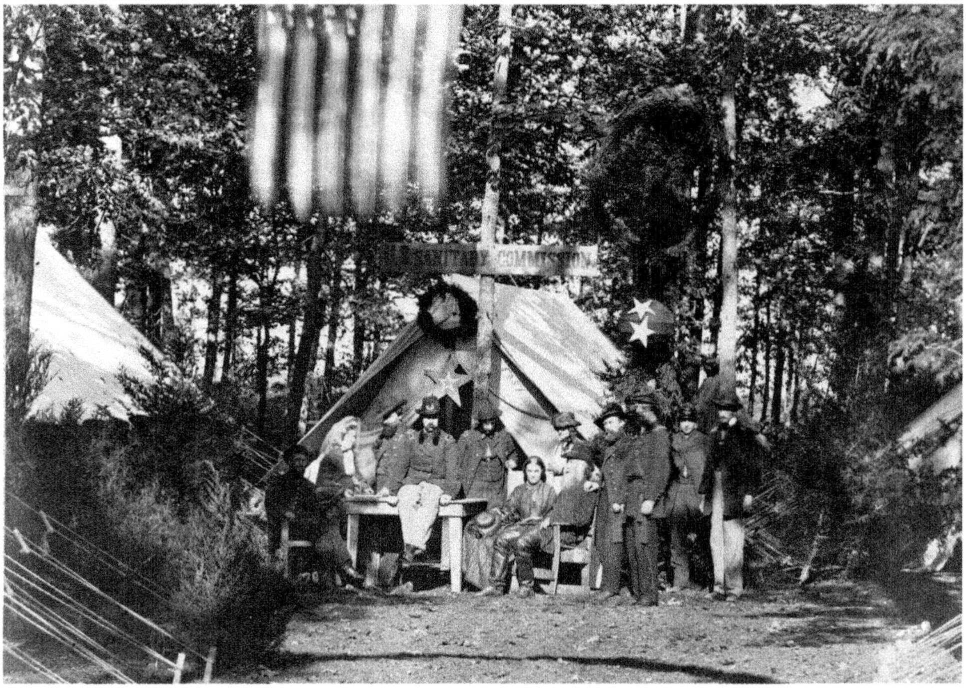

U.S. Sanitary Commission at Gettysburg General Hospital, August 1863. (*Library of Congress*)

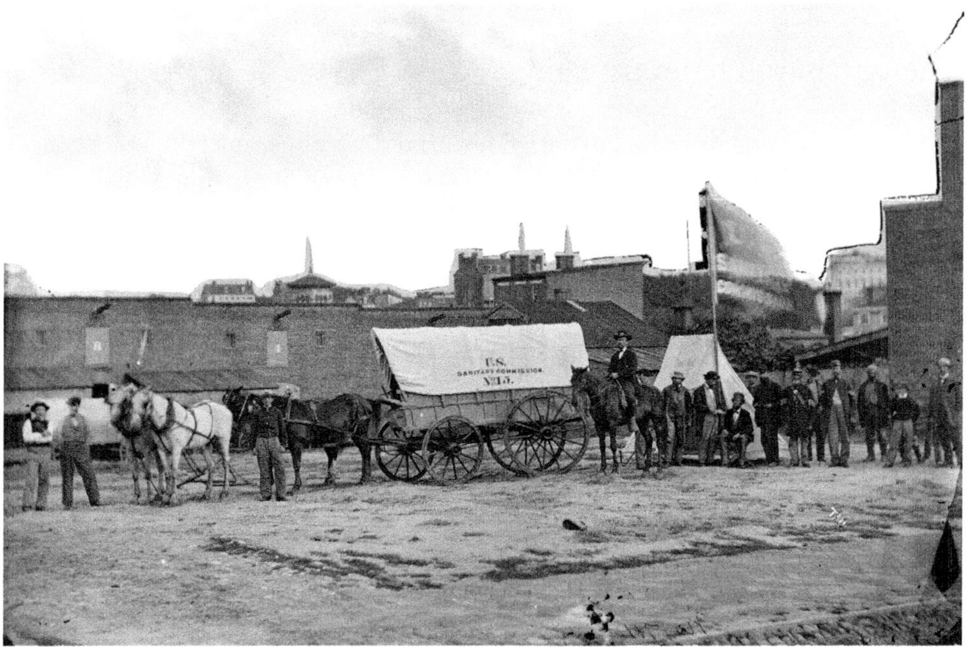

Washington, D.C., field relief wagons and workers of United States Sanitary Commission, 1865. (*Library of Congress*)

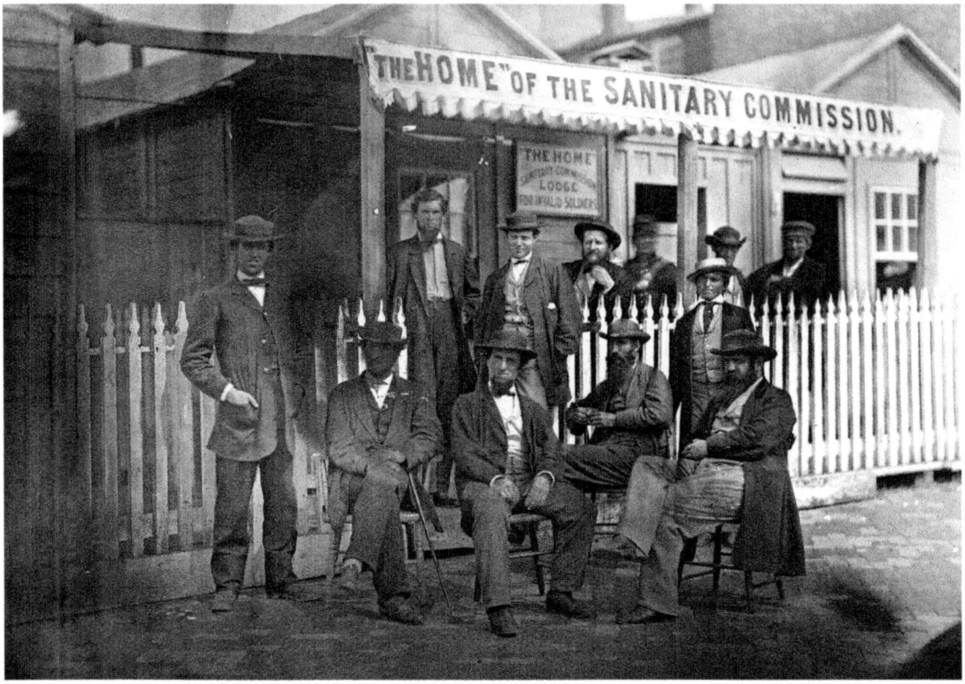

Group of United States Sanitary Commission workers at the entrance of the Home Lodge, Washington, D.C., 1861. (*Library of Congress*)

The Pittsburgh Sanitary Fair

In an article written in 1958, Pittsburgh historian Dorothy Daniel offered a concise overview of the challenges the federal government faced in providing medical care at the onset of the Civil War:

> At the beginning of the Civil War it became starkly plain to the Medical Corps of the Army of the Potomac that caring for a small national army in peace times was not the same problem either in application or scope as administering to the needs of hundreds of thousands of inadequately equipped volunteers. The Honorable Simon Cameron, who was then the heartily unpopular Secretary of War but a Pennsylvanian withal, at the suggestion of the medical bureau at Washington appointed the United States Sanitary Commission on the 9th day of June 1861. In his orders Secretary Cameron directed that the Sanitary Commission "direct its inquiries to the principles and practices connected with the inspection of recruits and enlisted men; to the sanitary condition of the volunteers; to the means of preserving and restoring the health, and of securing the general comfort and efficiency of the troops; to the proper provisions for cooks, nurses and hospitals; and to other subjects of like nature.[39]

Since the Sanitary Commission was not an agency of the government, it could not rely on governmental subsidy to operate. The commission preferred this arrangement since it precluded the interference of governmental control and political patronage. This separation, however, did require the commission to find alternate sources of revenue. The commission found its expenses running almost double its income by October 1863 and could not be counted upon to assist local chapters that provided the most relief. From that point forward, the local chapters tried to raise funds through lotteries, auctions, and cotillion but soon found a much more compelling vehicle with which to fund commission operations.

Mrs. A. H. Hoge of the Chicago chapter of the commission attempted something different and had been extremely successful. Her idea was to hold a fair near the Chicago courthouse. The fair displayed and sold sundry items, served hot dinners daily to 1,500 people, and exhibited rare relics and trophies from around the world. Mrs. Hoge's efforts met with immediate success, which caught the attention of other chapters across the county.

Mrs. Hoge was the wife of a leading Pittsburgh businessman and had been a long-term resident of the city before relocating to Chicago. At the invitation of Mrs. Hoge, Mrs. Rachel W. McFadden and Mrs. Felix R. Brunot traveled from Pittsburgh to Chicago to study her work. Upon returning to Pittsburgh, they informed Mr. Brunot that Pittsburgh should attempt such an undertaking and it was their opinion they could do better than the Chicago fair.

Mr. Brunot spoke with Thomas Bakewell, President of the Pittsburgh chapter of the Sanitary Commission, about sponsoring such a fair locally. Surprisingly, Bakewell was not interested and elected to remove his name from such an endeavor. Thankfully, the "Ladies Branch" of the local chapter saw the merit of McFadden's plans and chose to proceed with sponsoring a Pittsburgh fair. Felix Brunot was elected General Chairman. Among the planning committee were several Pittsburgh physicians, including, Drs. John Dickson, William Reiter, T. N. Shaw, and George D. Bruce.

Once it was agreed to go forward with a fair, a contingent of the planning committee was assigned to travel to Cleveland, Ohio, where the citizens of that city were just completing their fair. The purpose of the trip was to negotiate the purchase and removal of some or all of their buildings. James Park, Jr., John W. Chalfant, and Capt. Charles W. Batchelor were delegated to make the trip. Upon arriving in Cleveland, they completed the purchase of several buildings, tableware, and gas fixtures.

A general announcement was printed and distributed throughout the area informing citizens of the mission of the fair. Within a short period, a new committee was formed, and an office at 96 Water Street was selected to serve as headquarters. The committee made the most of their efforts in soliciting people from all ranks to take part in the planning and implementation of the fair. Businessmen, farmers, homemakers and school children readily complied with the committee's requests.

Every conceivable strategy was used to promote public acceptance and participation in this patriotic responsibility. Members of the planning committee informed the public of their plans by distributing the following message:

> ADDRESS.
> The Pittsburgh Sanitary Committee, a branch of the U.S. Sanitary Commission, established for the relief of the sick and wounded soldiers, announce to the public that a Great Fair will be held at Pittsburgh, Pa., commencing on such day as the Executive Committee will hereafter make known.
>
> The object of the Fair is to obtain money to enable the Sanitary Commission to proceed with their good work with increased energy and usefulness. The practical workings of the United States Sanitary Commission have been of such incalculable good, and have met such high approval from the entire people, that an enumeration of its claims is useless.
>
> Every one feels it a duty to succor the wounded, sick and disabled soldier. The promptings of every loyal heart speak clearly, that we, who do not bear the dint and turmoil of the battle, should provide liberally for the "war-worn sons of the Republic." Christian charity speaks trumpet-tongued to each and every one, telling us to tender to the wants of those who are sick, wounded and disabled in our country's glorious cause.
>
> The ranks of our armies are being rapidly filled, and several hundred thousand brave soldiers now stand "shoulder to shoulder" to uphold the lives (personal and political,) of the people of the Great Republic—to hold sacred our homes and our altars—to preserve our social, commercial and political prosperity; and shall we not succor and aid them when wounded, sick and disabled?
>
> This is no merely local matter. We cordially invite the donations, contributions, aid and co-operation, not only of Allegheny City, Birmingham, Allegheny County and the State of Pennsylvania, but of Ohio, and all the States of the Republic. The recipients of the care of the Sanitary Commission are the soldiers of the United States, without regard to what special State enlisted from, citizens or foreigners, old or young, and without respect to sect, creed, faith or color. All who fight and are disabled in the cause of our common country, are embraced in the management and care of the United States Sanitary Commission. We therefore ask the hearty co-operation and aid of all.
>
> Donations of money will be thankfully received by the Honorary Treasurer of the Fair, N. Holmes, Esq.
>
> Contributions of merchandise of every nature will be received by the Committees appointed for that purpose.[40]

Along with the address, "Calls were promptly issued to Western Pennsylvania particularly, and the whole North generally, for anything that could be eaten, worn, sold or was curious to look at."[41] The Fair, scheduled to open on 01 June 1864, would comprise many marvelous displays, entertainments, meals, and sundry items for sale.

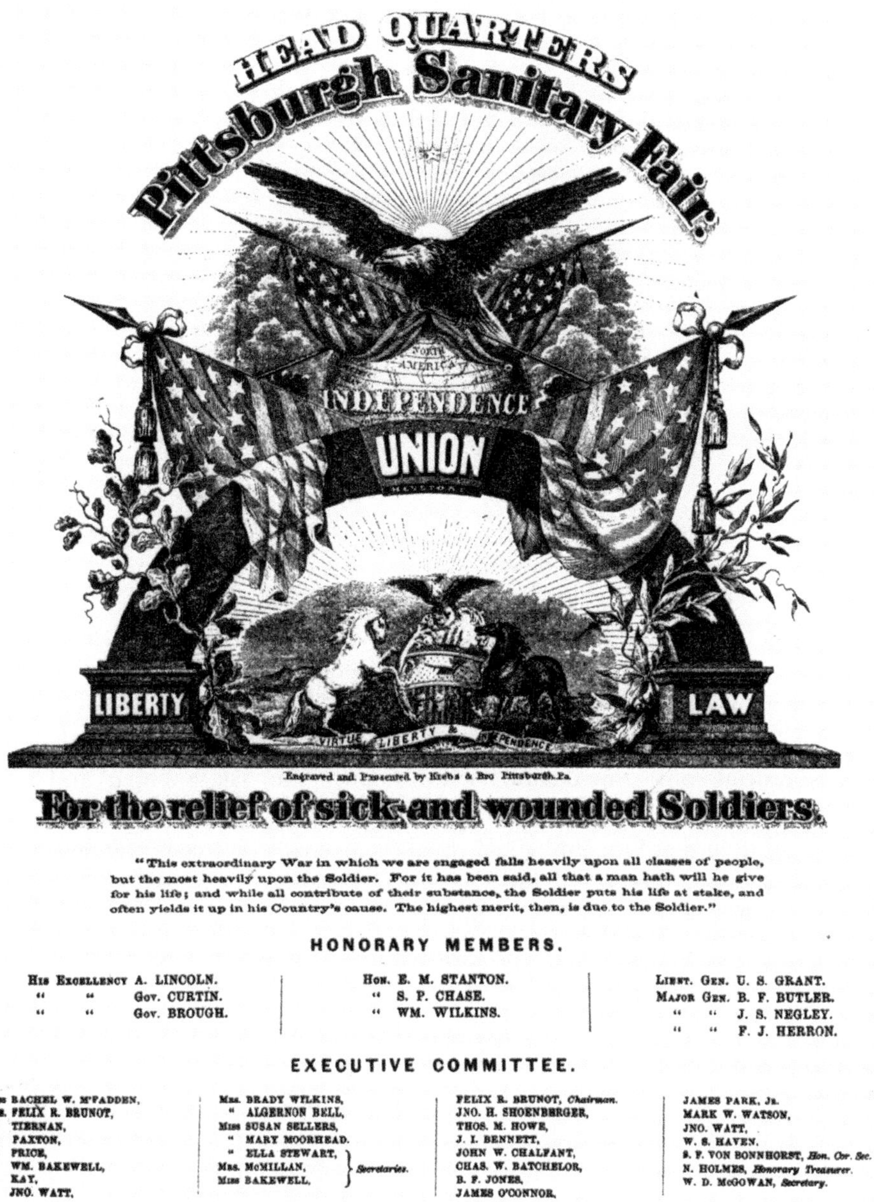

Pittsburgh Sanitary Fair Announcement, 1864. (*Library of Congress*)

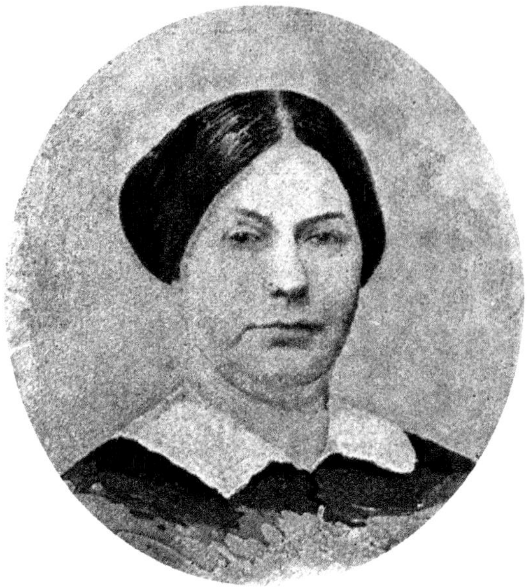

Miss Rachel McFadden, President of the Pittsburgh Sanitary Fair Executive Committee. (*Grand Army of the Republic 28th National Encampment program, Pittsburgh, 1894*)

In preparation for the fair, members of the Pittsburgh Sanitary Fair Committee corresponded with a variety of federal government officials to inform them of the group's plans, and to request their support. In the case of President Abraham Lincoln, they wrote on 15 April 1864: "We respectfully invite you to be present at the opening of the Fair, or at some time during its continuance, and ask you apart to lend your name in connection with it."[42] Several weeks later, on 20 May, they followed up with a letter indicating that Lincoln had declined their request, instead offering to send an "autographed letter" expressing his sympathy for their cause. In response, a letter was sent respectfully requesting the letter and other such "material aid" as he might offer.[43] Relative to the autograph, a large placard with photographs of President Lincoln and his Cabinet and their autographs was subsequently prepared and delivered to the Committee. On 02 June, Felix R. Brunot, chairman of the Pittsburgh Sanitary Fair Committee, sent Lincoln a telegram announcing the opening of the Fair.[44]

Opening day was filled with excitement and anxiety. Final deliveries continued to be made at the fair site. Complex parade routes were prepared, streets were cleared, and participating marchers organized. Dignitaries honed their speeches as crowds began arriving along the parade route early to claim a prime spot for viewing the festivities. Pittsburgh's businesses were closed for several hours that day to allow workers and their families to participate.

A few minutes after 4 p.m. on 01 June 1864, the fair's opening procession began from the Monongahela House and proceeded along Smithfield Street to Fifth, Market, and St. Clair Streets and on to the suspension bridge. After crossing the bridge, the procession traveled to Federal Street, and from there they went on to Ohio Street and the North Commons, which was the site of the fair.

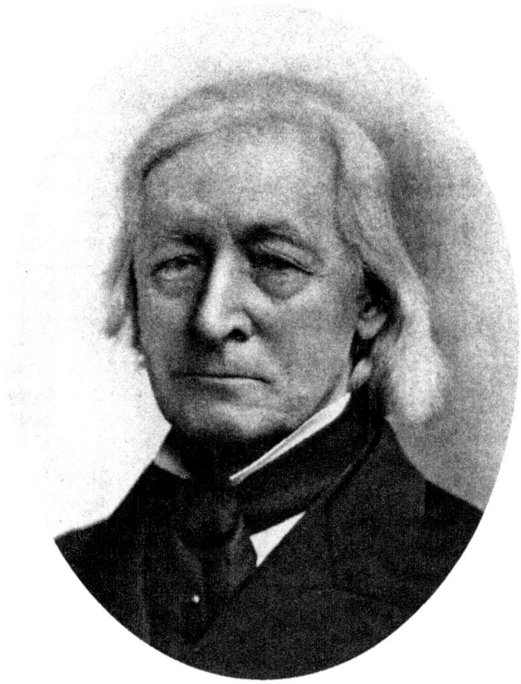

Rightt: Felix R. Brunot, Chairman of the Pittsburgh Sanitary Fair Executive Committee. (*Carnegie Library of Pittsburgh. All rights reserved. Unauthorized reproduction or usage prohibited*)

Below left: Letter to President Lincoln requesting "material aid" and autograph in support of the Pittsburgh Sanitary Fair. (*Library of Congress*)

Below right: Felix Brunot's letter to President Lincoln announcing the opening of the Pittsburgh Sanitary Fair. (*Library of Congress*)

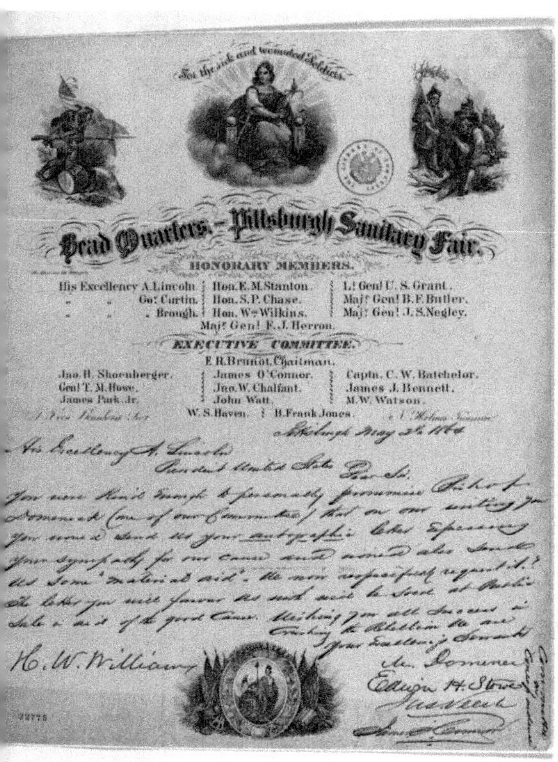

For the sick and wounded Soldiers

Head Quarters, — Pittsburgh Sanitary Fair.

HONORARY MEMBERS.

His Excellency A. Lincoln. | Hon. E. M. Stanton. | Lt Genl U. S. Grant.
" " Gov. Curtin. | Hon. S. P. Chase. | Majr Genl B. F. Butler.
" " Brough. | Hon. Wm Wilkins. | Majr Genl J. S. Negley.
Majr Genl F. J. Herron.

EXECUTIVE COMMITTEE.

F. R. Brunot, Chairman.

Jno. H. Shoenberger. | James O'Connor. | Captn. C. W. Batchelor.
Genl T. M. Howe. | Jno. W. Chalfant. | James J. Bennett.
James Park Jr. | John Watt. | M. W. Watson.
W. S. Haven. | B. Frank Jones.

Pittsburgh May 2d 1864

His Excellency A. Lincoln
President United States

Dear Sir,

[illegible] "material aid" [illegible]

H. W. Williams

32773

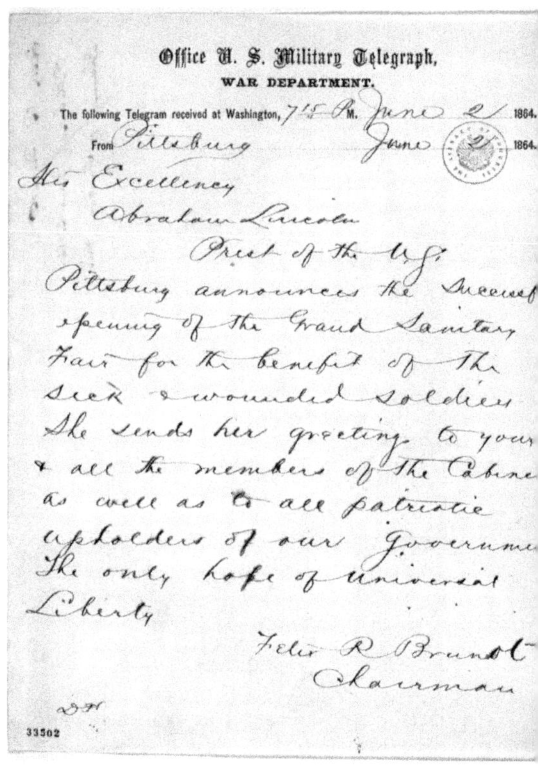

Office U. S. Military Telegraph,
WAR DEPARTMENT.

The following Telegram received at Washington, 7 15 PM. June 2 1864.
From Pittsburg June 2 1864.

His Excellency
Abraham Lincoln
Prest of the U.S.

Pittsburg announces the successful opening of the Grand Sanitary Fair for the benefit of the sick & wounded soldiers She sends her greeting to you & all the members of the Cabinet as well as to all patriotic upholders of our Government The only hope of Universal Liberty

Felix R Brunot
Chairman

33502

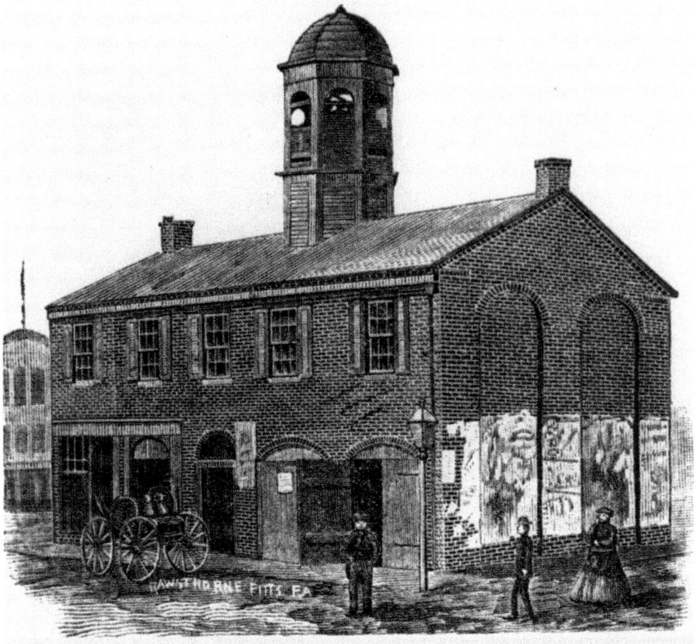

Old Allegheny City Town Hall torn down in 1862. The site and surrounding area was used for the Pittsburgh Sanitary Fair. (*Carnegie Library of Pittsburgh. All rights reserved. Unauthorized reproduction or usage prohibited*)

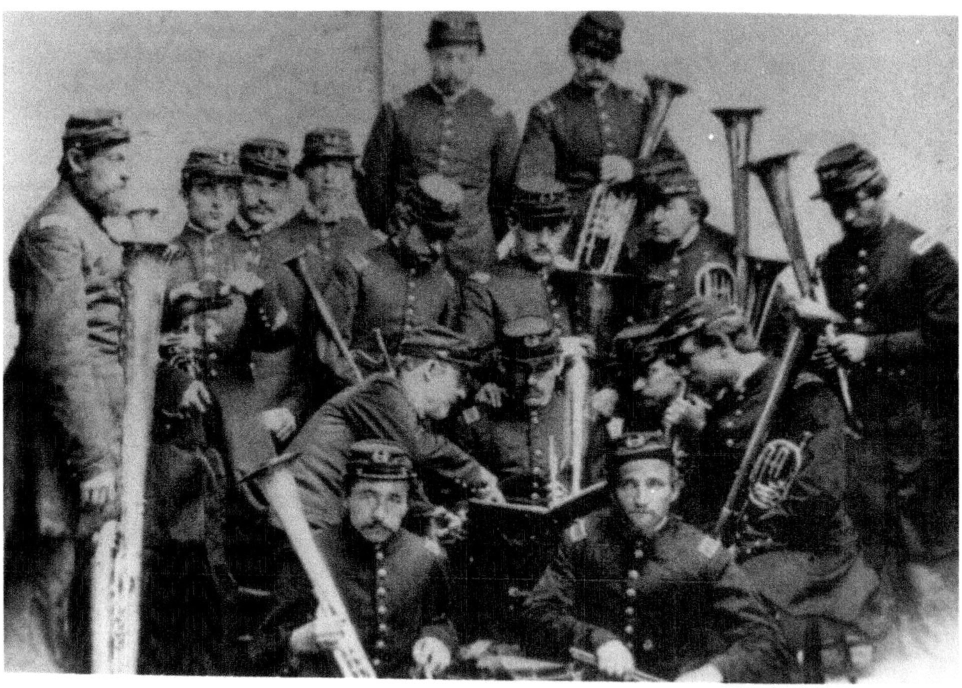

Pittsburgh Sanitary Fair Military Band, 1864. (*Carnegie Library of Pittsburgh. All rights reserved. Unauthorized reproduction or usage prohibited*)

Major-General James S. Negley served as chief marshal, accompanied by a chief assistant and a cadre of *aide-de-camps*. Judge James L. Graham served as chief civic marshal. A long list of assistants followed Graham, including a group of approximately twenty municipal, civic, and local military officers. Among the group was one of the city's leading physicians, Dr. John Dickson, and one of Pittsburgh's most prominent industrialists, Andrew Carnegie. It was noted: "The Chief Marshal of the Civic Marshal wore a red scarf and rosette. His assistant a rosette—red, white and blue—on the left breast."[45] Many thousands of local citizens filled the streets and cheered parade participants. Upon arriving at the Fairgrounds, the Auditorium was opened and filled immediately. Many who could not gain admittance filled the square surrounding the building.

Once all the officials had arrived and were seated, Felix R. Brunot called the assembly to order and introduced Rev. Dr. Preston, who led the opening prayer. After the prayer, Brunot introduced Pennsylvania Governor A. G. Curtin. After delivering a lengthy and laudatory speech, Curtin officially opened the Fair to the public. It was estimated that 5,000 people attended the ceremony.

There had never been anything in the city like the Pittsburgh Sanitary Fair. For eighteen days, the entire community focused its attention on making it a success. Descriptions of the various buildings and activities were highlighted in all of the city's newspapers. In its 02 June 1864 morning edition, The Pittsburgh Commercial newspaper offered an in-depth review:

> The Great Fair
>
> The Fair Buildings: The buildings erected for the use of the Fair are six in number, and are known as Floral Hall, Ladies' Bazaar, Dining Hall, Mechanics Hall, Monitor Hall, and Stock Department. Besides these, the City Councils of Allegheny have generously donated the use of their Council Chambers for the Art Gallery and "Old Curiosity Shop."
>
> Floral Hall.
>
> The crowning feature of the Fair is Floral Hall. Whether it is regarded as a beautiful creation of artificial scenery, or viewed as an assemblage or grouping together of several pictures so as to unite in harmony and symmetry a grand result, certain it is the accomplished artist has produced a work of surpassing loveliness.
>
> When you enter this temple of design and flowers, the eye is charmed, and the taste is pleased with the rare combination of rock, rough and tangled tufts of vegetation, old stumps and trees re-animated with living creepers, rustled arbors, flowers, fountains, cascades, dropping water, gurgling streams, evergreens, statuary, bowers, etc. What strikes the beholder first, as he comprehends the picture, is the singular unity and congruity of parts observable in the entire arrangement. Encircling the hall are a series of booths, of entirely different architecture, from the rude structure framed but of the native forestry, to the more advanced gothic style.

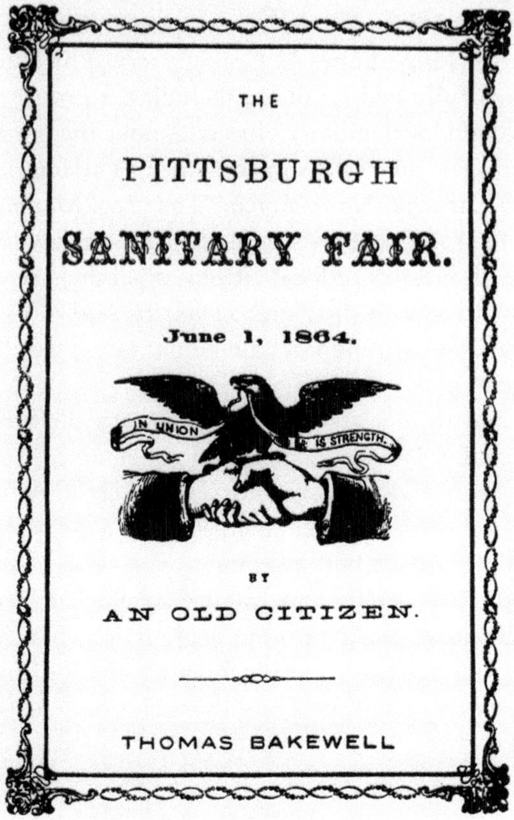

THE

PITTSBURGH

SANITARY FAIR.

June 1, 1864.

BY

AN OLD CITIZEN.

THOMAS BAKEWELL

Left: Pittsburgh Sanitary Fair program front page, 1864. (*Heinz History Center*)

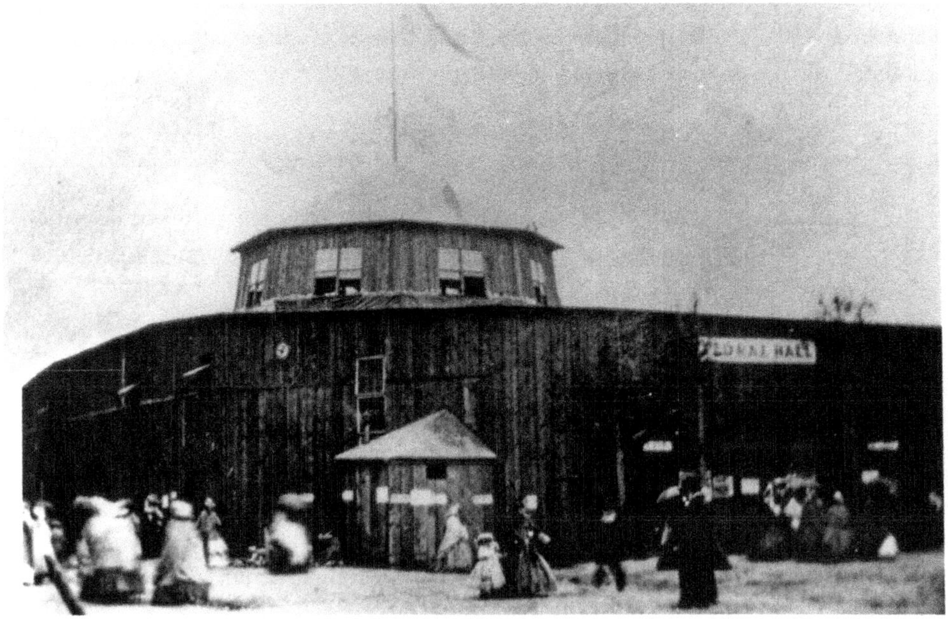

Below: Pittsburgh Sanitary Fair Floral Hall, 1864. (*Carnegie Library of Pittsburgh. All rights reserved. Unauthorized reproduction or usage prohibited*)

The Garden of Eden.
At the northern end of the hall stands the Garden of Eden. This is a combination of flowers, evergreens, jets of water, shells, patches of green turf, birds, and the peaceable animals of rare attraction. The artist has placed statues representing Adam and Eve, with the Serpent coiling and entwined around the tree of Knowledge of Good and Evil.

Ladies' Bazaar.
This building is situated on the corner of Ohio and Federal streets and forms the principal attraction of the Fair. At the main entrance, outside, is situated the ticket office. On the main floor, and appropriately arranged are the larger and more fanciful booths or buildings. These are all gotten up in a chaste and beautiful manner, and deserve more than a passing notice.

The first booth, on the left of the entrance, is set apart for the contributions from Chicago. There will be exposed a variety of articles, ornamental and useful, the gift of the ladies of the Garden City. In front of the East Liberty booth, and adjoining the Chicago booth, is the miniature skating pond. The Post-office is in an octagonal form, and is appropriately fitted up with letterboxes. It is beautifully decorated with red, white and blue. Here letters maybe had from the Army, and all parts of the country.

The most attractive looking building that next meets the eye is the Chinese Pagoda, which is appropriately decorated with red and yellow trimming. The ladies in charge of this beautiful feature will be clothed in Chinese costume, which will add to its uniqueness. Near the Pagoda, and in the center of the Bazaar, is erected a beautiful fountain. The fountain is beautifully decorated, and is surrounded with flowers from the members of the Agricultural Society. To the right of the fountain is the beautiful American booth. It is handsomely and appropriately decorated with flags. An immense canopy, formed by flags and evergreens is one of the largest in extent in the Bazaar, and is amply stocked with all that is useful and ornamental.

The next Grand attraction is Mrs. A. S. Bell's children's play-house. It is of cottage style of architecture, and is complete in every respect. The parlor is supplied with furniture, chandelier, etc., and these sleeping apartments are amply furnished with articles to delight children. It has a beautiful miniature garden attached, in which flowers and shrubbery have been planted. In the center of the garden is a small fountain. Adjoining the play-house is a handsomely fitted up and commodious ice cream saloon, which will no doubt be largely patronized during the continuance of the Fair. A large and handsomely decorated sewing-machine room is located immediately in front of the playhouse, where the contributions of sewing machines are for sale. The Union Booth is the next grand feature.

Mechanics' Hall.
This Department, which a week ago was supposed would be a failure, or at least present a meager show of the genius and mechanical skill of the citizens of Pittsburgh and the west generally, now bids fair to be the great center of attraction during the Fair. The

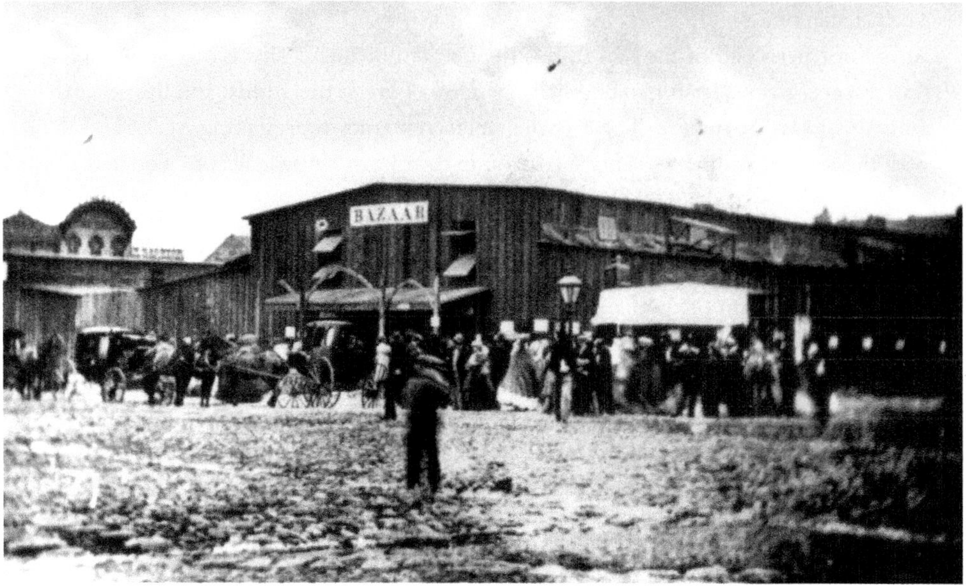

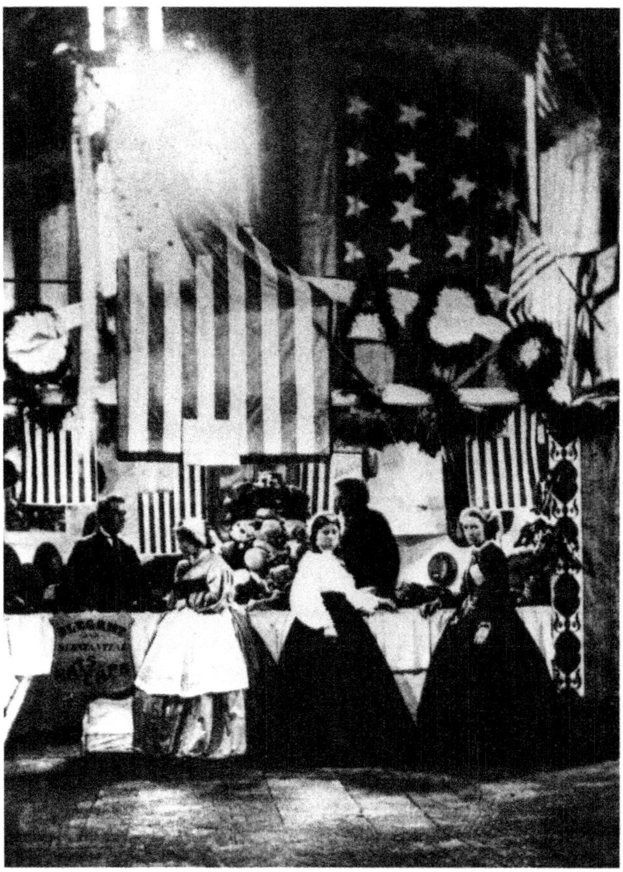

Above: Pittsburgh Sanitary Fair Ladies Bazaar building, 1864. (*Carnegie Library of Pittsburgh. All rights reserved. Unauthorized reproduction or usage prohibited*)

Left: Pittsburgh Sanitary Fair Ladies Bazaar hats and caps stand, 1864. (*Carnegie Library of Pittsburgh. All rights reserved. Unauthorized reproduction or usage prohibited*)

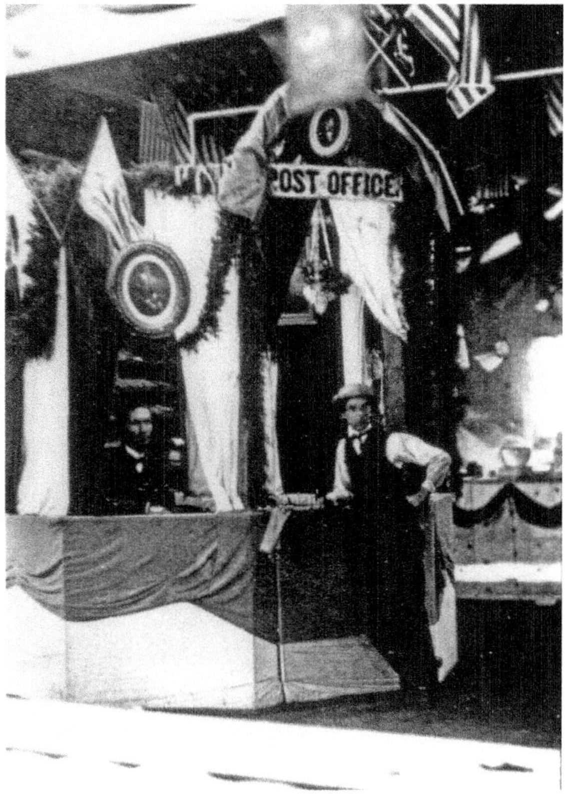

Right: Pittsburgh Sanitary Fair Ladies Bazaar Post Office, 1864. (*Carnegie Library of Pittsburgh. All rights reserved. Unauthorized reproduction or usage prohibited*)

Below: Pittsburgh Sanitary Fair Ladies Bazaar Bitters and Dyes booth, 1864. (*Carnegie Library of Pittsburgh. All rights reserved. Unauthorized reproduction or usage prohibited*)

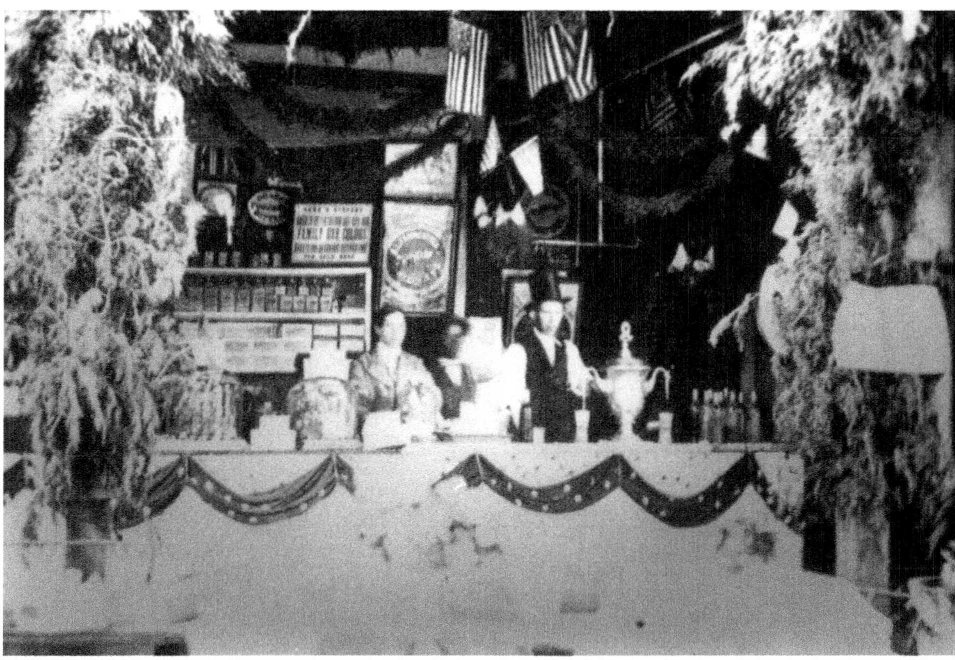

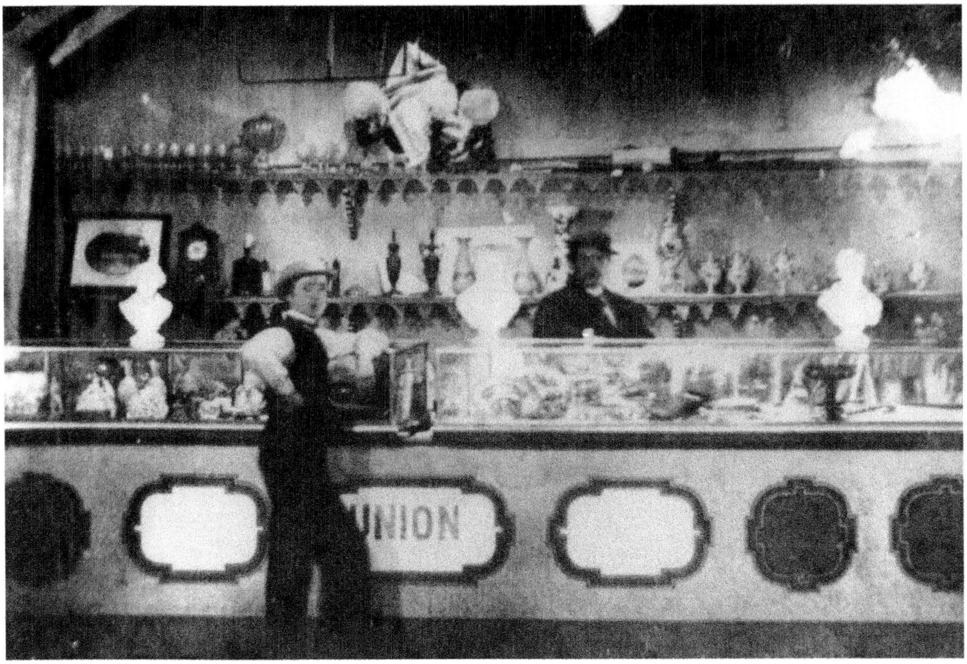

Pittsburgh Sanitary Fair Ladies Bazaar Union booth, 1864. (*Carnegie Library of Pittsburgh.*)

principal feature in Mechanic's Hall will perhaps, be the motive powered boiler, engine and line of shafting, furnished by the machinist and boilermakers in the city by joint contribution. The boiler, horizontal tubular, with fire-box attached, was built by Jared M. Bush. It is ten and a half feet long, and forty inches in diameter, substantially built and handsomely covered with imitation Russia sheet iron.

Monitor Hall.

This department will probably form the most novel and attractive feature of the Fair, as the people can, from a visit to it, obtain a better idea of the "art of war" than in any other way. The hall occupies the space between Floral Hall and the Auditorium, on Ohio street, and is enclosed and roofed on the four sides, the centre being uncovered. The centre of attraction is the miniature oval lake, and is the first object approached by visitors, and occupies that portion of the hall not under cover. It is sixty-five feet in length and thirty-two feet in width. In the centre is an island forty-five feet long and twelve feet wide, leaving ten feet of water surrounding it.

The lake bears several specimens of naval architecture, the most interesting of which is the model *Monitor*. The hull is made of copper; it is nine feet ten inches in length, twenty inches in width, and eight inches in depth, and has a revolving turret fourteen inches in diameter, mounting two model eleven-inch guns. The craft is propelled by steam being provided with a beautiful miniature brass engine, one and a quarter inches

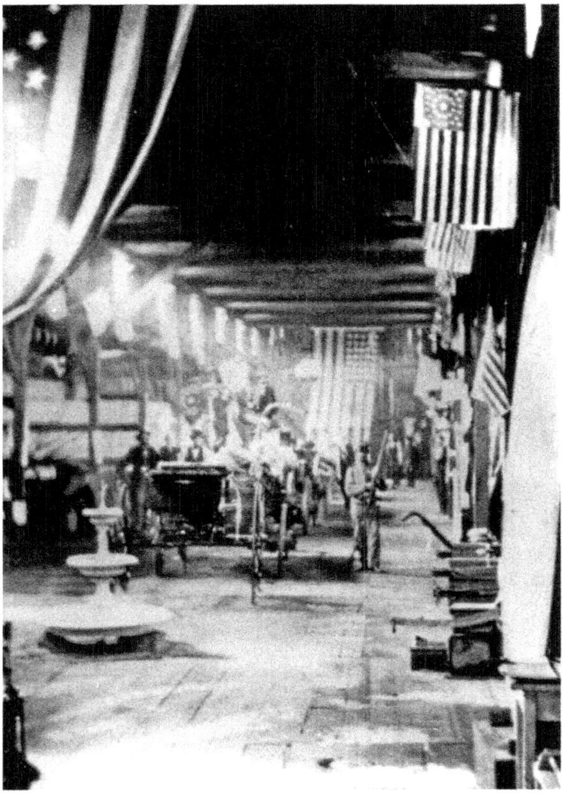

Right: Pittsburgh Sanitary Fair Mechanics Hall, 1864. (*Carnegie Library of Pittsburgh. All rights reserved. Unauthorized reproduction or usage prohibited*)

Below: Pittsburgh Sanitary Fair Mechanics Hall Heavy Machinery Display, 1864. (*Carnegie Library of Pittsburgh. All rights reserved. Unauthorized reproduction or usage prohibited*)

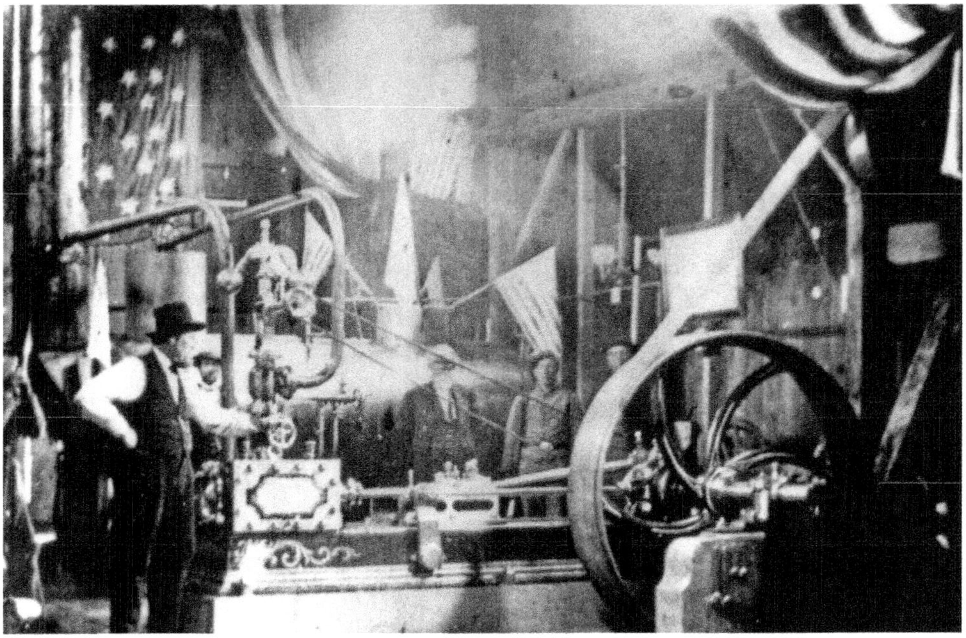

in diameter, and exactly as built by McElroy & Co. A novel boiler twenty-four inches long with safety valve, steam dome, and spirit lamps, by which the *Monitor* is propelled. The craft is the one-twenty-fourth size of the *Manayunk* now approaching completion at the south end of the Monongahela bridge, and in every respect except size, like her.

Next, and it natural contradistinction to the monitor, is an exact model of the rebel *Merrimac*, which requires no particular description. In addition to these also are to be seen two mortar schooners, to transport sloops, one Mississippi mortar boat, and two twenty-four gun full rigged ships. Near the furthest end of the island stands a very neat and tasteful Lighthouse.

In the centre of the island has been constructed a square fort, surrounded by a deep moat, on which is mounted one model twenty-inch gun, one-tenth size, and four ten-inch mortars, one-tenth size. The gun is supported on a "centre pintle," and moves easily and every direction. On the end of the island nearest the entrance is a very neat and formidable earthwork "water battery," mounting three fifteen-inch guns, one-tenth size (one navy and two army) and two ten-inch mortars, one-tenth size. These guns not requiring the same facility of movement as the gun in the fort, are mounted on models of the army iron casemented carriage.

To the rear of the lake is an enclosure containing many attractions, the chief of which are the patterns of the great twenty-inch and eight-inch Columbiads, side by side, illustrating the great advancement made in the manufacturer of heavy ordnance in the last few years. Twenty years ago the eight inch gun was considered a most remarkable achievement—the heaviest the services would ever require. Now the twenty inch gun has been successfully cast, and no one is at all surprised that a thirty inch gun is contemplated. In this enclosure is an elegant display of all kinds of ammunition, consisting of musket, rifle, shot, canister spherical case, from the smallest caliber to the one thousand pound solid shot of the twenty inch gun.

The Dining Hall.

This building which occupies a position on the south west corner of the Diamond Square extends the full length of the square. One of the principal objects of attention is a most beautiful Oriental Pa-g-o-d-a, which is situated in the center of the hall. A large Restaurant is attached to the rear of the Hall, where all who desire to revive the "inner man" can call and be satisfied. The hall is fitted up with tables where meals can be procured at "all hours," and from our knowledge of the ladies who have the culinary matters in charge, we are confident that everything will be done up to the best of style. Dinner will be served up during the continuance of the Fair from twelve o'clock till four o'clock P.M., after which ice cream etc., will be served up according to order.

Audience Hall.

This is one of the largest buildings of the entire collection, the auditorium having a capacity to seat two thousand persons. It is plainly and tastefully decorated, has four rows of seats, and has an ample stage, handsomely fitted up with scenery, curtain, etc.

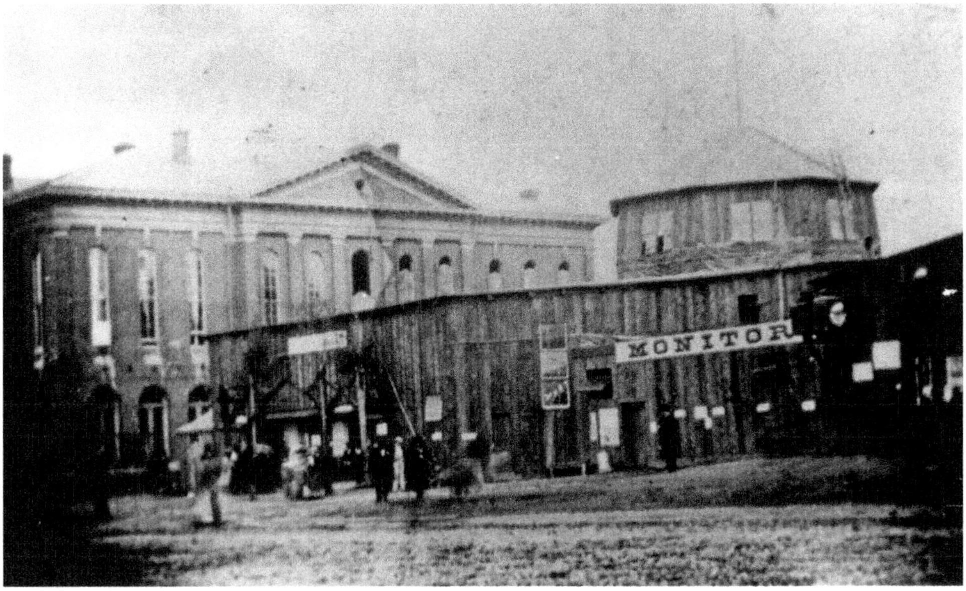

Pittsburgh Sanitary Fair Monitor Hall exterior with new Allegheny City Hall in background, 1864. (*Carnegie Library of Pittsburgh. All rights reserved. Unauthorized reproduction or usage prohibited*)

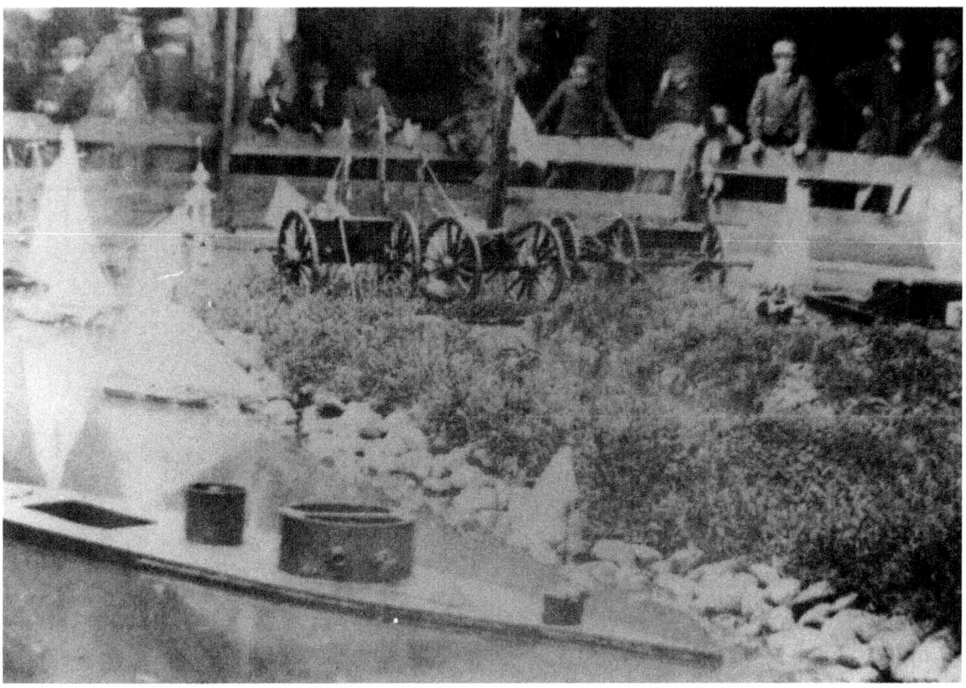

Pittsburgh Sanitary Fair Monitor Hall with model of the *Monitor*, 1864. (*Carnegie Library of Pittsburgh. All rights reserved. Unauthorized reproduction or usage prohibited*)

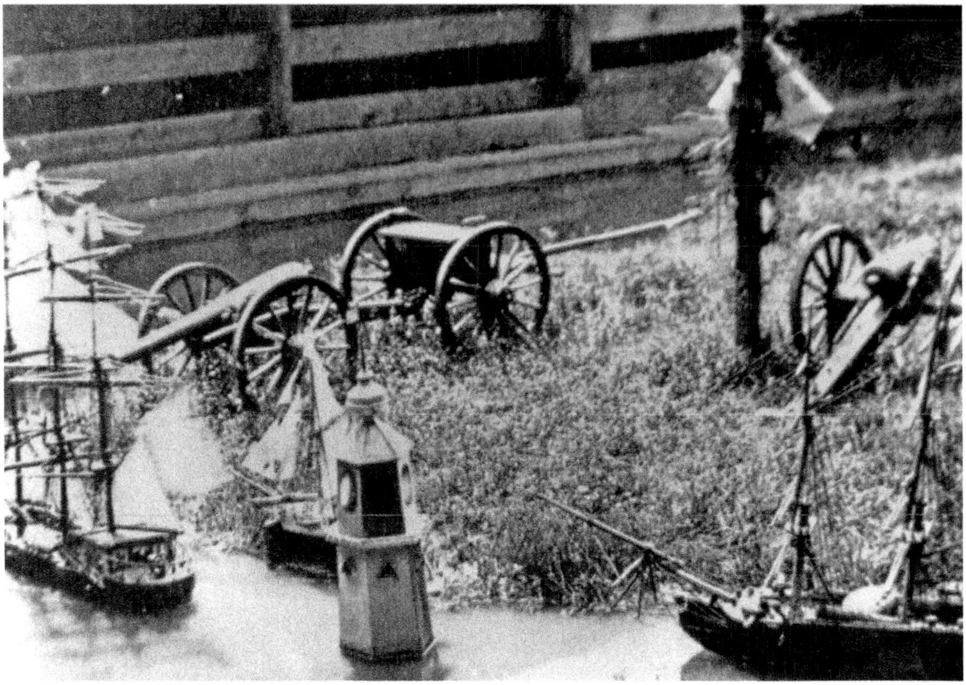

Pittsburgh Sanitary Fair Monitor Hall with model schooner, sloop, rigged ship, mortar boat, and small cannons, 1864. (*Carnegie Library of Pittsburgh. All rights reserved. Unauthorized reproduction or usage prohibited*)

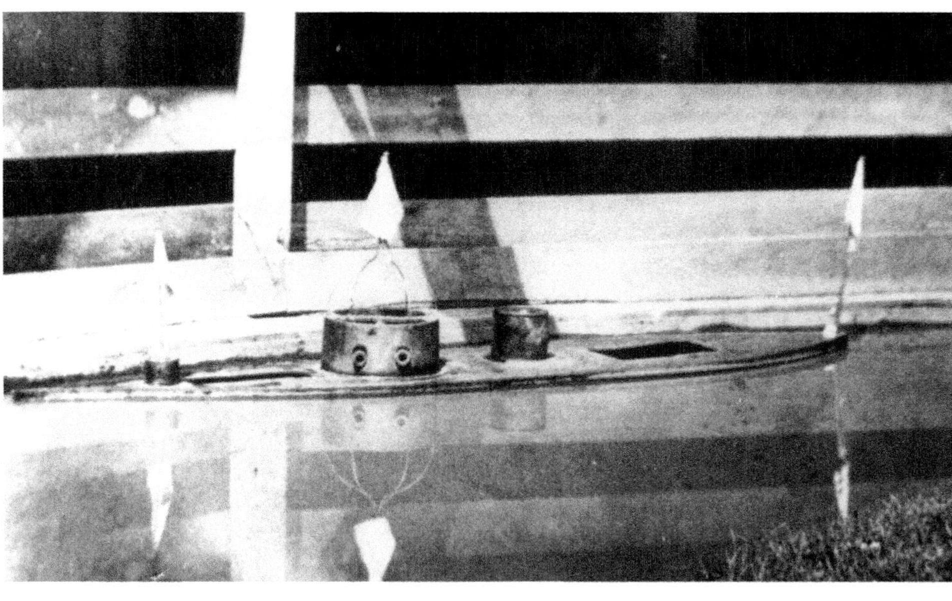

Pittsburgh Sanitary Fair Monitor Hall model of the *Monitor* in lake, 1864. (*Carnegie Library of Pittsburgh. All rights reserved. Unauthorized reproduction or usage prohibited*)

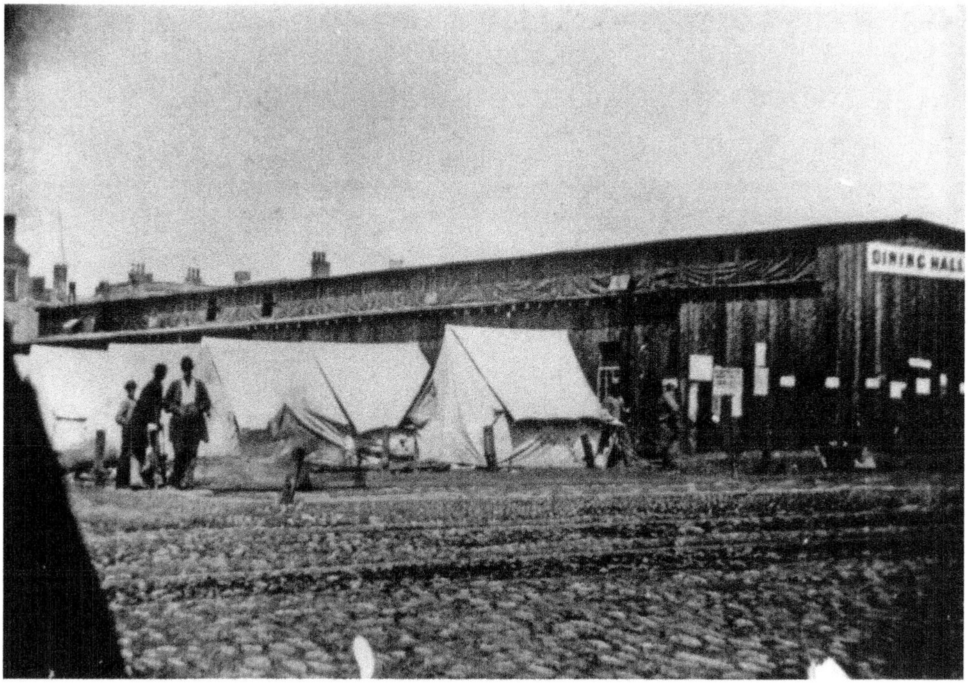

Pittsburgh Sanitary Fair Dining Hall exterior view with tents, 1864. (*Carnegie Library of Pittsburgh. All rights reserved. Unauthorized reproduction or usage prohibited*)

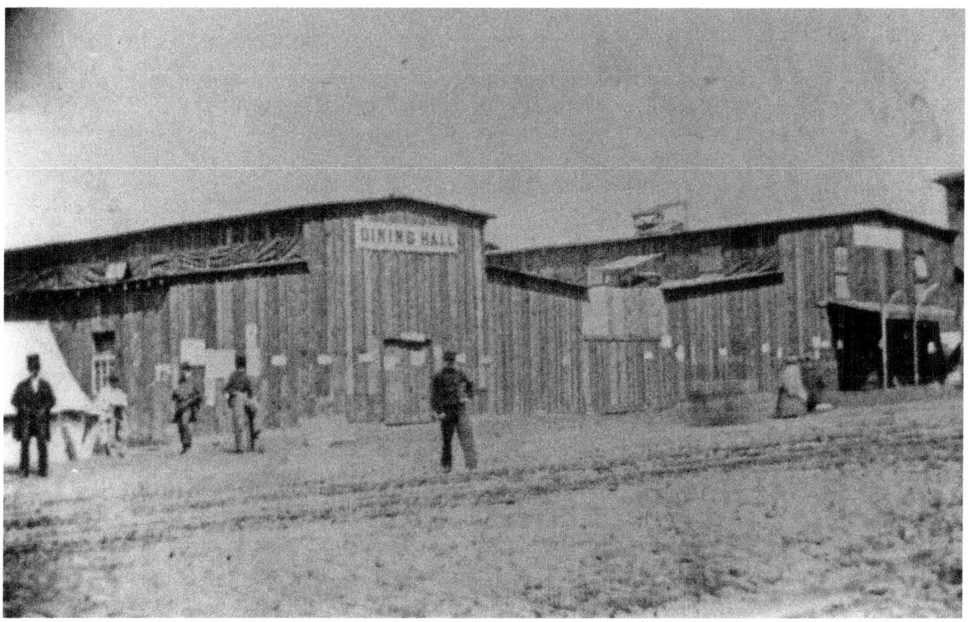

Pittsburgh Sanitary Fair Dining Hall exterior view, 1864. (*Carnegie Library of Pittsburgh. All rights reserved. Unauthorized reproduction or usage prohibited*)

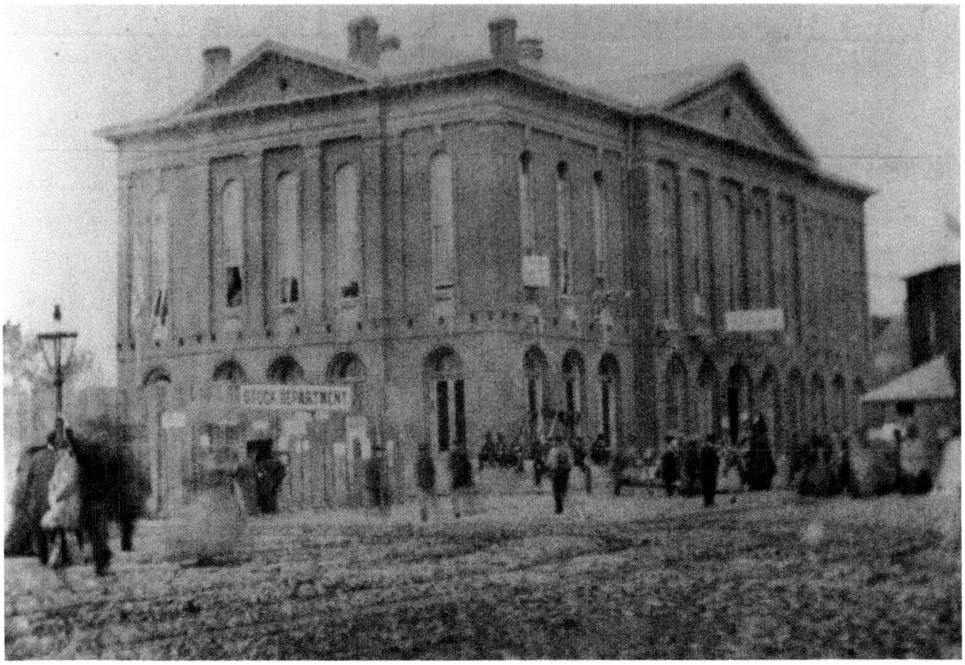

Pittsburgh Sanitary Fair Stock Department exterior view next to new Allegheny City Hall, 1864. (*Carnegie Library of Pittsburgh. All rights reserved. Unauthorized reproduction or usage prohibited*)

The scene at the rear of the stage is a representation of the old frigate "*Constitution*" above which is painted a spread eagle, surrounded by flags.

Stock Department.
The building for the exhibition of the Cashmere goats has been erected in front of the new City Hall. The only animals yet placed in the building are the aforesaid goats, which in themselves would form a centre of attraction; when the entire menagerie of domesticated and useful animals are congregated, the show will be highly interesting and worth ten times the admittance fee.

Art Gallery.
Owing to the indefatigable exertions of the Committee, the Art Gallery will be a decided success. The Halls being unfinished, it required great labor and no little exercise of ingenuity to hide the rough, unplastered walls, but that has been accomplished creditably, and the pictures are now being hung upon a background that relieves the eye. Notwithstanding, some have withheld their Works of Art from the Exhibition, enough have been sent by others to make it the finest collection ever gathered here, and one that our community may be proud of. We had no idea that so many splendid paintings were owned about Pittsburgh. It speaks highly for the cultivation of aesthetic taste here—that so many gems of Art has

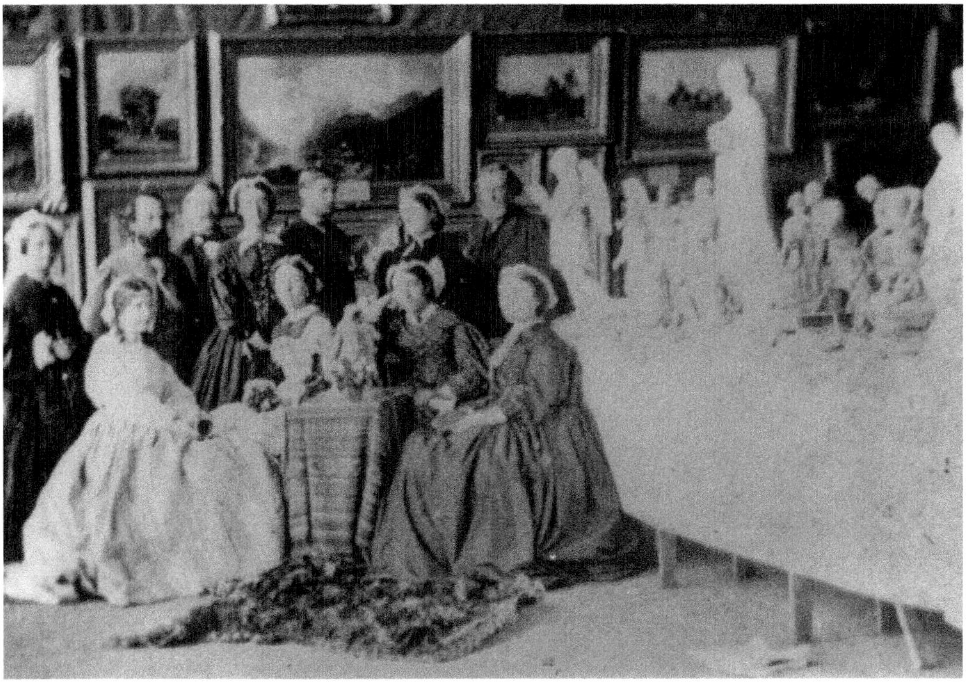

Pittsburgh Sanitary Fair Art Gallery view, 1864. (*Carnegie Library of Pittsburgh. All rights reserved. Unauthorized reproduction or usage prohibited*)

been obtained by our citizens. We will mention only a few of the distinguished artist works represented: Achenbach, Verboeckoven, Holl, Ferdinand de Brackerleer, Herzog, etc.

Old Curiosity Shop.
This department abounds in relics which awaken mingled feelings of joy and sorrow, as we contemplate the memories connected with each. All the influence of War which Southern barbarity or inhuman ingenuity could contribute were represented, and one feels the horrors of the strife which we are engaged in understanding when viewing the savage productions of a so-called chivalric race.

The Indian genius is displayed here to perfection: the simple contrivances of our red brethren presents a strange contrast to the daily implements of society, afforded by the enlightenment of the eighteenth century, and yet they awake a feeling of sympathy for their peculiar history. Nor are the productions of the orient missing, but scattered throughout our many antique and curious specimens of that opium-eating and dreamy land of indolence. Books, whose dates carry us back the stream of centuries, are profusely scattered, and whose mouldering pages inspire none but holy feelings. The language of the Hebrews, Greeks, Romans, etc. are all here. Coins, busts, models, weapons, cherished and patriotic relics are seen in countless numbers affording the richest food for reflective minds.

> We desire now particularly to call attention to some relics which will possess great value in the eyes of every true and loyal American. They were presented by Mrs. Agnew, relics of the late Dr. James Agnew, a well-known physician, and one of the high standing in this city, who died here some years since. The first article presented is a piece of the coffin of Washington. Attached to it, in the handwriting of the venerable lady whose recollections go back to the time when, as a little girl, she strewed flowers in the pathway of the great and good Washington as he passed under the triumphal arch erected at Trenton New Jersey, when on his way to New York to be inaugurated first President of the United States, is the following: a fragment of the first coffin in which the body of Washington, the Father of his Country, was deposited immediately after his death.[46]

By all accounts, there were many amazing things to see and do at the fair. On the last few days of the event, several auctions were held. Some of the most notable auction items included books written by Longfellow with his autograph, autographed copies of poems by Oliver Wendell Holmes and Goethe, David Gilmour Blythe's *Old Virginia Home* painting, and those of many other notable artists. Other items included photographs and autographs of Henry Clay, General U. S. Grant, Abraham Lincoln, his cabinet officers, and some Senators and Representatives. Bidding on

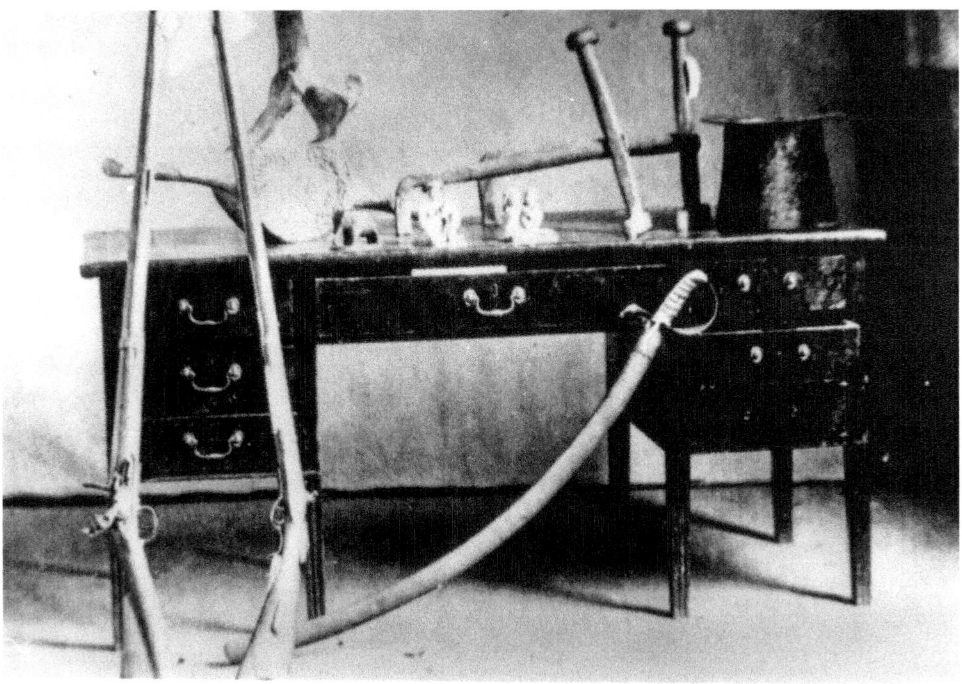

Pittsburgh Sanitary Fair Old Curiosity Shop items, 1864. (*Carnegie Library of Pittsburgh. *)

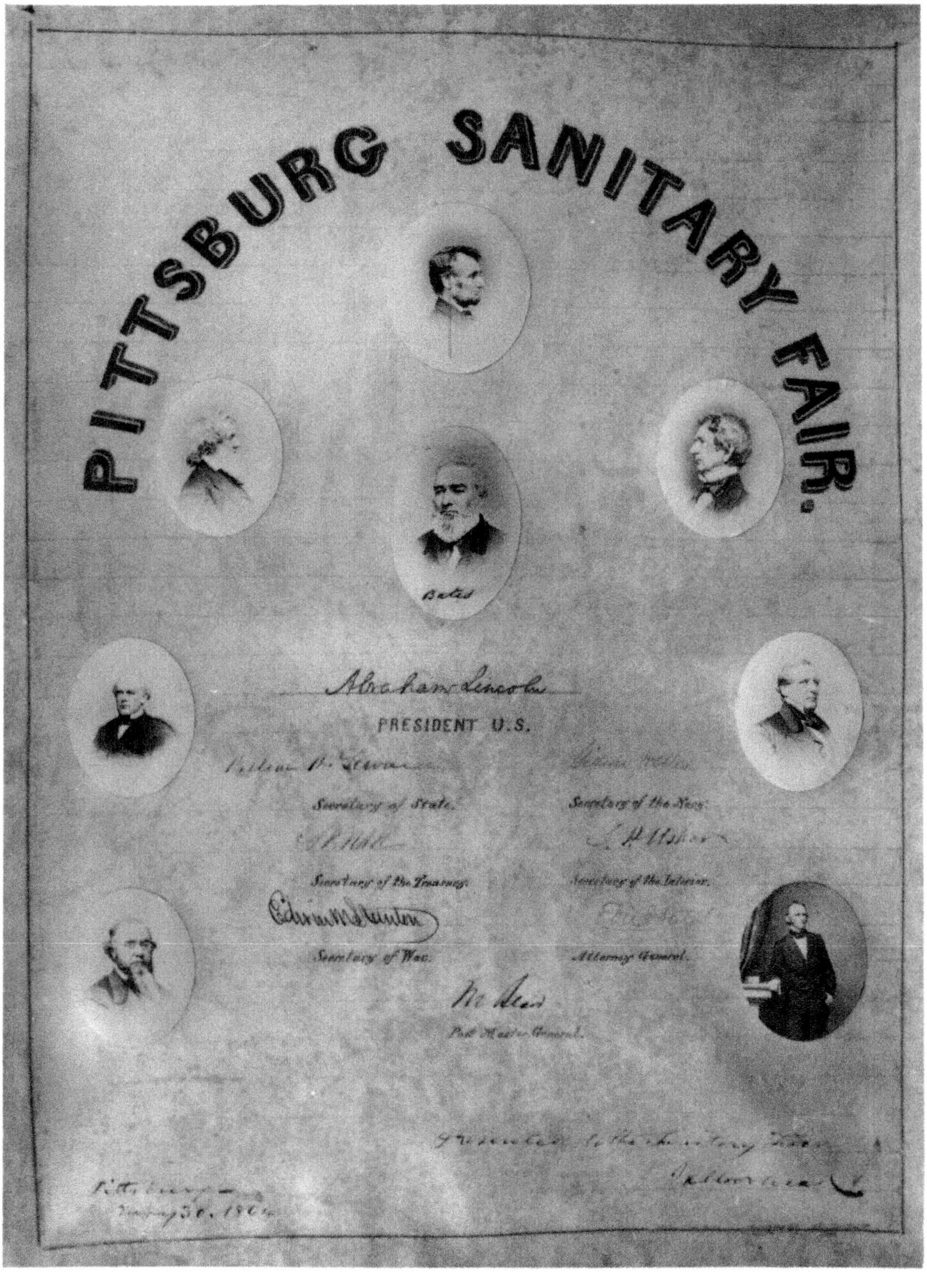

Pittsburgh Sanitary Fair board with autographs of President Lincoln and cabinet, 1864. (*Heinz History Center*)

these and numerous other items produced a significant amount of money that added greatly to the fair's proceeds.

A biographical account of Felix Brunot's life described the outcome of the Fair:

> For eighteen days this Fair was the busiest spot in western Pennsylvania, and at the close it was found that $320,000 had been cleared for the sick and wounded soldiers. This was accomplished without diminishing gifts from other sources, for the fortnight before the Fair opened the committee sent $50,000 to Philadelphia for the Christian Commission. Of the receipts from the Fair $80,000 were set aside to establish a soldiers' home after the war. When the war was over, the funds remaining on hand were added to this sum, making an aggregate of $183,000. "The Pittsburgh Sanitary Soldiers' Home" was immediately established with this endowment, and there Mr. Brunot, one day in February 1867, on behalf of the people of Pittsburgh, received the Senate and Representatives of the State of Pennsylvania, and spoke to them of the part which Pittsburgh had played in the great war.[47]

Dorothy Daniel also offered favorable remarks on the impact of the Fair:

> Pittsburgh's Sanitary Fair was not the first of its kind, nor the last, nor the greatest, nor the one to receive the most national publicity. But when all the quarters and dimes had been counted and all the costs deducted Pittsburgh's donation to the cause was $3.47 per capita. In this, we were first. No other community gave so much.[48]

Indeed, a final tally of profits indicated the Pittsburgh Fair had generated the fourth largest amount of money raised from such events in the Union.

Other Civilian Support

The Civil War saw other innovations developed solely in response to military need. Two of the major accomplishments were nursing care and dietary intervention. Nursing care, which had been heretofore relegated mainly to men and almost entirely composed of convalescent or undesirable soldiers, invalids, prisoners, those too young or too old to serve, or relatives, could not possibly meet the challenge of maintaining care at the front and at the numerous hospitals built by the Army or converted to military use. As the war progressed, there were never sufficient numbers of nurses to handle the need. The Pittsburgh Sisters of Mercy became one of the earliest groups of women to be enlisted into military service as nurses. In reality, the various Catholic and Protestant orders were the closest to a professional nursing service the country could muster. This situation would change once Dorothea Dix arrived in Washington, D.C.

As noted earlier, Dix was appointed Superintendent of Female Nurses of the Army on 19 April 1861, after considerable politicking by her and members of the United

States Christian Commission. With her appointment, she had the responsibility and authorization to recruit nurses. War Department Order Number 351 stated: "Women nurses will be assigned only on appointment to the General Superintendent (Dix) unless they are specifically appointed by the Surgeon General." Her success did not come easily since changing the opinions of the "old regime" of medical men, and frankly, that of public perceptions toward women caring for ill men they were not related to, was a considerable achievement. The physicians who comprised the medical establishment had long felt that a "professional" nursing service was unwarranted and many actively fought the interjection of women into the hospital setting. Before Dix's appointment, there were on average five male nurses to every one female. Many physicians preferred the old "tried and true" methods of nursing and at best preferred the services of nuns since they could always be counted upon to remain unquestioning and obedient.

It is estimated between 3,000 and 4,000 women eventually served as nurses in Union hospitals. This figure does not include the countless women who served in nursing capacities at the front and in field hospitals under the auspices of the United States Christian Commission or the United States Sanitary Commission. Dix's achievement changed the complexion of hospital care that remains with us today.

The other civilian innovation was the "low diet," a nutritional intervention created for use in military hospitals. The diet was reportedly initiated by Pittsburgh resident, Mary E. Moorhead, under the auspices of the Christian Commission. Miss Moorhead was the daughter of Pennsylvania Congressman J. K. Moorhead. Moorhead's "low-diet" was a modification of the typical army authorized meal plan that reduced portion sizes of meats and whole bread and added things like rice and farina to maximize digestion. Miss Moorhead established her first low-diet in the Cumberland Military Hospital at Nashville, Tennessee.

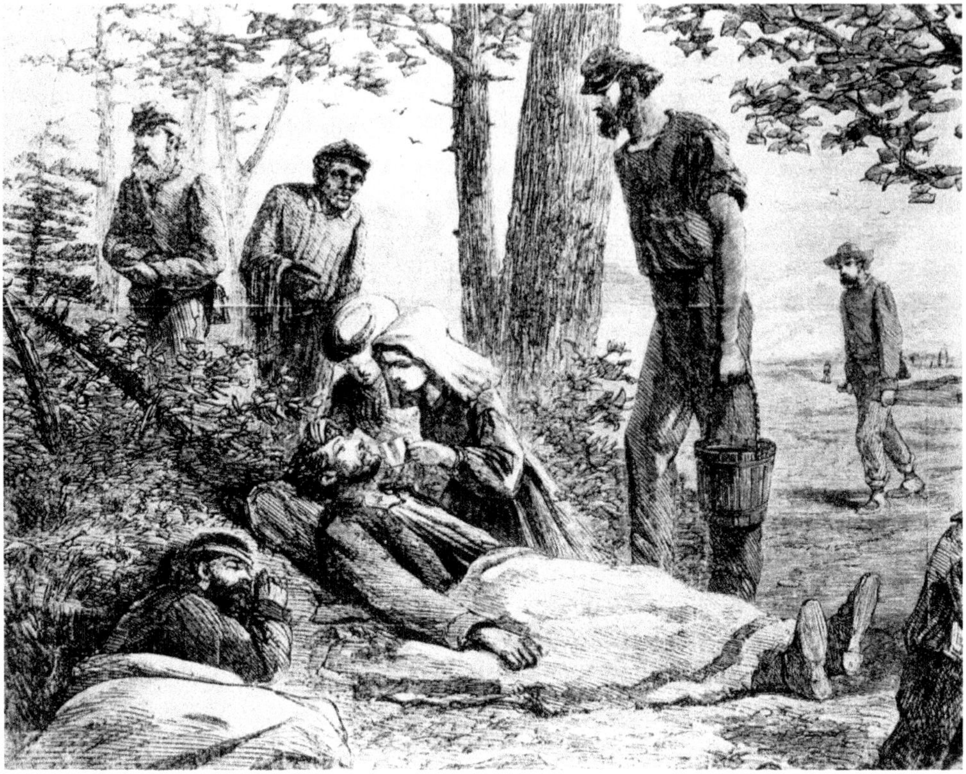

Nursing in the Civil War. (*National Library of Medicine*)

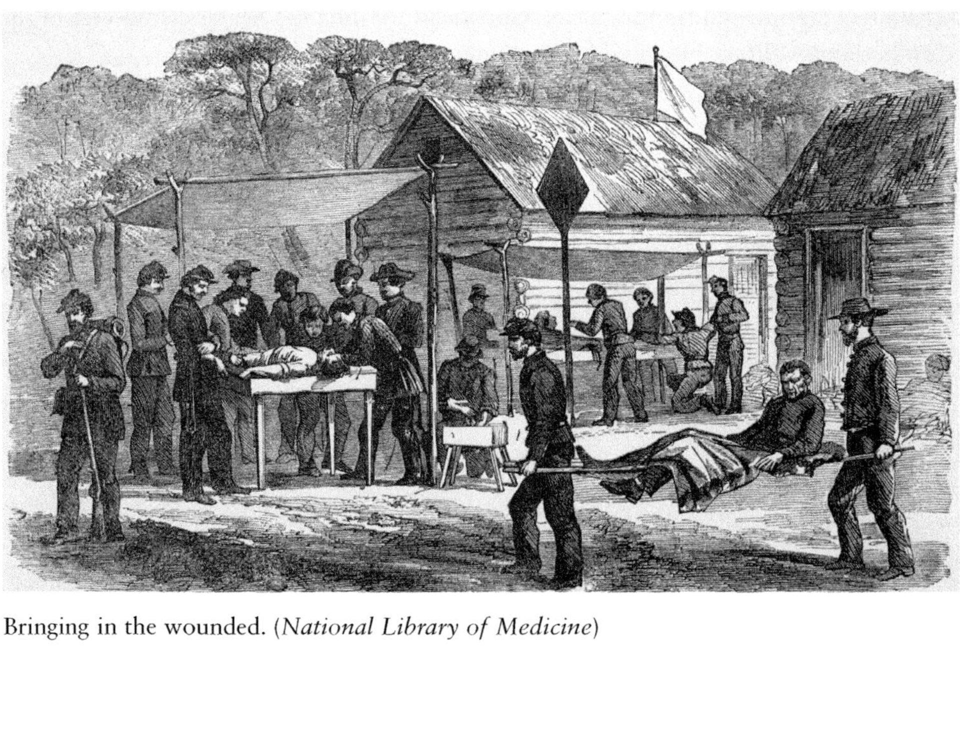

Bringing in the wounded. (*National Library of Medicine*)

6

Yet Another War: The State of Military Medical Affairs

The opening of the Civil War in April 1861 changed everything in the country—in cities and countryside where the battles were being fought—and on the home front were soldiers were being treated for their wounds and illnesses. Soon after the first battles occurred, Pittsburgh's citizens reacted. Thousands of raw recruits from the city and surrounding areas rapidly volunteered for service. Businesses and manufacturers moved quickly to ramp up production of weapons, munitions, and materials needed to support the war effort. Private citizens organized civic organizations to provide food, medical care, and sundry items that conscripted soldiers were not provided by the inadequately prepared and rapidly overextended federal government. Pittsburgh's doctors—whether as private individuals donating their skills or as physician-soldiers serving at the front or in newly emerging federal hospitals—were thrust into war. Collectively, they were unprepared for what was to come. The lessons learned along the way would, in a few short years, leave an indelible mark.

At the outbreak of the hostilities, the state of medicine was grossly inadequate for the necessities of staging a sustained war. Brooks in his treatise of Civil War Medicine stated the Federal Government entered the war with "Medical capabilities below those of Imperial Rome."[1] For the ordinary man, the existence of hospitals was of little concern since "hospitals were dirty, smelly and contaminated ... a good place to stay out of—especially when sick."[2] For the Federal Government, the provision of hospitals became a necessity for the survival of the Union Army.

The Federal Government entered the war without a major military hospital in the country. The largest military medical facility at the time held but forty-one beds and was located at Fort Leavenworth, Kansas. It was not until the spring of 1862 that new military hospitals were being built. By early 1863, the Union had built or taken control of enough civilian hospitals to provide 58,715 beds. In total, the government controlled 151 hospitals. By the end of the war, they operated 704 hospitals, which comprised 136,894 beds with most averaging 500 beds each. Satterlee Hospital in Philadelphia was the largest with 3,500 beds.

Public sentiment quickly began to change regarding hospital care—mainly in response to the horrible battles that left sick, wounded, and mutilated bodies strewn across the battlefields without access to ample medical care. Significantly, it was after the Battle of Second Bull Run, in late August 1862, that the poor perception of hospitals appears to have mitigated most of the fear of hospital care by ordinary citizens. There were still many problems to overcome in providing this care, but new ideas were now being promoted, and some even implemented, by the Army Medical Department.

The old unchallenged modes of medical care, which had not significantly changed since the Revolution, now gave way to necessity. In total, the war cost more than 600,000 men their lives (current estimates suggest 750,000). There were 360,000 northern deaths out of 1,556,678 enlistments. Three out of every five Union soldiers died from diseases such as typhoid, chronic diarrhea, or inflammation of the lungs. Typhoid alone killed one-quarter of the victims during the first year of the war.

While disease was a major cause of death during the war, it was not always a product of battle. Sometimes it was brought to camp and field with improperly screened volunteers who, particularly early in the conflict, arrived from the cities and rural farms unprepared for the exigencies of war. Dr. A. J. Phelps, Surgeon United States Volunteers, described the situation:

> The plan of voluntary enlistment, relied upon by our government for raising its army, brought to the recruiting office all sorts of men who were anxious and determined to go into the service. The surgeon was influenced in the examination by the prevailing impression that for the volunteer service it was not necessary to be as severe as if examining for the regular army.[3]

His description of the shape in which the volunteers arrived illustrates the challenges facing the examiners. He reported:

> Feeble boys, toothless old men, consumptives, asthmatics, one-eyed, one-armed men, men with different length of legs, clubfooted and ruptured, and, in short, men with every variety of disability, and whose systems were replete with the elements of incipient disease, were accepted as recruits, and started to the field only to become a tax upon the government, and to encumber the movements of its armies.[4]

The unprepared and overworked army surgeons who were tasked with quickly examining thousands of recruits were as culpable as the overeager and unsuspecting "raw" recruit. But not all of the deaths caused by disease were a result of a lack of proper screening or medical attention. Many were caused as a consequence of the long marches, poor food, ill-suited clothing, adverse weather, unsafe sanitary

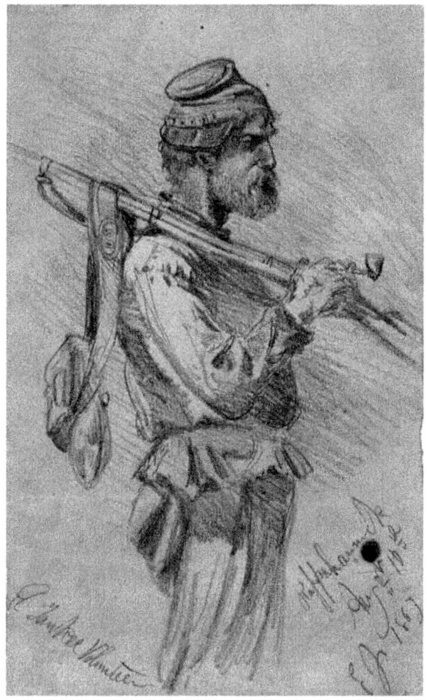

A Yankee Volunteer by Edwin Forbes, 1863. (*Library of Congress*)

conditions in the camps, and the intermixing of recruits with immunity to some diseases they had previously acquired with those who had never before been exposed.

To further emphasize his point about the effect of illness and disease on the troops, Dr. Phelps cited Major General Thomas J. Wood, who reported:

> That statistics derived from the observations of the closest observers, lineal and medical officers, disclose the startling fact that, as a rule, throughout the entire war, not more than thirty-five per cent of the muster-roll strength of the armies of the Union appeared on the battle-field bearing muskets![5]

Battle wounds were equally as destructive and cost the lives of approximately 110,000 Union soldiers throughout the war. It is an anomaly that Dr. Samuel Guthrie, whose invention of a new form of percussion powder and his innovative punch lock system for igniting it, would make the Minié ball (developed by French army officer Claude-Étienne Minié) a more deadly projectile, while his discovery of chloroform as a new form of anesthesia would help save countless lives.

The Medical Department of the Union Army began the war with far too few doctors and a very limited number of hospitals beds. In Washington, D.C., the city's only hospital at the outbreak of war was a two-story building with six rooms that had recently been used for isolating smallpox patients. While the hospital bed situation was dire, the physician shortage was even more consequential. With a core

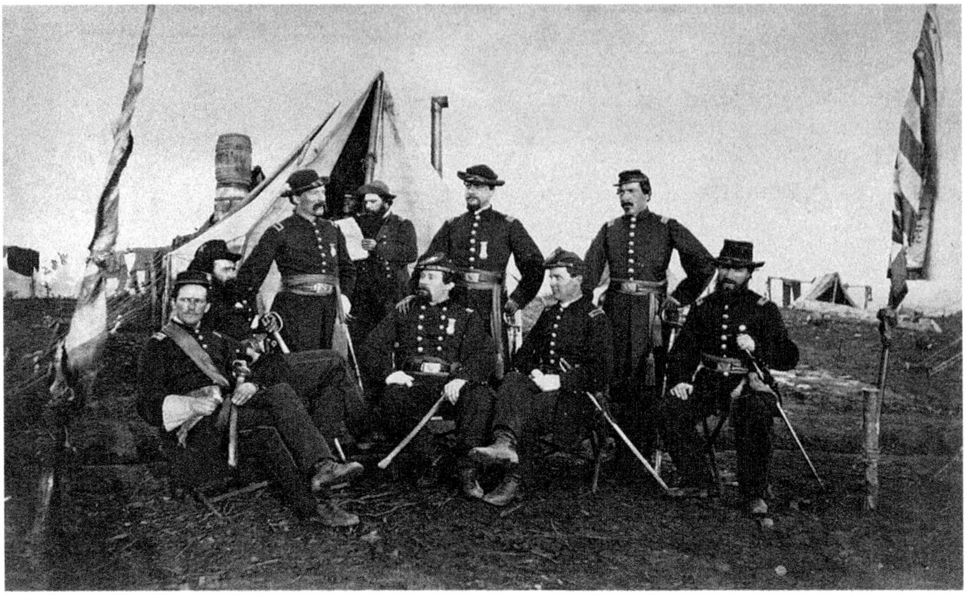

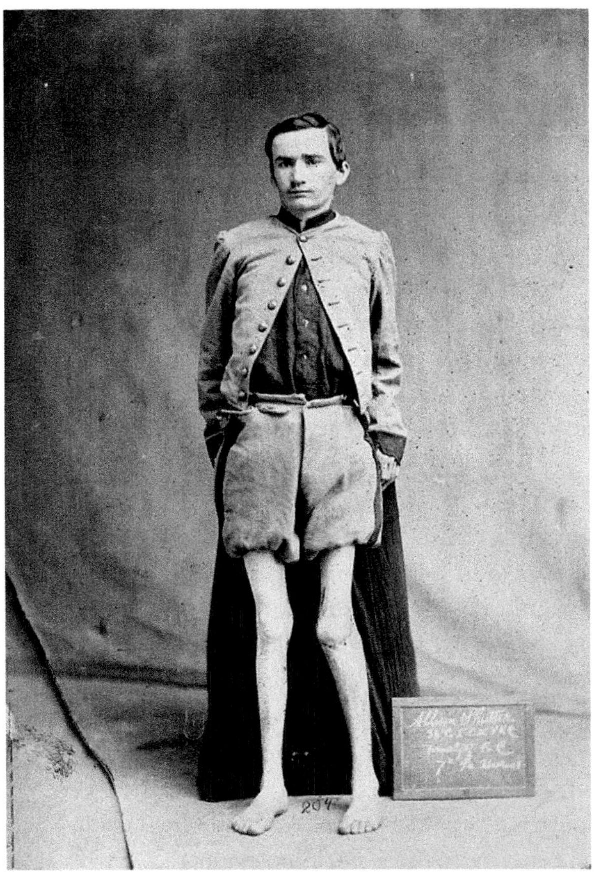

Above: Officers of 139th Pennsylvania Infantry. (*Library of Congress*)

Left: Allison Shutter, Drummer Company "C," 7th Pennsylvania Reserves, surgical photo. (*Library of Congress*)

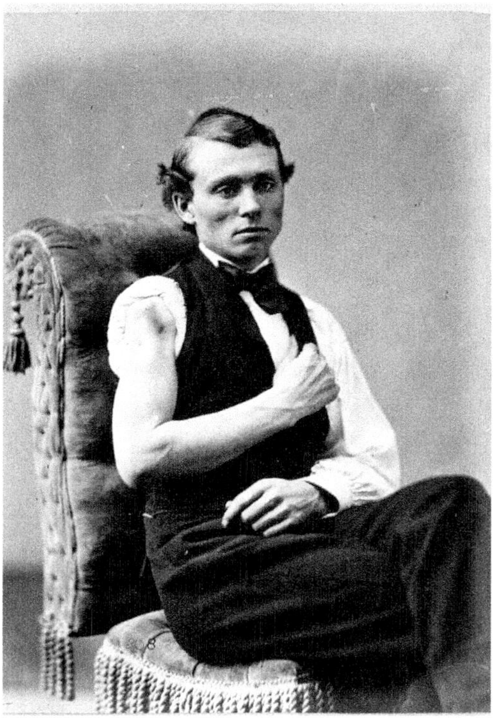

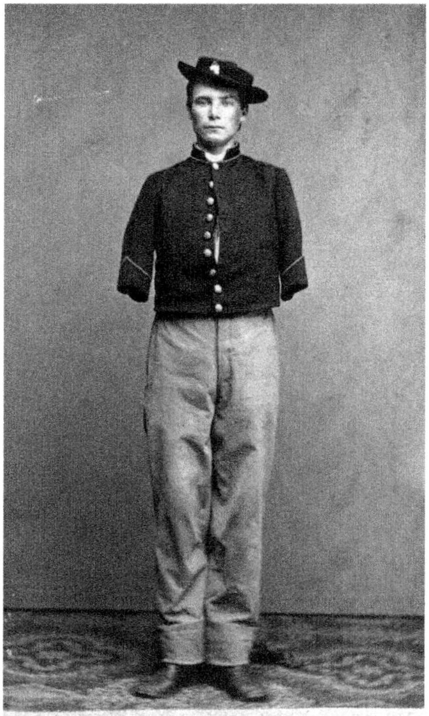

Above left: John Brink, Private Company "K," 11th Pennsylvania Cavalry surgical photo. (*Library of Congress*)

Above right: Private William Sergent, Company "E," 53rd Pennsylvania Infantry Regiment after the amputation of both arms. (*Library of Congress*)

Right: Samuel H. Decker, Private Company "I," 9th U.S. Artillery, surgical photo. (*Library of Congress*)

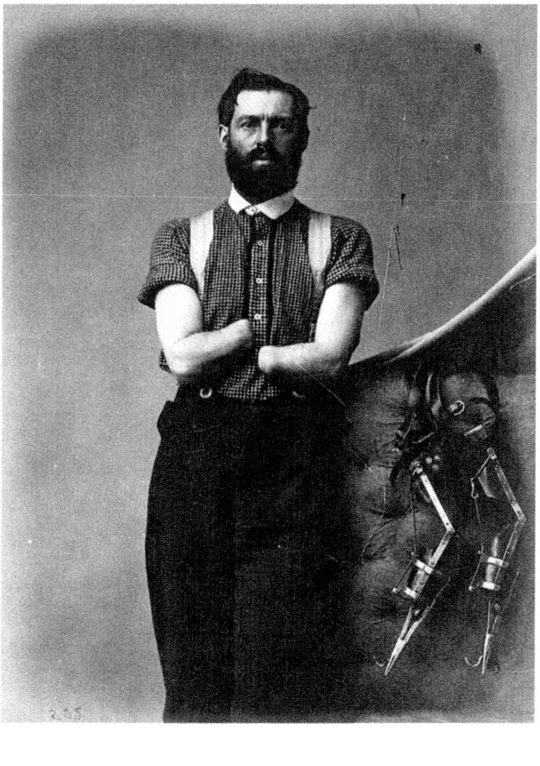

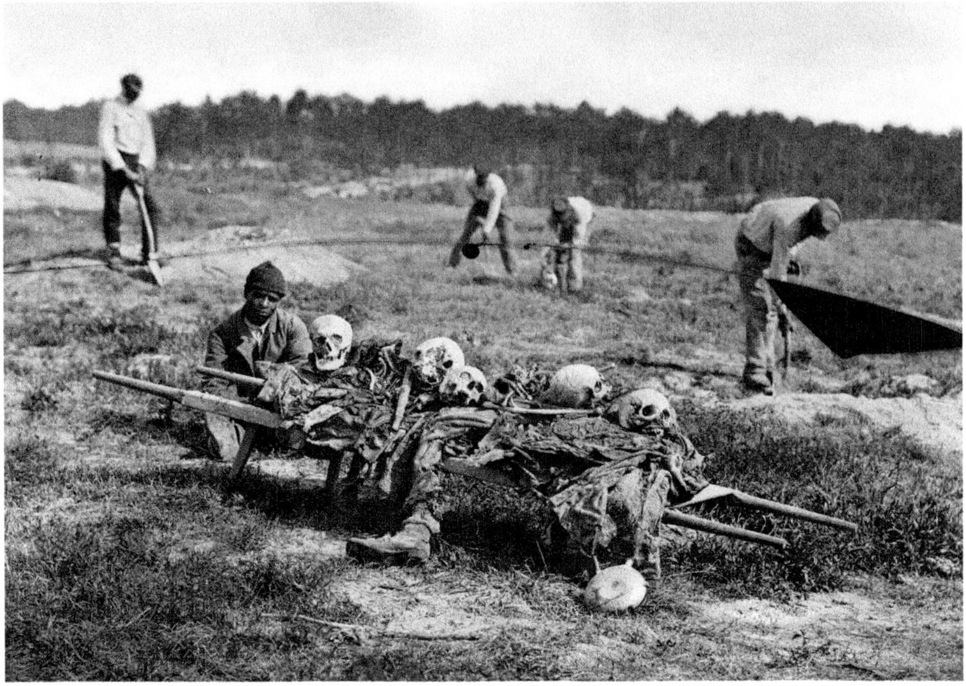

Collecting bones of soldiers killed during the Battle of Cold Harbor, Virginia, 1864. (*Library of Congress*)

of approximately 100 physicians supporting a peacetime army of about 16,000 men, there was an immediate need for massive recruitment.

When war broke out, Surgeon General Thomas Lawson, a veteran of the War of 1812, led the physicians in charge of the Medical Department. The group was comprised of older men surviving through patronage and corruption, and they fought a fierce battle to stave off any changes to their antiquated modes of operation. Most of these physicians had received their training through apprenticeship, exactly in the same manner as their predecessors. Fortunately, the "old guards" resistance to change was futile. The introduction of new blood into their organization was necessitated by the demands of war. By the end of the war, almost 13,000 doctors had served in various capacities in the battlefields and hospitals of the Union Army. A new breed of young physicians, with many having some medical school training in addition to their apprenticeship, would soon comprise the majority of army doctors.

Unfortunately, not all physicians were created alike. The clarion call for physicians early in the war was answered by an influx of both trained and ill-trained recruits from major cities and the backwoods. Initially, and particularly among those seeking to join as volunteers or those recruited to fill the various state organized regiments, little effort was made to determine suitability for service as no testing or standards were then in place. That would change later in the war, but the initial

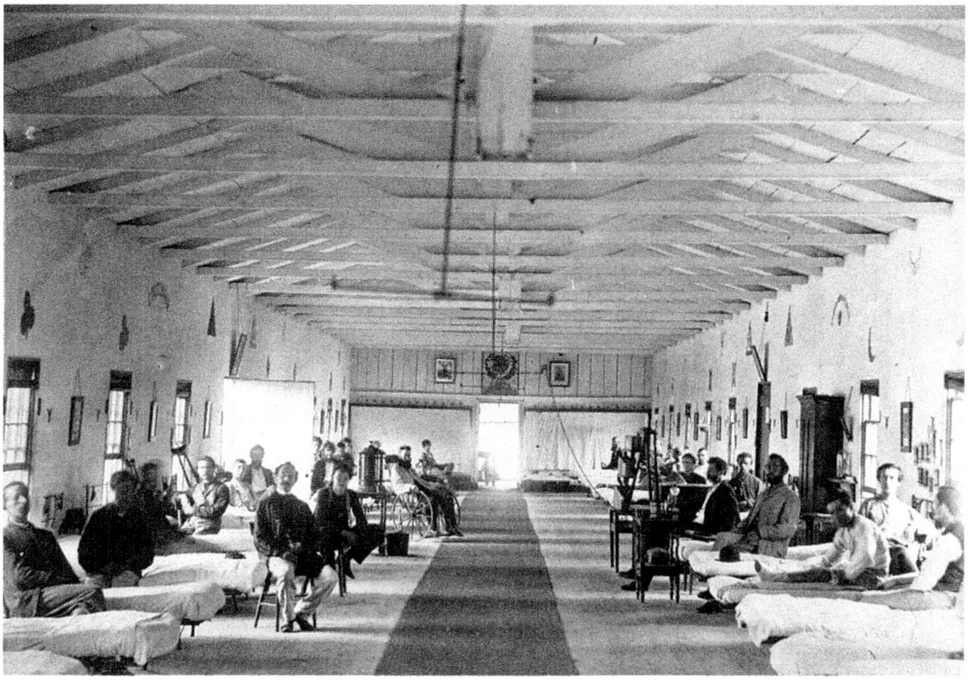

Patients in Ward "K," Armory Square Hospital, Washington, D.C., 1865. (*Library of Medicine*)

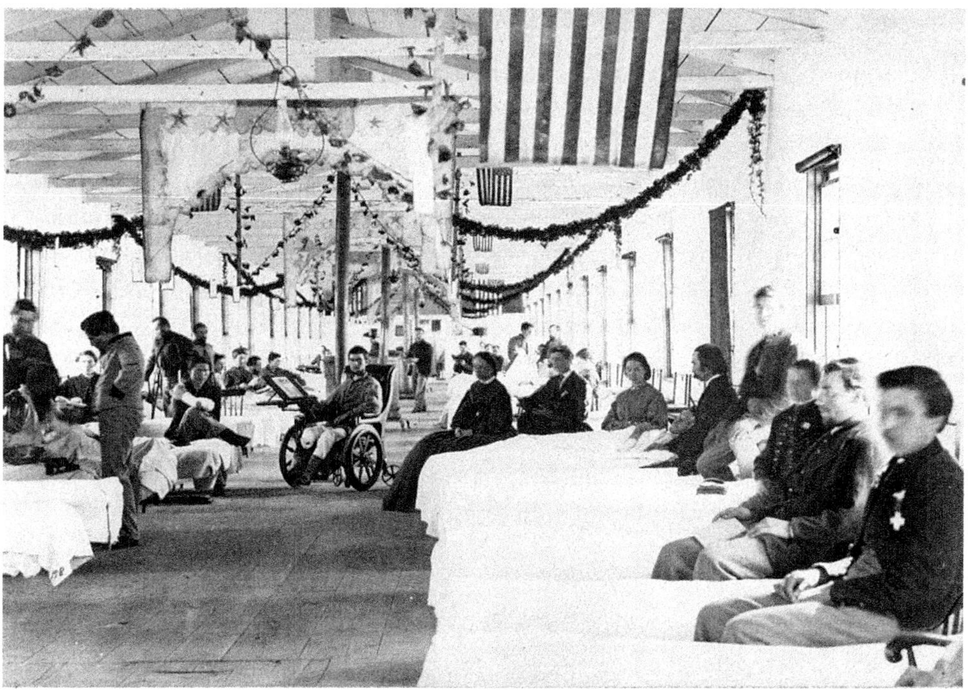

A ward in Armory Square Hospital, Washington, D.C. (*Library of Medicine*)

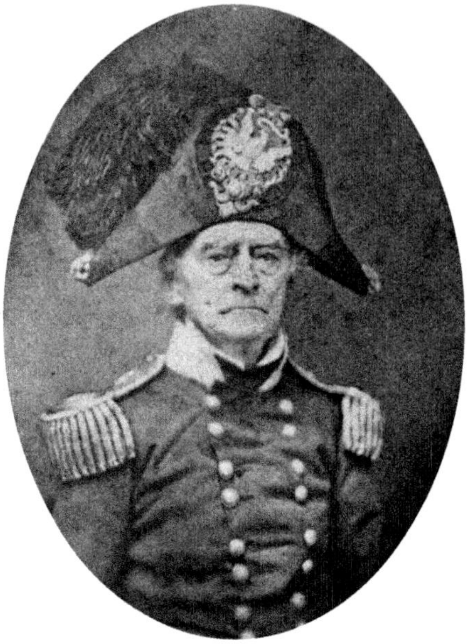

Thomas Lawson, Surgeon General of the Army 1836–1861. (*National Library of Medicine*)

influx of inexperienced and under qualified physicians proved detrimental to the army. Thousands of soldiers, unfortunately, lost their lives or limbs as a result of the malfeasance of many ill-prepared surgeons. In September 1862, the situation was still not under control as an editor of the *American Medical Times* noted:

> But it must be admitted that the class of persons who volunteer for such service [surgical aid] are not always, if, indeed, they are in a majority of instances, qualified to discharge the duties which we have briefly noticed. Large numbers of practitioners, influenced by patriotic and humane feelings, but who have no knowledge of surgery or practical experience, obey the summons. Others from mere curiosity accept the gratuitous transportation of Government and heedlessly seek the scene of conflict. Still others, who are aspirants for surgical distinction, but who have never had an opportunity for practice, especially in operative surgery, rush frantically to the battlefield as the great theatre where they may operate without stint or hindrance. On every field where a sanguinary battle has been fought these different classes of volunteers have been found, and the results which have followed have been deplorable. The unnecessary sacrifice of limbs, the failure to perform proper and necessary operations, and the injury needlessly inflicted in the search for missiles, are the legitimate results of the labors of such incompetent surgeons.[6]

At the beginning of the war, many physicians had not seen or used a stethoscope, thermometer, syringe, ophthalmoscope, laryngoscope, or any other advanced instruments widely utilized in Europe. Although many were unacquainted with these modern diagnostic tools, things changed quickly. Ultimately, they were capable of bringing about significant changes in medical care for soldiers during the war, and for the civilian population afterward. These "nouveau surgeons" needed to learn quickly. General battlefield conditions offered a quick education. The seemingly endless hands-on surgical experience they gained became the great equalizer between those educated in medical schools and those who were trained through apprenticeship. The urgency of war provided an education like no other available across the globe:

> Surgery After a Battle
> The following passage from a recent letter written after one of the late battles, presents a striking picture of the surgeons duties on the field:
>
> Day before yesterday some 300 Rebel wounded fell into our hands. Of these, 21 required capital operations. They were placed in a row, a slip of paper pinned to each man's coat collar telling the nature of the operations that have been decided upon. Dr. Morton first passes along with a towel saturated with ether puts every man beyond consciousness and pain.
>
> The operating surgeon follows and rapidly and skillfully amputates a leg or an arm, as the case may be till the 21 have been subjected to the knife and saw without one twinge of pain. A second surgeon ties up the arteries; a third dresses the wounds. The men are taken to tents nearby and wake up and find themselves cut in two without torture, while a winrow of lopped off members attest to the work. The last man has been operated upon before the first awakened, nothing could be more dramatic and nothing could more perfectly demonstrate the value of anesthetics. Besides, men fight better when they know that torture does not follow a wound, and numberless lives are saved that the knife would lose to their friends and the country. Honor, then, to Morton and Jackson, the men who so opportunely for the war placed in their hands an agent that relieves the soldier from untold misery, and his friends from untold anguish.[7]

All physicians who served in the army throughout the war were referred to as surgeons—whether they liked it or not. Generally, physicians were exempt from the draft, but based on the number who responded to the call to arms, there were as many driven by patriotism as those by vanity. There was a range of different classifications under which a physician could serve, all but one of which incorporate "surgeon" in their title. They included regular surgeon; regular assistant surgeon; volunteer surgeon; volunteer assistant surgeon; regimental surgeon; regimental assistant surgeon; acting assistant surgeon; reserve surgeon; veteran corps medical officer; acting staff surgeon; colored troop surgeon; and colored troop assistant surgeon.

Regular surgeons with commissions held the rank of major; assistant surgeons held the rank of captain or lieutenant. Most surgeons who served were regimental surgeons appointed by the Governor of the State to accommodate the regiments formed in the State. The typical alignment in a regiment allocated one surgeon and

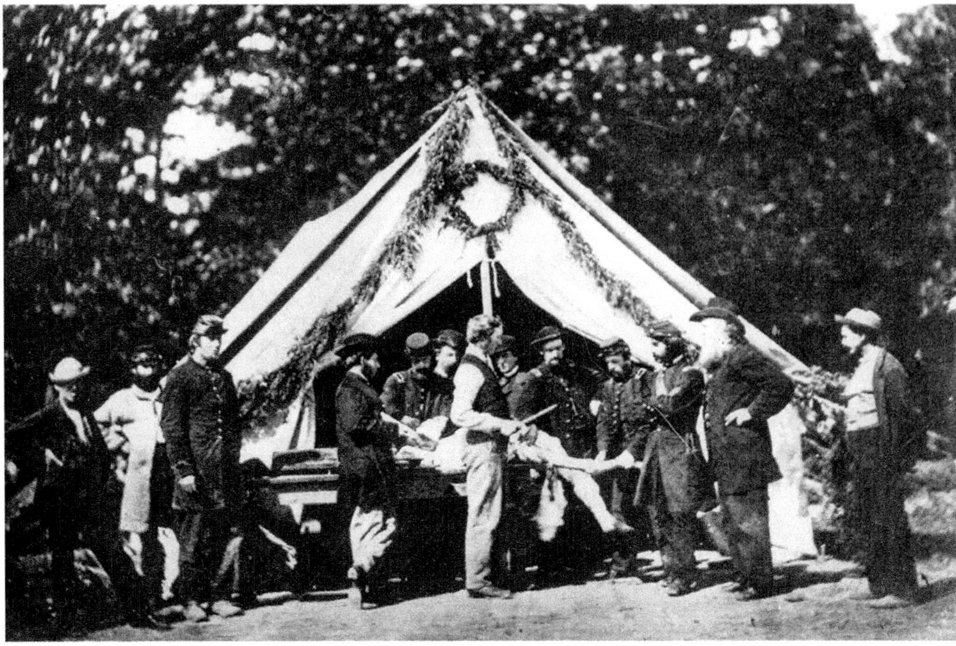

Amputation being performed, Gettysburg, July 1863. (*National Library of Medicine*)

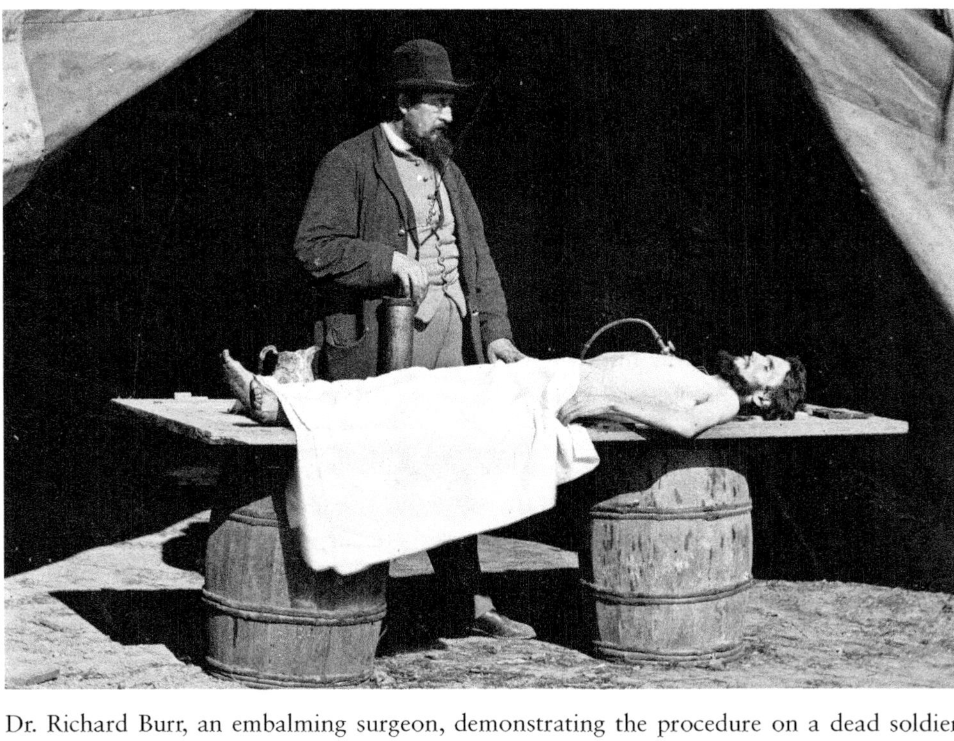

Dr. Richard Burr, an embalming surgeon, demonstrating the procedure on a dead soldier. (*Library of Congress*)

two assistant surgeons to each. Acting assistant surgeons were not commissioned but were considered "contract surgeons." As the war progressed, contract surgeons comprised approximately 5,500 of the 13,000 physicians who served. Contract surgeons customarily held the rank of lieutenant and generally split their time between hospitals and private practice. Army regulations of 1861–1863 that covered contract surgeons are interesting to note. A few example regulations include:

> Regulation #1304
> When it is necessary to employ a private physician as medical officer, the commanding officer may do it by written contract, conditioned as in Form 18, at a stated compensation not to exceed $50 a month when the number of officers and men, with authorized servants and laundresses, is 100 or more; $40 when it is from 50 to 100, and $30 when it is under 50,
>
> Regulation #1305
> But when he is required to abandon his own business and give his whole time to the public service, the contract may be not to exceed $80 a month; and not to exceed $100, besides transportation in kind, to be furnished by the Quartermaster's Department, where he is required to accompany troops on marches or transports.
>
> Regulation #1306
> And when a private physician is required to furnish medicines, he will be allowed, besides the stipulated pay, from 25 to 50 percent, on it, to be determined by the Surgeon-General.[8]

Regiments typically were comprised of 800 men and between two and five regiments served in each brigade (approximately 2,600 soldiers); two to four brigades served in each division (approximately 8,000 soldiers); two to three divisions comprised a corps (approximately 26,000 soldiers); and three corps made up a full army group (approximately 80,000 soldiers).[9] Keeping the troops in a healthy battle-ready state was a major challenge to officers and surgeons alike. The sheer magnitude of injuries and illnesses that occurred during the war are displayed in the tables below.

Sicknesses in the Union Army

SICKNESS[10]

Of 5,825,480 admissions to sick report there were:

Cases	Illness	Deaths
75,368	Typhoid	27,050
2,501	Typhus	850
11,898	Continued Fever	147
49,871	Typho-Malarial Fever	4,059

1,155,266	Acute Diarrhea	2,923
170,488	Chronic Diarrhea	27,558
233,812	Acute Dysentery	4,084
25,670	Chronic Dysentery	3,229
73,382	Syphilis	123
95,833	Gonorrhea	6
30,714	Scurvy	383
3,744	Delirium Tremens	450
2,410	Insanity	80
2,837	Paralysis	231

Wounds and Amputations of the Union Army

WOUNDS TREATED[11]	
Shot wounds	245,790
Sabre and bayonet wounds	922
TOTAL	246,712

AMPUTATIONS[12]

	Total	Deaths	% Fatality
Hands or Fingers	7,902	198	2.9
Wrist Joint	68	7	10.4
Forearm	1,761	245	14.0
Elbow Joint	40	3	7.6
Upper Arm	5,510	1,273	23.8
Shoulder Joint	866	245	29.1
Foot or Toe	1,519	81	5.7
Ankle Joint	161	40	25.1
Leg	5,523	1,790	33.2
Knee Joint	195	111	57.5
Thigh	6,369	3,411	54.2
Hip Joint	66	55	83.3
TOTAL	29,980	7,459	26.3

The typical military hospitals developed early in the war were of the "pavilion type" where each ward was detached, usually on three sides, or the "isolation" type where each ward was housed in a separate building.[13] The underlying premise dictating this design was the teaching of a nurse, Florence Nightingale, who almost singlehandedly changed the course of military hospital care during the Crimean War. Her achievements in hospital design were not dismissed by the U.S. Army Medical

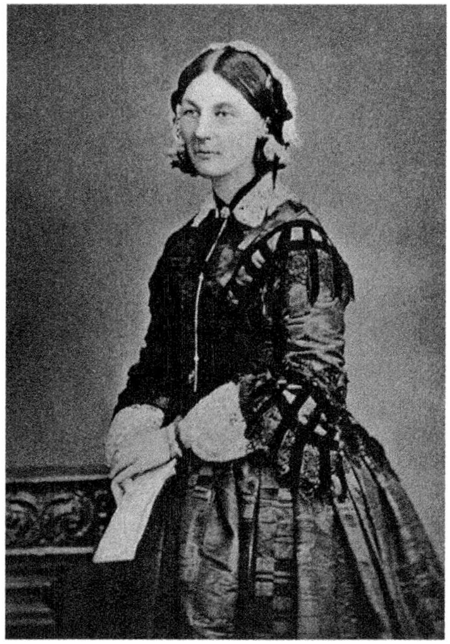

Florence Nightingale. (*Library of Congress*)

Department. Nightingale's teaching of cleanliness and ventilation was, at the outset of the war, uppermost in everyone's mind even though the state of medicine still indicated "the patient might on occasion know as much about medical science as the people treating him."[14]

The Medical Department was soon able to confirm the benefit of Nightingale's "fresh air" doctrine. It was quickly proven that "by 1862, the mortality among the sick and wounded housed in tents and other breezy installations was significantly lower than among those held in more elaborate but poorly ventilated infirmaries."[15] The army later specified in a circular distributed in July 1864 exact specifications for newly established hospital wards:

> Each ward will be a ridge-ventilated pavilion, one hundred and eighty-seven by twenty-four (187 X 24) feet. At each extremity two small rooms, nine by eleven (9 X 11) feet, one on each side of the passage, six (6) feet wide, will be partitioned off. The space remaining for patients will be one hundred and sixty-five by twenty-four (165 X 24) feet. The wards will he fourteen (14) feet high from floor to eaves – the pitch of the roof to vary in accordance to the materials composing it. The floor to be elevated at least eighteen (18) inches from the soil, with free ventilation beneath it. A ward thus constructed will accommodate sixty (60) patients, allowing more than one thousand (1,000) cubic feet of air space to each.[16]

The hospital administrative command developed under the army would also prove to become a role model for civilian hospitals, including Pittsburgh's, long after the war had ended. The typical hospital chain of command: Medical Director of Hospitals to Surgeon In-charge to Regular Army or Contract Surgeon (approximately one per 70 patients) to Matron to Assistant Matron to Nurses, Cooks, Laundresses, etc.

Other typical hospital staff members included the wardmaster who was responsible for looking after the personal effects of patients, hospital furniture, and cooking utensils, and the hospital steward who supervised stores and drugs, kept medical records, and was responsible for maintaining sanitary measures. The steward held the rank of warrant officer and normally had been a medical student or apothecary before military service.

After the war, Surgeon General William Hammond is attributed with stating that the Civil War "took place at the end of the medical middle ages." For all practical purposes, he was correct since basic scientific discoveries relative to bacteriology and aseptic surgical technique had yet to be applied. The Civil War did, however, offer several advances in the practice of medicine. These advances were implemented successfully in Pittsburgh and other cities across the nation.

The most significant was the establishment of well-run general hospitals with strictly demarcated chains of authority, elaborate attention to record keeping, and the development of the field-relief system. Other important improvements included the development of specialty practices and hospitals, integration of professional nursing, drastic improvements in the overall sanitary conditions of hospitals in general, and initial steps toward dietary control and intervention.

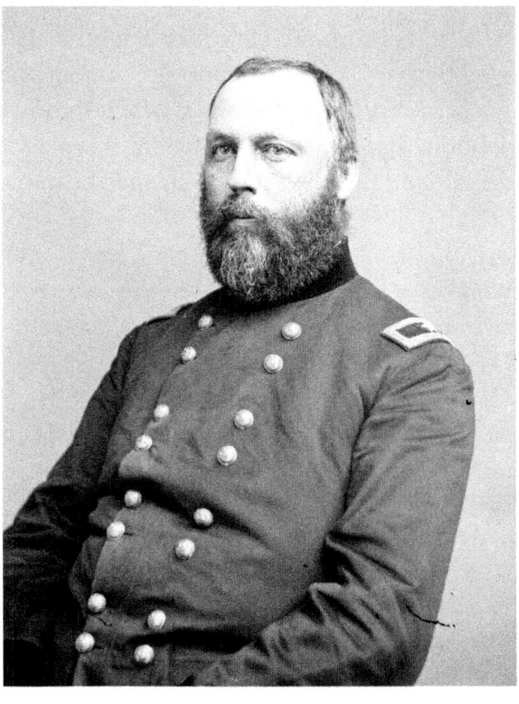

Brigadier General William A. Hammond, Surgeon-General, 1860. (*Library of Congress*)

Shortly after the firing on Fort Sumter, Secretary of War Edwin M. Stanton issued a plea for medical support to hospitals throughout the Union. Pittsburgh was of particular interest since it was his recent place of residence and he had a large number of friends and supporters there. His longtime friend, John Harper, then Vice President and Treasurer of Western Pennsylvania Hospital, along with its president, Thomas Bakewell, had an intriguing offer. Since the hospital had recently just completed the construction of the area's first specialized hospital for treatment of the insane, Dixmont Hospital, they asked the Secretary if he would be interested in converting the original hospital to military use for the duration of the war. Stanton's answer was affirmative. In December 1862, the hospital officially became the U.S.A. General Hospital Pittsburgh, under control of the federal government and the local authority of the U.S. Army Department of the Monongahela.

Seven months earlier, the first wounded soldiers arrived in the city soon after the Battle of Shiloh where approximately one-third of the 77,000 Union soldiers participating were shot or captured. Sixty-eight wounded Union and Confederate soldiers were brought to the city. Thousands more would make the trip to Pittsburgh over the next four years. U.S.A. General Hospital Pittsburgh would ultimately provide the majority of care.

In one of U.S. Surgeon General Hammond's reports, he noted as of 17 December 1864, capacity at the U.S.A. General Hospital Pittsburgh was 723 beds. He further indicated 584 beds were occupied and 139 beds were vacant.[17] At the time of the report, Surgeon James Bryan USV (United States Volunteers) was in charge of the hospital.

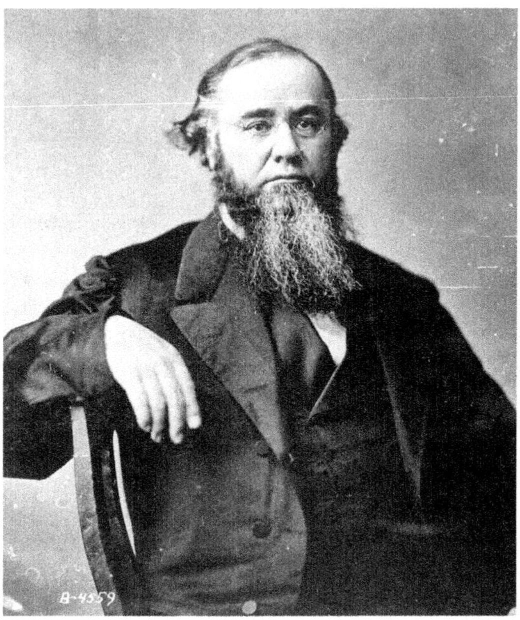

Edwin M. Stanton, U.S. Secretary of War. (*National Archives and Records Administration*)

Contracts obligating private physicians to military service were standard. Depending upon the circumstance, contracts would last for a period of three months to three years. John Rae, M.D., was one such physician. He was appointed acting assistant surgeon at the U.S.A. General Hospital Pittsburgh, and served from December 1862 until December 1864. He was expected to bring his own instruments or otherwise be charged for those provided to him by the Army Medical Department. By joint agreement between Western Pennsylvania Hospital and the Federal Government upon transfer of the institution to the U.S. Army, Dr. Rae was paid by the hospital board of directors with an agreement he would "attend to the preservation of the property and keeping it in order."[18]

U.S. Army Medical Director and Surgeon L. H. Holden signed Dr. Rae's contract. At the time of the contract, Dr. Rae was expected to possess a signed copy of an

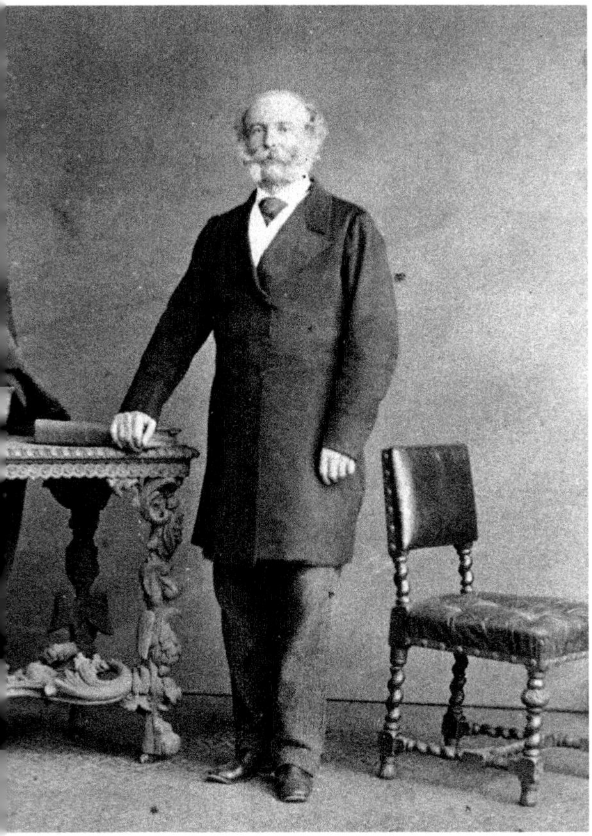

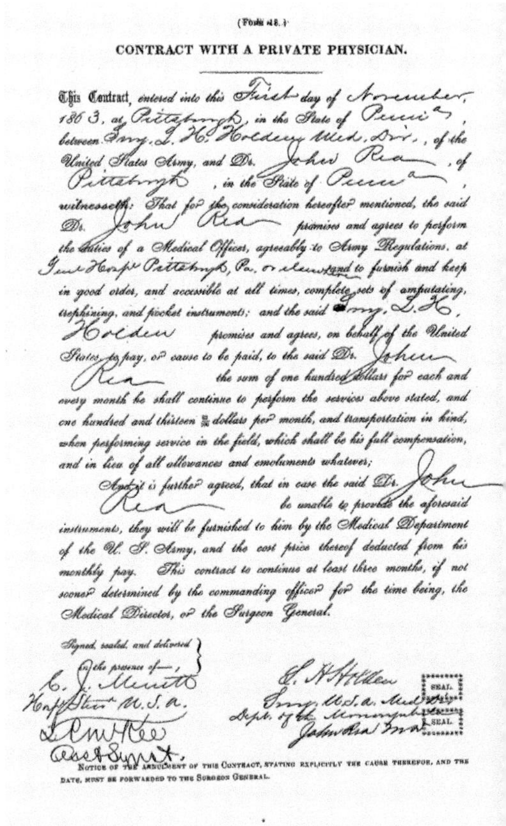

(Form 48.)

CONTRACT WITH A PRIVATE PHYSICIAN.

This Contract, entered into this First day of November, 1863, at Pittsburgh, in the State of Penn^a, between Surg. L. H. Holden Med. Dir., of the United States Army, and Dr. John Rea, of Pittsburgh, in the State of Penn^a, witnesseth: That for the consideration hereafter mentioned, the said Dr. John Rea promises and agrees to perform the duties of a Medical Officer, agreeably to Army Regulations, at Genl Hosp^l Pittsburgh, Pa. or elsewhere and to furnish and keep in good order, and accessible at all times, complete sets of amputating, trephining, and pocket instruments; and the said Surg. L. H. Holden promises and agrees, on behalf of the United States, to pay, or cause to be paid, to the said Dr. John Rea the sum of one hundred dollars for each and every month he shall continue to perform the services above stated, and one hundred and thirteen dollars per month, and transportation in kind, when performing service in the field, which shall be his full compensation, and in lieu of all allowances and emoluments whatever;

And it is further agreed, that in case the said Dr. John Rea be unable to provide the aforesaid instruments, they will be furnished to him by the Medical Department of the U. S. Army, and the cost price thereof deducted from his monthly pay. This contract to continue at least three months, if not sooner determined by the commanding officer for the time being, the Medical Director, or the Surgeon General.

Signed, sealed, and delivered in the presence of—,

SEAL.

SEAL.

NOTICE OF THE ANNULMENT OF THIS CONTRACT, STATING EXPLICITLY THE CAUSE THEREFOR, AND THE DATE, MUST BE FORWARDED TO THE SURGEON GENERAL.

Above left: Civil War surgeon John Rae, M.D. (*National Library of Medicine*)

Above right: Civil War surgeon John Rea's contract. (*National Archives and Records Administration*)

oath of allegiance to the U.S. government. Rae signed his oath, which was also countersigned by Holden, on 19 August 1863.

Between August 1861, when the Army Department of the Monongahela began supervising local medical care for the wounded in Pittsburgh, and October 1865, when the hospital was officially returned to civilian administration, the Army appointed a total of thirty-seven surgeons to the hospital. Several of the surgeons originated from Pittsburgh, others subsequently relocated permanently to the city. A register of the medical staff that served during this period includes:

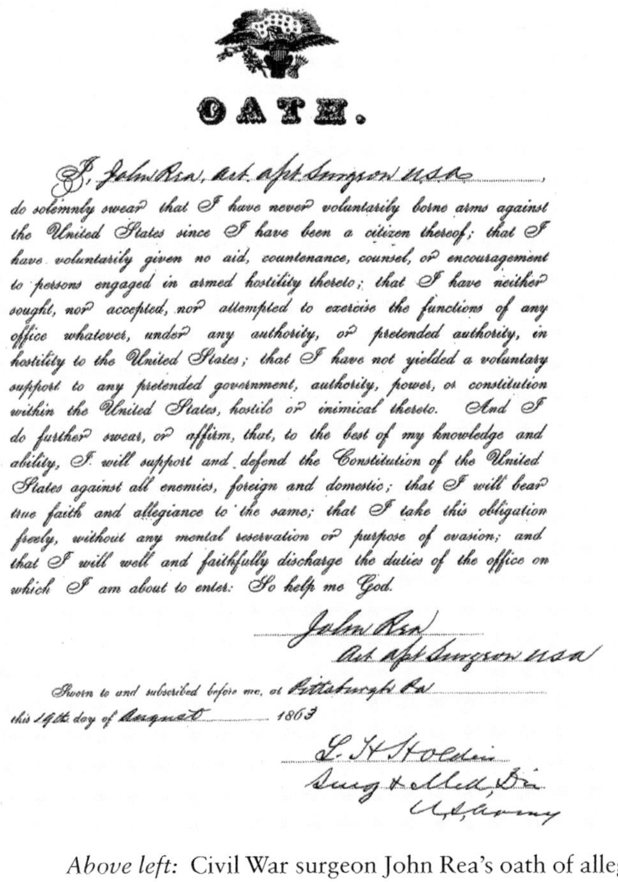

OATH.

I, John Rea, Act. Asst Surgeon USA, do solemnly swear that I have never voluntarily borne arms against the United States since I have been a citizen thereof; that I have voluntarily given no aid, countenance, counsel, or encouragement to persons engaged in armed hostility thereto; that I have neither sought, nor accepted, nor attempted to exercise the functions of any office whatever, under any authority, or pretended authority, in hostility to the United States; that I have not yielded a voluntary support to any pretended government, authority, power, or constitution within the United States, hostile or inimical thereto. And I do further swear, or affirm, that, to the best of my knowledge and ability, I will support and defend the Constitution of the United States against all enemies, foreign and domestic; that I will bear true faith and allegiance to the same; that I take this obligation freely, without any mental reservation or purpose of evasion; and that I will well and faithfully discharge the duties of the office on which I am about to enter: So help me God.

John Rea
Act. Asst Surgeon USA

Sworn to and subscribed before me, at Pittsburgh Pa
this 19th day of August 1863

L. H. Holden
Surg & Med Dir
U.S. Army

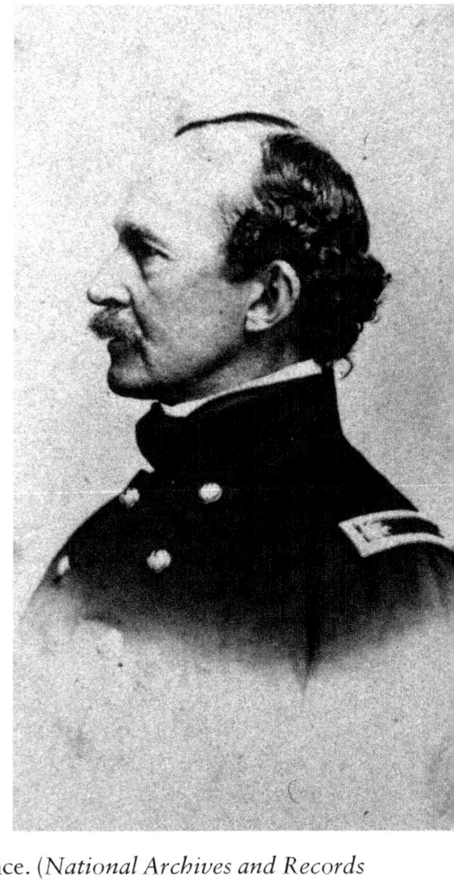

Above left: Civil War surgeon John Rea's oath of allegiance. (*National Archives and Records Administration*)

Above right: L. H. Holden, surgeon and Medical Director of the U.S. Army, Department of the Monongahela, Pittsburgh. (*National Library of Medicine*)

MEDICAL STAFF—U.S.A. GENERAL HOSPITAL—PITTSBURGH[19]

Pittsburgh, Pennsylvania Post and General Hospital, Western Pennsylvania Hospital

Name	Rank	In Service Date	Out Date	Notes
Irish, Franklin	A.A.S.	Aug 5, 1861	Sept 2, 1861	Recruits
Wood, Charles	A.A.S.	Aug 28, 1861	Oct 28, 1861	Recruits 105 PA
Wagenseller, B.	A.S.	Sept, 1862	Not recorded	139 PA
Stiles, Richard C.	A.A.S.	Nov 4, 1862	Dec, 1862	
Reiter, William C.	A.A.S.	Sept 19, 1862	June, 1863	
Simpson, Robert B.	Dft. Surgeon	Apr 18, 1863	June 15, 1865	22 Dist. PA
Authurs, Addison	A.A.S.	July 18, 1863	Oct 15, 1863	Recruits
Levis, John C.	A.A.S.	Dec 1, 1863	July 9, 1865	Drafted Men
Rea, John	A.A.S.	Dec 8, 1862	Dec 10, 1864	
Heaney, Patrick	A.A.S.	Dec 5, 1862	Feb 9, 1863	
McKee, James C.	A.S. USA	July 19, 1863	Dec 2, 1863	Charge
White, Charles B.	A.S.	Apr 8, 1863	July 18, 1863	Charge
Murdoch, Andrew C.	A.A.S.	June 26, 1863	Aug 26, 1863	
Winne, Charles K.	A.S. USA	Sept, 1863	Oct 6, 1863	
Bowen, Charles H.	A.A.S.	Oct 4, 1863	Feb 29, 1864	
Beust, Bernard	S. USV	Nov 23, 1863	Mar 23, 1864	
Marand, Alfred L.S.	A.A.S.	Mar 2, 1864	Dec 10, 1864	
Curtis, Henry R.	A.A.S.	Mar 6, 1864	Oct 2, 1864	
Bryan, James	S. USV	Mar 16, 1864	Dec 29, 1864	
Minassian, Simon G.	A.A.S.	Mar 24, 1864	Jun 2, 1865	
Duncan, James	A.A.S.	Mar 24, 1864	Apr 23, 1864	
Sargent, Gorham P.	A.A.S.	Apr 26, 1864	Sept 10, 1864	
Rankin, David N.	A.A.S.	June 25, 1864	Apr 24, 1865	
Beal, George F.	A.A.S.	Aug 3, 1864	Mar 10, 1865	
Riggs, David W.	A.A.S.	Aug 3, 1864	Jan 14, 1865	

Sargent, Rufus	A.A.S.	Sept 10, 1864	Mar 9, 1865	
Downs, Thomas A.	A.A.S.	Sept 13, 1864	Feb 3, 1865	
Rankin, Andrew H.	A.A.S.	Sept 26, 1864	Feb 3, 1865	
Miller, Samuel J.F.	A.A.S.	Dec 10, 1864	Jun 8, 1865	
Silliman, Henry R.	A.S. USA	Dec 29, 1864	Dec 8, 1865	
Young, Peter B.	A.A.S.	Jan 14, 1865	Feb 5, 1865	
Cox, George H.	A.A.S.	Mar, 1865	July 13, 1865	
Bartram, Thomas S.	A.A.S.	Apr 7, 1865	May 6, 1865	
Hanna, Edmund S.	A.A.S.	May 14, 1865	May 20, 1865	
Van Duyn, John	A.S. USA	May 26, 1865	July 1, 1865	
Campbell, William	S.	July 1, 1865	Aug 8, 1865	202 PA
Upton, George	A.S. USVV	Aug, 1865	Oct, 1865	

KEY:

A.S.: Assistant Surgeon	USA: U.S. Army
A.A.S.: Acting Assistant Surgeon	USV: U.S. Volunteers
S.: Surgeon	USVV: U.S. Veteran Volunteers

The responsibilities of the senior medical officer at a hospital are interesting. Among their many duties, regulations called for them to do the following:[20]

> Regulation #1277
> The senior medical officer of a hospital will distribute the patients, according to convenience and the nature of their complaints, into wards or divisions, under the particular charge of the several assistant surgeons, and will visit them himself each day, as frequently as the state of the sick may require, accompanied by the assistant, steward, and nurse.
>
> Regulation # 1280
> Senior medical officer of a hospital will enforce the proper hospital regulations to promote health and prevent contagion, by ventilated and not crowded rooms, scrupulous cleanliness, frequent changes of bedding, linen, etc.
>
> Regulation #1290
> The senior medical officer of each hospital, post, regiment, or detachment, will keep the following records, and deliver them to his successor: a register of patients; a prescription book; a diet book; a case book; a meteorological register; copies of his requisitions, annual returns, and quarterly reports of sick and wounded; and an order and letter book, in which will be transcribed all orders and letters relating to his duties.

By 1864, physicians entering service were much better screened. Charlatans, quacks, eclectics, and other pretenders were turned away. Only those with sound training and discernable skill were enlisted. Veteran surgeons, particularly those who remained in service for months or years and served at the front, were now among the most highly trained and experienced military surgeons in the world. An unnamed surgeon summed up the situation well when he wrote:

> American military surgery is yet in its infancy. Our Revolutionary war produced hardly anything on the subject, and we have been such a peaceful nation ever since that civil surgery has far outstripped its warlike sister. There is an immense amount of facts and statistics accumulating during the present rebellion, which coming man may develop into reliable landmarks for future guidance. But, more important, there is a large body of intelligent and careful observers throughout the loyal States, who find now a rich field of experience which they otherwise could never have enjoyed.[21]

Indeed, those intelligent and careful observers would return to their cities and towns with new knowledge and superior skill sets.

7
Civil War Physician-Soldiers

Pittsburgh physicians were as likely to volunteer, as were doctors in other cities. Whether they lived in the North or South, in large metropolitan cities or small rural towns, they sought positions in the regular army or volunteer regiments. By the end of the Civil War, Pennsylvania added approximately 1,000 surgeons and assistant surgeons to the Union Army. Hundreds of others served in adjunct medical roles as ordinary civilians.

Pittsburgh physicians left their mark serving the ill and wounded—whether on the battlefield or behind the lines in the hospitals. More than 150 years after the end of the war, new information continues to be discovered about their service and exploits, and many of those who participated have not yet been documented. The following descriptions of the military service and professional accomplishments of those known to have served in the military or outside the military in a role supporting the war effort are included below.

The list is not presented as an all-inclusive history of Pittsburgh physician-soldier service during the war, but rather as a representative account of what is known about those who have thus far been identified. In some instances, military records incorporate service histories slightly outside the Civil War period. They are included since they relate to doctors who are known to be in Pittsburgh during or immediately after the Civil War and were therefore motivated by the physicians and soldiers returning from the front. They were also affected by the myriad organizations supporting the war effort. Besides the military service-related information that follows for each physician, an effort has been made to include other biographical details, where available.[1]

ARTHURS, Addison

Military Service: Arthurs served as Acting Assistant Surgeon at U.S.A. General Hospital Pittsburgh from 18 July 1863 until 15 October 1863.

ARTHUR, H. W.

Military Service: Dr. Arthur served in Company "O" of the 9th Regiment of the Maryland Infantry.

General Background: Arthur spent much of his childhood in the Baltimore, Maryland, area. Shortly after beginning training in dentistry, his studies were interrupted by the Civil War. After military service, he returned to his studies at the Baltimore College of Dental Surgery, where he received his D.D.S. degree. He came to Pittsburgh in 1868 to establish his dental practice. He was a member of the prominent professional dental organizations, including the American Dental Association, the Pennsylvania Dental Association, and the Pittsburgh Dental Association. Arthur served as president of the Odontological Society of Western Pennsylvania for several years.

BARTRAM, Thomas S.

Military Service: Bartram served as Acting Assistant Surgeon at U.S.A. General Hospital Pittsburgh from 07 April 1865 until 06 May 1865.[2]

BATTEN, John Mullin

Military Service: Batten served as U.S. Medical Cadet at U.S. Army Hospital Christian Street, Philadelphia. On 22 March 1864, he became acting assistant surgeon in the U.S. Navy. During his service, Batten saw considerable action. He was discharged from the Navy on 22 March 1866.

General Background: Batten was raised on a farm in Brandywine, Pennsylvania. After completing his early academic education, he worked as a teacher. During the winter of 1856, he began the study of medicine. In 1864, he graduated with a medical degree from University of Pennsylvania. Before graduation, he served in the military for eighteen months. After discharge from the Navy, he moved to Pittsburgh and established a successful medical practice. Batten belonged to a wide range of professional medical organizations, including the American Medical Society, the Pennsylvania Medical Society, the Allegheny County Medical Society, and the Mott Medical Club. He held an officer position in several state and local organizations, and in 1887, he served as a delegate to the Ninth International Medical Congress that met in Washington, D.C.

BEAL, George F.

Military Service: Beal served as Acting Assistant Surgeon at U.S.A. General Hospital Pittsburgh from 03 August 1864 until 10 March 1865.

BENHAM, S. N.

Military Service: Benham served as a surgeon during the Civil War.

General Background: Benham was an original organizer of the Pittsburgh Free Dispensary. He was also the youngest physician participating in founding the Allegheny County Medical Society in 1865.

BEUST, Bernard

Military Service: Beust served as Volunteer Surgeon at U.S.A. General Hospital Pittsburgh from 23 November 1863 until 23 March 1864.

BOGGS, J. N.

Military Service: Between August 1861 and January 1862, Boggs served as a physician in Company "D" of the 4th Alabama Infantry. He later transferred to Banner Hospital in Richmond, Virginia, where he served as assistant surgeon. He was subsequently commissioned assistant surgeon serving with the Third Alabama Hospital, Richmond, Virginia, until December 1863. After Richmond, he was assigned assistant surgeon to the Third Division of Camp Jackson. In March 1864, he was promoted to the Surgical Reserve Corps of the Army of Virginia. In that capacity, he served at all battles fought between Generals Grant, Lee, Sheridan, and Early until the end of the war.

General Background: Boggs was born in South Carolina on 05 December 1828. After completing preparatory school, he attended the Medical College of Atlanta, Georgia, and graduated in 1861. After graduation, he joined the Confederate Army. After the war, he practiced in Richmond, Virginia, for a brief period before relocating to Pittsburgh in October 1865.

BOWEN, Charles H.

Military Service: Bowen served as acting assistant surgeon at U.S.A. General Hospital Pittsburgh from 04 October 1863 until 29 February 1864.

BRYAN, James

Military Service: Bryan served as surgeon at U.S.A. General Hospital Pittsburgh from 16 March 1864 until 29 December 1864.

BURCHFIELD, John P.

Military Service: Burchfield served as assistant surgeon with the Pennsylvania 3rd Reserves Infantry (32nd Volunteers). He mustered out of service on 17 June 1865.

General Background: Following his service, Dr. Burchfield maintained his practice on Penn Avenue in Pittsburgh.

CAMPBELL, *William*

Military Service: Campbell served as Surgeon at U.S.A. General Hospital Pittsburgh from 01 July 1865 until 08 August 1865. He was a member of the 202nd Pennsylvania Regiment.

CHAPMAN, *Millie Jane*

Military Service: Chapman was prohibited from serving in the military; however, she contributed to the war effort as a volunteer to the local home guard organizations, including the local branch of the U.S. Christian Committee and the Pittsburgh Subsistence Committee. She was an active volunteer and prepared bandages and accouterments for soldiers passing through the city.

General Background: Chapman was one of the earliest woman physicians to establish a medical practice in the city. She was born in July 1845 in Edinboro, Pennsylvania, where she received her early academic education. In 1874, she graduated from the Cleveland Homeopathic Hospital College with an M.D. degree. After graduation, she moved to Pittsburgh and established a practice specializing in treating diseases of women and children. Chapman was a staff member of the Pittsburgh Homeopathic Hospital and the city's Children's Temporary Home. She was a regular contributor of articles to professional homeopathic medical journals, and she held memberships in, and read papers before, the leading national, state, and local professional homeopathic societies. Dr. Chapman was elected chairperson of the Institute of Homeopathy's Bureau of Obstetrics.

COFFEE, *H. T.*

Military Service: During the war, Coffee served as a private volunteer surgeon. He is known to have been present and performed heroically attending the wounded at Belle Plain and Fredericksburg, Virginia in early May 1864.

General Background: Coffee was a founding member of the Allegheny County Medical Society in 1865.

COX, *George H.*

Military Service: Cox served as acting assistant surgeon at U.S.A. General Hospital Pittsburgh from March 1865 until 13 July 1865.

CURTIS, Henry R.

Military Service: Curtis served as acting assistant surgeon at U.S.A. General Hospital Pittsburgh from 06 March 1864 until 02 October 1864.

DALY, William Hudson

Military Service: Daly served in both the Confederate and Union armies. His initial service was with the Confederate Army where he served as a Private in Company "B" of the 15th Virginia Volunteers. Under the Confederate flag, he fought in a number of battles from Big Bethel to Lee's Mills. After being captured and released through a prisoner exchange in 1863, he enrolled at Jefferson Medical College. Shortly afterward, he swore allegiance to the United States and began work as Medical Cadet at the Germantown Hospital in Philadelphia. He subsequently served as acting assistant surgeon in the Union Army at White Hall Army Hospital and was later detailed to Savannah, Georgia, where he served at the Hilton Head Hospital. He later served as post surgeon Hilton Head, South Carolina, and in August 1865 was sent to Jacksonville, Florida, to assist in the reception of the last 5,000 prisoners who had been liberated from Andersonville Prison. In 1871, Daly was commissioned lieutenant colonel and surgeon-in-chief of the 18th Division PA National Guard. At the outbreak of the Spanish-American War, he was appointed surgeon-in-chief of the Pennsylvania Volunteers. His relationship with General Nelson A. Miles afforded him opportunities to visit and inspect military medical institutions in this country and Europe. Daly ended his military career after instigating a national investigation into the poor quality of preserved meat furnished to the Army.

General Background: Daly was born on 11 September 1842 in Blairsville, Pennsylvania. In 1859, Daly was orphaned, and he moved to Richmond, Virginia. Upon discharge from the Union Army, Daly resumed his medical education at the University of Michigan in Ann Arbor, where he received his M.D. degree in early 1866. Following graduation, Daly moved to Pittsburgh where he established a private practice and became affiliated with Western Pennsylvania Hospital and Pittsburgh Free Dispensary. During his career, Daly maintained memberships in all of the most prominent professional medical organizations. He traveled extensively throughout Europe visiting many of the leading hospitals and major medical organizations to further his study of medicine and his specialty of laryngology, which he commenced in the late 1870s. Daly is considered Pittsburgh's pioneer in that specialty. In 1870, Daly became recording secretary of the Allegheny County Medical Society and was recognized there as the city's first throat specialist. He held the secretary position for eleven years, until 1881, when elected president of the Society.

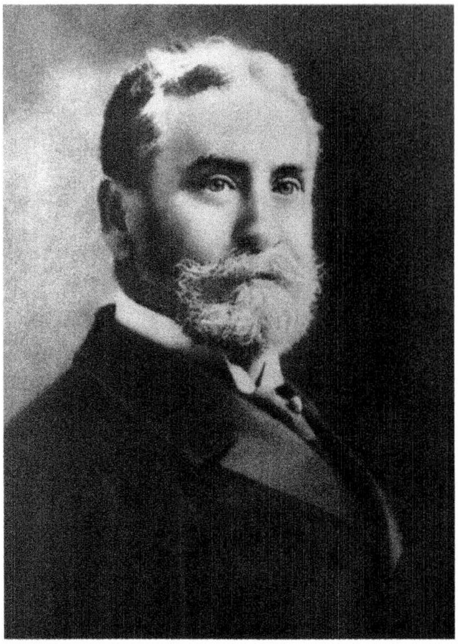

William H. Daly, M.D. (*Allegheny County Medical Society*)

DAVIS, Thomas B.

Military Service: At the age of sixteen, Davis joined the army as a private in Company "F" of the 133rd Pennsylvania Volunteer Infantry. He served for ten months.

General Background: Davis graduated from Jefferson Medical College in Philadelphia in 1870. His early academic education took place in Morgantown, West Virginia, and Monongahela, Pennsylvania. He matriculated at Jefferson College in Canonsburg, Pennsylvania, and graduated in 1866. After graduation, Davis served a one and one-half year residency at Blockley Hospital in Philadelphia. He then moved to Dayton, Ohio, where he was affiliated with the Soldier's Home and Pension Board. In 1877, he moved to Pittsburgh and established a practice. Davis held memberships in the American Medical Association and the Pennsylvania and Allegheny County Medical Societies. He regularly contributed to professional medical publications. He was a Fellow of the American Academy of Medicine and held staff positions at St. Francis and Mercy Hospitals. For a time, Davis also held the position of Lecturer on Physiology and Hygiene at the Pennsylvania Female College (now Chatham University).

DELANY, Martin R.

Military Service: Delany was not a physician, but he came close and should be better recognized for his accomplishments. He was commissioned as major in the Union Army, 104th Regiment of the United States Colored Troops, on 27 February 1865. His was the first such commission of an African-American. During his tenure, he served as a recruiting agent for U.S. Colored Troop regiments and was later assigned to Freedman's Bureau on 15 July 1865. He was discharged from the Army on 18 September 1868.

General Background: Delany was born a free black male in Charleston, Virginia on 06 May 1812. In 1822, he moved to Chambersburg, Pennsylvania. At the age of nineteen, he moved to Pittsburgh. A few years afterward, he read medicine with Dr. Andrew N. McDowell, who trained him as an assistant performing various duties, including cupping and leeching. In 1837, Delany established his own business and advertised "cupping, leeching and bleeding" services from a business location on Fifth Avenue near Wood Street. Advertisements for those services appeared in the city's directories up until 1847, the year in which he appears to have begun offering his services as a "galvanizer" as well. Between 1843 and 1847, Delany was involved in writing, editing and publishing *The Mercury* and *The Mystery* newspapers. It was around this time that Delany resumed his medical studies and apprenticed under two of Pittsburgh's leading physicians, Drs. Joseph P. Gazzam and F. Julius LeMoyne. During his years in Pittsburgh, Delany was actively involved in the abolitionist movement and Underground Railroad. Between 1847 and 1849, he worked with Frederick Douglas in editing the *North Star*, a prominent anti-slavery newspaper. In 1850, hoping to complete his medical studies, Delany applied to the Berkshire Medical School at Pittsfield, Massachusetts. He was not admitted due to his reluctance to agree with an admission condition that required he leave America and practice in Liberia. After failing to enroll at Berkshire, Delany set his sights on attending Harvard. There he met with more success and was admitted for the 1850–1851 term. His achievement was short-lived, as he was not permitted to return after the other students protested. Between then and the beginning of the Civil War, Delany continued to hone his abolitionist messages; he provided support to the Underground Railroad, and traveled to Liberia to explore the possibility and benefit of establishing a new and independent black nation in Africa. At the age of fifty-one, he abandoned the idea of a new free nation and began to consider how he might become involved in the war effort at a time when the federal government was hesitant to allow African-American participation. In 1863, he began recruiting for black regiments in Massachusetts, Rhode Island, and Connecticut. His efforts were so successful that he began constructing a proposal for the development of an African-American army to be led by black officers. In February 1864, he obtained a meeting with President Lincoln to advance this plan. Lincoln balked at the idea, but later engaged Secretary of War Stanton on how to better use African-American volunteers in the federal army. The outcome of those deliberations led to Delany being offered a commission as major in the U.S. Army. He was recognized for the excellent work that he accomplished. In 1884, he attempted to return to the practice of medicine. His efforts, however, were brief. He died the following year in 1885.

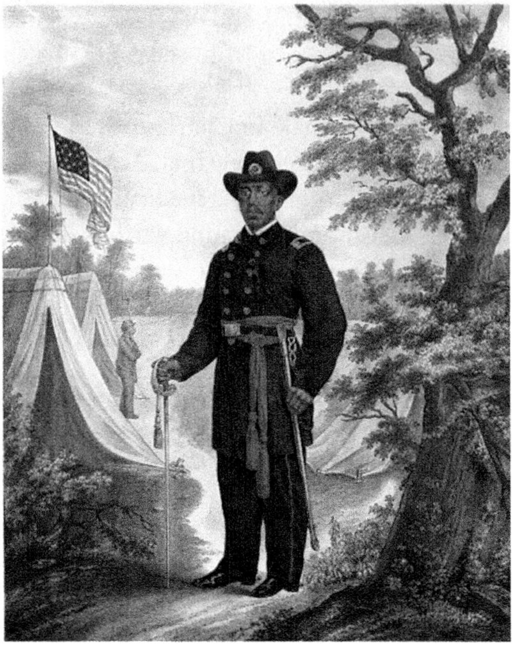

Martin Robison Delany. (*National Portrait Gallery, Smithsonian Institution*)

DICKSON, *John M.*

Military Service: Dickson served as assistant surgeon in the 93rd Regiment and surgeon in the 203rd and the 213th Pennsylvania Infantry Regiments during the Civil War. Immediately after the battle of Shiloh (Pittsburg Landing) in April 1862, together with Dr. McCook, he left Pittsburgh with two hospital-boats on the "Expedition to the Tennessee River" to retrieve wounded soldiers and transport them to hospitals in the city. His passionate care of the wounded from that battle and numerous others including the battle of Gettysburg was well documented.

General Background: Dickson was born in Cecil County, Maryland, in May 1812. He and his family moved to the Pittsburgh area in 1821. Dickson began the study of medicine under Dr. Leatherman, a prominent physician in Canonsburg, Pennsylvania. He graduated from the University of New York Medical School in 1830. He started his practice in Sewickley, Pennsylvania, at the age of twenty-eight. Later, he traveled extensively to attend medical lectures in the major cities of Europe. In 1843, Dickson moved his office to Allegheny City, and later into Pittsburgh. He was one of the earliest physicians to establish a dissecting room, in which he trained many aspiring physicians who otherwise had little access to anatomical studies. He is credited with developing numerous surgical instruments when the needed tool could not otherwise be found. Dr. Dickson was a hunter, zoologist, and avid botanist who reportedly could name over four thousand species of Pennsylvania plants. He died in January 1888.

DICKSON, John Shields

Military Service: John S. Dickson enlisted in the army at the age of sixteen. He served as a private in Company "G," 28th Pennsylvania Volunteer Infantry from 01 July 1861 to November 1862, when he was discharged due to disability. Dickson was one of the volunteer physicians participating in Pittsburgh's "Expedition to the Tennessee River" and later in an effort to relieve wounded soldiers at Belle Plains and Fredericksburg, Virginia in April 1862.[3]

General Background: Dickson was born in Allegheny City in April 1844. He was the oldest son of Dr. John M. Dickson. He graduated from Jefferson Medical College in Philadelphia in 1868 and practiced medicine with his father for one year. He then left for extended study at hospitals in Europe. In 1870, he was appointed as surgeon on the staff of Mercy Hospital, a position he held for more than a decade.

DICKSON, Joseph

Military Service: Joseph Dickson was among the group of physicians that accompanied members of the U.S. Christian Commission's Pittsburgh branch in volunteering their services at the front immediately after the Battle of Gettysburg.

DICKSON, Thomas

Military Service: Thomas Dickson, brother of Joseph and John Dickson, was among the group of physicians who joined members of the United States Christian Commission's Pittsburgh branch as a volunteer at the battlefront. While at the battlefront with McClellan's army during its siege of Richmond, he contracted typhoid fever and died.

DONNELLY, Edward J.

Military Service: From November 1864, he served as surgeon in the 1st Provisional Cavalry, and the 2nd and 5th Regiment Reserves. He mustered out of service on 13 July 1865.

DOWNS, Thomas A.

Military Service: Downs served as acting assistant surgeon at U.S.A. General Hospital Pittsburgh from 13 September 1864 until 03 February 1865.

DUFF, James Henderson

Military Service: Duff passed his examination for the United States Navy after graduation from medical school in 1848. He was responsible for raising a regiment of emergency volunteers during the Civil War. Duff served at various hospitals around Washington, D.C., and later organized a company of emergency volunteers. After refusing the position of regimental colonel, he moved to Pittsburgh in 1866.

General Background: Born in 1824 of Scotch-Irish heritage, Duff graduated from Jefferson Medical School in 1848. His early years were spent on a farm in Westmoreland County. His grandfather, John Duff, first settled there after the Revolutionary War. Upon completion of his studies, James Duff took the examination for the United States Navy and passed. He was an avid abolitionist and volunteered early for service in the Civil War. He raised a family of six children, including John Milton Duff, who also became a prominent physician in Pittsburgh.

DUFF, *John Milton*

Military Service: John Milton Duff served as private in the 107th Pennsylvania Volunteer Infantry. He enlisted at the age of fifteen and was wounded twice. Duff was promoted by special order for meritorious conduct at the Battle of Dabney's Mills (Rowanty Creek) on 05–07 February 1865.

General Background: Born in Westmoreland County, Pennsylvania, in 1849, Duff began his academic education locally and subsequently graduated from Pittsburgh's Western University. He attended and graduated from Jefferson Medical College in Philadelphia in 1874. After graduation, he moved to Pittsburgh's South Side where he established a private practice and remained there until his death. Duff was consulting surgeon at Passavant Hospital and gynecologist and surgeon at South Side Hospital. Duff assumed a professorship in obstetrics at the Western Pennsylvania Medical College upon its opening in 1886 and remained in that position for several years. During his career, he was a member of the Pennsylvania, Pittsburgh, and Allegheny County Medical Societies. He was also a fellow of the American Academy of Medicine.

DUNCAN, *James A.*

Military Service: Duncan participated as a volunteer surgeon in Pittsburgh's "Expedition to the Tennessee River." He also volunteered at Belle Plains and Fredericksburg, Virginia. He later served as acting assistant surgeon at U.S.A. General Hospital Pittsburgh from 24 March 1864 until 23 April 1864.

FISHER *(first name unknown)*

Military Service: Fisher is recorded as participating in Pittsburgh's "Expedition To The Tennessee River" to treat wounded soldiers in April 1862.

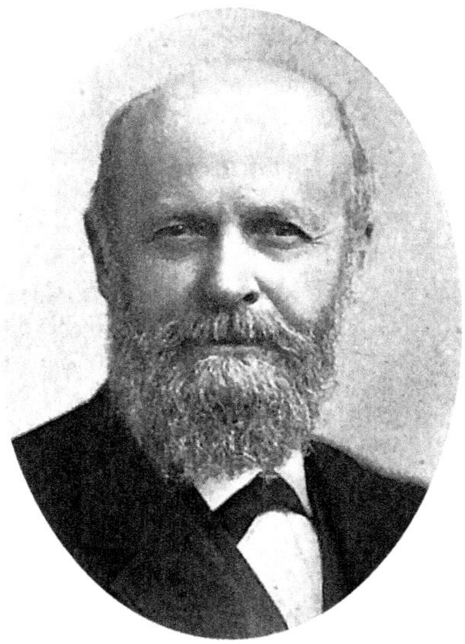

Andrew Fleming, M.D. (*Carnegie Library of Pittsburgh. All rights reserved. Unauthorized reproduction or usage prohibited*)

FLEMING, Andrew

Military Service: Fleming did not serve in the military during the Civil War. He did, however, support the war effort as an untiring volunteer treating sick and wounded soldiers at the Pittsburgh Subsistence Committee's Soldiers' Home throughout the war.

General Background: Fleming was born in Pittsburgh on 03 July 1830. He was an apprentice of Dr. Joseph P. Gazzam and graduated from Jefferson Medical College in 1855. Following graduation, he served an internship at the Pennsylvania Hospital in Philadelphia. He established his practice in Pittsburgh in 1857 in partnership with his mentor, Dr. Gazzam. Fleming was a member and officer of the city's Bedford Medical Society and prolific writer who authored more than forty medical studies. He is perhaps best known for a monograph he authored in 1858, entitled *Blood Stains in Clinical Trials*. He was a founding member of the Allegheny County Medical Society in 1865.

FOSTER, William S.

Military Service: Foster held the rank of second lieutenant and adjutant in the 2nd Battalion of the 1st Pennsylvania Reserve Cavalry.

General Background: Born in Pittsburgh in 1842, Foster received his early academic training in Juniata County, Pennsylvania. After that, he attended Jefferson College in Canonsburg, Pennsylvania, and later enrolled at Jefferson Medical College in Philadelphia. Upon graduation in July 1866, he moved to Pittsburgh to establish his private practice specializing in diseases of women and children. During his career, he was a member of the American Medical Association and the Pennsylvania and Allegheny County Medical Societies. Foster held staff positions at both Passavant and Allegheny

General hospitals. He also held positions at various times at the Home for the Destitute of Pittsburgh, the Pittsburgh Fire Department, and Pittsburgh Home for Aged Women.

FULTON, Henry W.

Military Service: Fulton was among the "three months' men" who enlisted at the outbreak of the Civil War. He later reenlisted with 53rd Pennsylvania Volunteers and was subsequently transferred to the Signal Corp Army of the Potomac, serving under General's McClellan and Grant.

General Background: Born in 1838, Fulton was raised in Westmoreland County. After serving in the military for most of the war, he returned to Westmoreland County and married. Shortly after that, he began the study of medicine with Dr. L. H. Willard in Allegheny City and subsequently attended Hahnemann College in Philadelphia. He graduated in 1872 and traveled to Pittsburgh to establish a practice. He was a member of the medical staff of the Pittsburgh Homeopathic Hospital and the leading national, state and local homeopathic medical societies.

FUNDENBERG, W. F.

Military Service: During the Civil War, Fundenberg served as a surgeon in the 136th Pennsylvania Volunteer Infantry and the 176th Pennsylvania Volunteer Infantry. He also participated in Pittsburgh's "Expedition to the Tennessee River."

General Background: Fundenberg graduated from Washington University of Maryland in 1852 and relocated to Pittsburgh. He was a member of the American Medical Association, Allegheny County Medical Society, American Dental Association, Pennsylvania Dental Society, and the Pittsburgh Dental Association. He served as president of the Pennsylvania Dental Society in 1888, and of the Pittsburgh Dental Society in 1874–79 and 1881.

GAZZAM, Edward D.

Military Service: Gazzam did not have a military career, but he is nonetheless remembered for his leading role in challenging the distribution of guns and powder, intended for shipment to the Confederate states, from the Allegheny Arsenal immediately before the outbreak of the Civil War.

General Background: Born in Pittsburgh in 1803, Gazzam studied law under Hon. Richard Biddle. Due to poor health, he abandoned law after two years and took up the study of medicine. An opponent of slavery, he was active in state and local political matters, and in 1848, he changed political parties by joining the "Free-soil" movement from which the Republican Party originated. He was the Free-soil party's first candidate for governor of Pennsylvania, and in 1855, he was the party's candidate for state senator. He lost both elections, but the failure would be short-lived. The following year, his candidacy was again advanced for the office of state senator as a representative of the Union Republican party. This time he won, thereby becoming the first Republican state senator from Allegheny County.

GRAHAM, *Samuel*

Military Service: Graham served as assistant surgeon in the Pennsylvania 174th Infantry from January 1863 until December 1864, after which he served as assistant surgeon in the 81st Infantry. He mustered out of service on 29 June 1865.

GREEN, *John*

Military Service: Green served as a private in the 167th Pennsylvania Volunteer Infantry and later in Company "C" of the 4th Pennsylvania Cavalry. During his military career, he served in various branches of detached service, including the Headquarters Fifth Army Corps as a courier and color-bearer.

General Background: Green spent some years in the academic teaching profession before engaging in the practice of medicine. He was born in Murrysville, Pennsylvania, in May 1845. After his military service and teaching for several years, he took up the study of medicine and served an apprenticeship under several prominent physicians near his home and in Cleveland, Ohio. He attended Western Reserve Medical College for three years and graduated in February 1870. He then moved to Pittsburgh to set up practice. Green associated himself with the Pittsburgh Board of Health, St. Francis Hospital, and Pittsburgh Free Dispensary. He held memberships in the American Medical Association, the Pennsylvania Medical Society, Allegheny County Medical Society, and Obstetrical Society of Pittsburgh.

GROSS, *Augustus H.*

Military Service: Gross helped form one of the city's independent military companies. He served as a surgeon during the Civil War.

General Background: Gross arrived in America from Germany in 1833. In 1840, he established a medical practice in Indiana. In 1848, he came to Pittsburgh and began a practice in the East Liberty section of the city. Gross took an active role in both medicine and public affairs. In the public realm, he served in the Pennsylvania House of Representatives and on the Pittsburgh Select Council. He was a founding member of the Allegheny County Medical Society in 1865.

HAMILTON, *William*

Military Service: Hamilton participated in Pittsburgh's "Expedition to the Tennessee River" in April 1862.

HANNA, Edmund S.

Military Service: Hanna served as acting assistant surgeon at U.S.A. General Hospital Pittsburgh from 14 May 1865 until 20 May 1865.

HAZZARD, Thomas L.

Military Service: Hazzard attended Chester Military Academy and afterward became assistant surgeon with the Pennsylvania 18th Infantry Militia Regiment.

General Background: Born in Monongahela City in April 1855, Hazard traced his roots to relatives who traveled from England and arrived in America in 1639. After completing his local academic education, he attended Chester Military Academy. He next attended Washington and Jefferson College from 1875 until 1878. He entered medical school at the University of Pennsylvania in Philadelphia and graduated in 1881. Afterward, he moved to Pittsburgh and established a private practice in Allegheny City. Hazzard practiced both medicine and surgery and served for several years as a physician of the Allegheny Poor Board and as Professor of Physiology at Western Pennsylvania Medical College. He was an assistant physician on the medical staff of Western Pennsylvania Hospital; surgeon on the medical staff of Allegheny General Hospital; and life (service) member of the Pittsburgh Free Dispensary. He was also a member of the Allegheny County Medical Society.

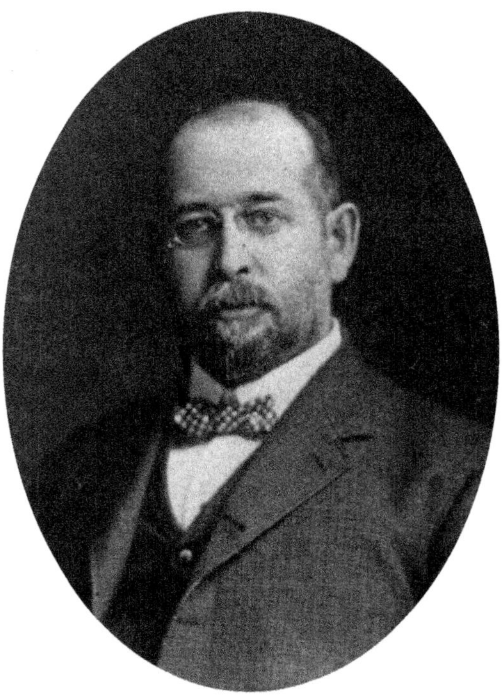

T. L. Hazzard, M.D.

HEANEY, *Patrick*

Military Service: Heaney served as Acting Assistant Surgeon at U.S.A. General Hospital Pittsburgh from 05 December 1862 until 09 February 1863.

HECHELMAN, *Herman W.*

Military Service: During the American Civil War, Hechelman served as acting assistant surgeon and later as surgeon with the U.S. Volunteers. He later served in the German Army as a surgeon during the Franco-Prussian War (1870–71).

General Background: Born in Bavaria 1848, Hechelman came to America in 1860. He was the son of a noted local brewer, Marlin Hechelman. In 1865, he returned to Germany and completed his academic education. He returned in 1867 and studied medicine at Jefferson Medical College in Philadelphia. In 1869, he received his medical degree and departed for Europe to further his medical studies at leading universities in Munich and Vienna, focusing his attention on diseases of the eyes and ears. He moved back to Pittsburgh in 1871 and established a practice in Allegheny City. Dr. Hechelman was appointed surgeon at Allegheny General Hospital in 1885. A year later, he became a professor of diseases of the eye and ear at Western Pennsylvania Medical College. Hechelman was a member of the Allegheny County Medical Society and served as Ophthalmologist and Otologist at Western Pennsylvania Hospital, an eye and ear surgeon at Pittsburgh Home for the Friendless, and physician and surgeon at the Benedictine Convent.

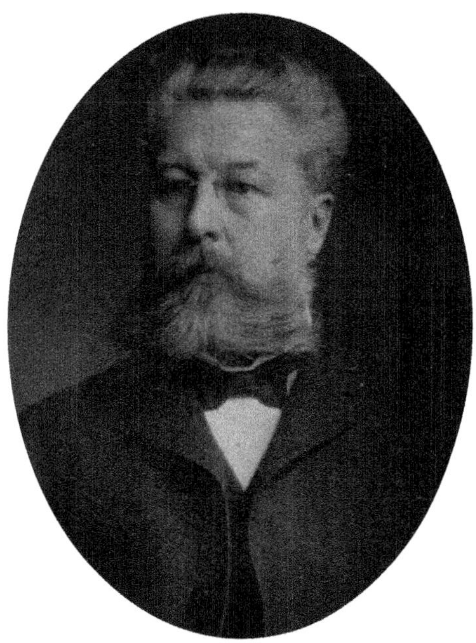

H. W. Hechelman, M.D.

HERRON, J. B.

Military Service: Herron participated in the Pittsburgh "Expedition to the Tennessee River" in April 1862.

HEZLEP, William B.

Military Service: Hezlep served as Surgeon with the 6th Pennsylvania Heavy Artillery from October 1864 until being reassigned to the 7th Pennsylvania Cavalry on 27 June 1865. He mustered out of service on 23 August 1865.

HUSELTON, W. S.

Military Service: Huselton entered the U.S. Army in August 1862 as acting assistant surgeon. He then passed the medical board exams and became a surgeon of the Volunteers. He was offered but declined an officer's commission in the Volunteer Army.

General Background: Born in Wilkes-Barre, Pennsylvania, Huselton and his family moved to Butler, Pennsylvania, during his teenage years. After completing his early academic education, he commenced work as a teacher but later decided to take up medicine at Jefferson Medical College in Philadelphia. He subsequently moved to Georgetown University in Washington, D.C., to complete his medical degree. After service in the Civil War, he returned to Butler for a short period. In April 1867, he moved to Allegheny City to establish a new practice. Dr. Huselton served on the surgical staff of Allegheny General Hospital, was the medical director of the P&W Railroad, and held numerous other professional medical positions. Huselton was also an active businessman involved in a range of private business ventures, including the Huselton Automatic Car Coupler Company, which manufactured and sold railroad car coupling devices. It was a lucrative business as indicated by an advertisement for the device published in an 1890 edition of the Railroad Gazette. It read:

> This coupler is made of malleable iron and in different sizes and can be put on old or new cars without changing existing carriers. The Huselton company says that over 10,000 of these couplers are now in use on different roads, and the letters which accompany the circular issued by the company commend it highly.[4]

IRISH, Franklin

Military Service: Irish served as acting assistant surgeon at U.S.A. General Hospital Pittsburgh from 05 August until 02 September 1861.

General Background: Irish was a member of the Allegheny County Medical Society from 1865 until his death in 1869.

KEARNS, William Dickey

Military Service: Kearns served as acting assistant surgeon under General McClelland. He was among the group of volunteer surgeons who participated in Pittsburgh's "Expedition to the Tennessee River."

General Background: On 08 January 1831, William Dickey Kearns was born in the Coal Hill area of Pennsylvania. He attended Duquesne College. After leaving Duquesne, he enrolled at Jefferson College where he received a degree in 1851. He left the city for several years before returning in 1854 to study medicine under Dr. John Dickson. Kearns later enrolled at the Medical University of New York and graduated in 1857. During spring 1858, he returned to the city and established a private practice. Kearns maintained membership in a range of leading national and local medical professional organizations, including the American Medical Association, Pennsylvania Medical Society, Allegheny County Medical Society, and Pittsburgh Obstetrical Society. He was also an active member of various local education-related organizations, including the board of education.

KING, Cyrus B.

Military Service: King entered the Union Army as assistant surgeon the day after graduating from medical school on March 8, 1863. He was later promoted to surgeon. From 1863 to 1865, he was assigned to a hospital in Philadelphia. Between 1865 and 1871, he served as Superintendent of the Pittsburgh Soldiers' Home at Western Pennsylvania Hospital.

General Background: King was the child of Samuel M. and Maria King of Monongahela City, Pennsylvania. He was born in February 1839. His father was a physician. After completing his early academic education, he attended Columbia College in Washington, D.C., and later studied medicine at Jefferson Medical College in Philadelphia and graduated in 1862. In 1865, immediately after the Civil War, he joined the surgical staff of Western Pennsylvania Hospital. In 1871, he established a private practice in Allegheny City and served on the medical staff of Western Pennsylvania Hospital, Allegheny General, and the Children's Hospital of Pittsburgh. He also served as a consulting physician to McKeesport Hospital. At Western Pennsylvania Hospital, he was appointed the superintendent. In 1886, when Western Pennsylvania Medical College opened, he served as President of the Board of Trustees and professor of orthopedic surgery. He was a member of the American Medical Association and Pennsylvania and Allegheny County Medical Societies. In 1876, he was named a delegate to the International Medical Congress in Philadelphia. King regularly contributed to leading American medical journals.

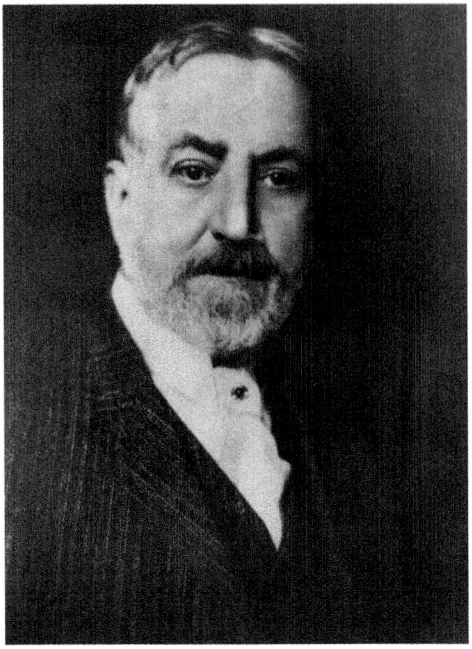

C. B. King, M.D. (*Allegheny County Medical Society*)

KING, James

Military Service: At the outbreak of the Civil War, King joined the army as a surgeon at Camp Curtain and was later named Medical Director of Pennsylvania Reserves until mustering out of service after the Battle of Antietam in 1862 at the request of Governor Curtin. He was subsequently named Surgeon General of Pennsylvania and served in that role until August 1864. As Surgeon General, he was responsible for executing rigorous medical officer examinations for all Pennsylvania physicians being sent into the field. He served as one of the first members of the State's Examining Board. A physician who was among those treating the wounded at Belle Plains and Fredericksburg, Virginia, and on a steam transport from Fredericksburg to Washington, offered this account of King:

> Surgeon General James King was constantly with his volunteer corps in the great emergency about which you and your readers are already sufficiently acquainted. But he was not with them merely for the purpose of ordering, but for the solid work of this occasion. He was busy day and night operating, dressing, nursing and arranging for the comfort of wounded under our care. His ear was open to the call of everyone, and his hand was ever ready to the willing dictates of his own noble heart. No soldier ever appealed to him in vain, and no angry look ever darkened his brow, or cruel word ever emanated from his lips. His work was both Herculean and Protean, and was performed with the greatest good will and kindness. Dr. King has all through the scenes of this

> infamous rebellion done good work. The hearts of numerous soldiers will bless him for the manner in which he has discharged his arduous duties towards them.[5]

General Background: King was born in Bedford County, Pennsylvania, in 1816. He received his medical education as a student of Dr. Benjamin W. Dudley, a noted lithotomist and ovariotomist associated with the University of Lexington, Kentucky. King graduated from Transylvania University in 1838 and then established his practice in Hollidaysburg, Pennsylvania. In 1844, upon his election as Professor of Anatomy, Physiology, and Hygiene at Washington College, he moved to Washington, Pennsylvania. In 1850, he moved to Pittsburgh and established a practice. Upon resigning as Surgeon General of Pennsylvania in August 1864, he resumed his practice in Pittsburgh, joining in partnership with Dr. Francis Le Moyne. In April 1865, he was one of the founders of the Allegheny County Medical Society. He served as president of both the Pennsylvania Medical Society and Allegheny County Medical Society. He was also an Associate Fellow of the College of Physicians in Philadelphia.

KIRKER, John

Military Service: During the period 1862–63, Kirker served as surgeon-in-charge of U.S.A. General Hospital in Grafton, West Virginia. From 1864 until the close of the war, he served as surgeon-in-charge of U.S.A. General Hospital in Wheeling, West Virginia.

General Background: Kirker was born in Harmony, Pennsylvania, in February 1835. He attended Allegheny College in Meadville before enrolling at Bellevue Medical College in New York. After completing his military service in the Civil War, he moved to Pittsburgh to establish a general practice. By the late 1880s, he was credited with having one of the largest practices in Allegheny City. He was a member of the American Medical Association and the Pennsylvania and Allegheny County Medical Societies.

LANGE, Charles C.

Military Service: In 1861, Lange entered the army as hospital steward of 103rd Pennsylvania Volunteer Infantry. He held that position until mustered out in 1865. Between April 1864 and March 1865, he was held as a prisoner at Andersonville Prison in Georgia.

General Background: Lange was born on 10 June 1843 in Pittsburgh, where he received his early education. He graduated from Pittsburgh Central High School in 1860 and began reading medicine with Dr. A. Lange. After the war, he resumed his medical studies at the University of Pennsylvania. Upon receiving his medical degree in March 1867, he returned to Pittsburgh where he established a general practice.

During his career, Lange served on the medical staffs of Passavant Hospital and the Pittsburgh Free Dispensary. He held membership in the Allegheny County Medical Society and several other professional organizations.

LEE, *J. M.*

Military Service: At the age of thirteen, Lee served as an orderly to General Lane. He served in that capacity until the end of the war, after which U.S. Congressman Columbus Delano appointed him to the U.S. Naval Academy. Lee resigned the commission to study medicine.

General Background: Lee established his practice of medicine and surgery in Pittsburgh in 1876 after graduating from the College of Physicians and Surgeons in New York City. He served as a physician at the Pittsburgh Free Dispensary and Mercy Hospital. Lee specialized in the study of climate and its influence on pulmonary diseases. During his career, he was published widely in a variety of prominent medical journals and held memberships in all of the leading local professional medical organizations.

LEMOYNE, *Francis*

Military Service: LeMoyne served as assistant surgeon in the 9th Pennsylvania Reserves Infantry. He was later transferred and named surgeon of the 16th Pennsylvania Cavalry (161st Volunteers) in January 1864. He mustered out of service on 11 August 1865.

General Background: A graduate of the University of Pennsylvania Medical School, LeMoyne joined the army, rising to the rank of brevet lieutenant colonel. After the war, he returned to Pittsburgh and formed a partnership with Dr. James King. Together they opened an office on Fourth Street near Grant Avenue. He served as a surgeon at Western Pennsylvania Hospital and was a driving force in establishing Pittsburgh Children's Hospital. He also served as president of the Allegheny County Medical Society and chairman of the Pittsburgh Water Commission.

LEVIS, *John C.*

Military Service: Levis was drafted and served as acting assistant surgeon at U.S.A. General Hospital Pittsburgh from 01 December 1863 until 09 July 1865.

MARAND, *Alfred L. S.*

Military Service: Marand served as acting assistant surgeon at U.S.A. General Hospital Pittsburgh from 02 March 1864 until 10 December 1864.

MARTIN, William J.

Military Service: Martin served as private in Company "A" of the 193rd Pennsylvania Volunteer Infantry.

McCANN, James

Military Service: After a brief period in private practice, McCann joined the U.S. Army and served as assistant surgeon in the 5th Pennsylvania Heavy Artillery Regiment (204th Volunteers). His service as assistant surgeon began at the Battle of Gettysburg in July 1863. He served until the end of the war.

General Background: McCann was born in Allegheny County's Penn Township in 1836. He was a grandson of Thomas McCann, who served in the Revolutionary War under General Anthony Wayne. Upon completion of his early education, he served as an apprentice under Dr. John Dickson. In 1858, he attended New York University but transferred to the University of Pennsylvania in 1863, from which he graduated with a medical degree. After the war, he returned to the city and briefly entered into an association with Dr. W. C. Reiter. After that, McCann established a private practice and became a surgeon with the Pennsylvania and Lake Erie Railroads. In 1870, he joined the surgical staff of Western Pennsylvania Hospital, and in 1883, he was one of the original promoters and stockholders of Western Pennsylvania Medical College. Upon its official opening in 1886, he was named the first faculty president and professor of surgery and clinical surgery. He was a

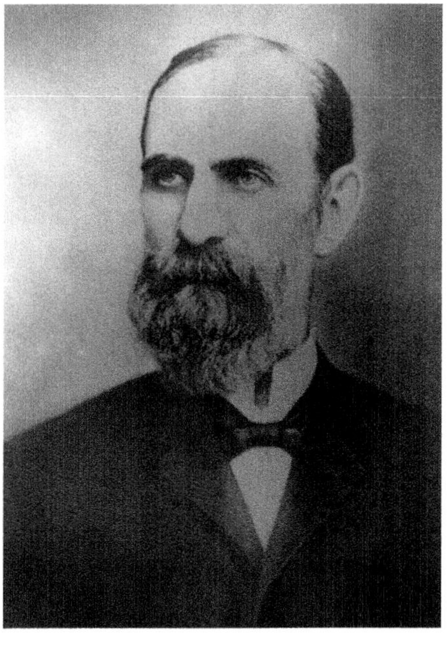

James McCann, M.D. (*Allegheny County Medical Society*)

member of the leading national, state and local professional medical societies. In 1891, he represented the American Medical Association as a delegate to the British Medical Association's meeting in London. He was a prolific writer and published many articles on surgery. He died as one of Pittsburgh's most esteemed physicians in July 1893.

McCANDLESS, J. Guy

Military Service: McCandless served as assistant surgeon in the 52nd Pennsylvania Infantry Volunteers for two years. He was later appointed surgeon at Cotton Factory Hospital in Harrisburg. He served in that post for one year.

General Background: McCandless was born in 1839 in Perrysville, Pennsylvania, just north of Pittsburgh. He was a descendant of that area's earliest settlers, and today, a township there continues to carry the family name. McCandless initially studied medicine under his father, A. G. McCandless, who was a leading physician in the area. After studying with his father, he enrolled at Jefferson Medical College in Philadelphia, from which he received his medical degree. He was a member of the Allegheny County Medical Society and served as a physician to the Pittsburgh Board of Health. During his career, he held many civic positions.

McCLELLAND, J. B.

Military Service: McClelland served for three years in Hampton's Pennsylvania Battery.

General Background: McClelland was born in 1843. He read medicine with Dr. J. H. McClelland and later attended and graduated from Hahnemann Medical College in Philadelphia. After graduation, he established a practice in Pittsburgh and served as an obstetrician with the Pittsburgh Homeopathic Hospital.

McCOOK, George L.

Military Service: McCook served as a special medical inspector for enrollment of short-term physicians during the Civil War. McCook was among the physicians who volunteered at the front immediately after the Battle of Gettysburg. In their regimental history, members of the 155th Pennsylvania Regiment later praised his service and that of the other surgeons who accompanied him. "No corps of surgeons labored more devotedly in the field hospitals on the battlefield and in the town of Gettysburg, than did the patriotic members of the Pittsburgh delegation, and too much praise cannot be awarded the noble deeds and acts of the surgeons named."[6]

General Background: Born in 1824 to a family in Lisbon, Ohio, McCook came to Pittsburgh in 1851 after graduating from Jefferson Medical College. Before coming to the city, he had taught in the Baltimore Medical College. McCook was one of the original members of the Committee on Munitions of War, a subcommittee of

Pittsburgh's Committee of Public Safety. His role in working with Dr. Edward D. Gazzam to restrict the movement of contraband weapons and munitions from the Allegheny Arsenal to the Confederate states before the war was invaluable to the ultimate success of the Union Army. McCook was among the founding members of the Allegheny County Medical Society in 1865.

McKEE, James C.

Military Service: McKee served as acting assistant surgeon at U.S.A. General Hospital Pittsburgh from 09 July 1863 until 02 December 1863. During this service, he was in charge of the hospital.

METZGAR, S. R.

Military Service: Metzgar was among the volunteer surgeon group in Pittsburgh's "Expedition to the Tennessee River" in April 1862.

General Background: Metzgar was a member of the Allegheny County Medical Society from 1868 until his resignation in 1872.

MILLER, J. Edwin

Military Service: On August 1, 1862, Miller enlisted in Hampton's Independent Battery after graduation from medical school. He was discharged on 28 June 1865.

General Background: Miller was brought to the area by his parents in November 1846 when they settled in McKeesport, Pennsylvania. He stayed in that area until he enlisted to fight in the Civil War. After the war, he decided to pursue a medical degree and enrolled in the Jefferson Medical College. After graduating in March 1870, he moved to Pittsburgh to establish his practice. In 1872, he reenlisted in the military and spent the next two years in the U.S. Navy. In the Navy, Miller was a senior medical officer at the Pensacola Navy Yard. After leaving service, he spent some months living in the Piedmont, Florida area before returning to Pittsburgh.

MILLER, Samuel J. F.

Military Service: Miller served as acting assistant surgeon at U.S.A. General Hospital Pittsburgh from 10 December 1864 until 08 June 1865.

MILLER, William Newlon

Military Service: Miller was a member of the U.S. Christian Commission during McClellan's Richmond campaign. He later became an assistant surgeon in the 193rd Pennsylvania Volunteer Infantry.

General Background: Miller established his medical practice in Murrysville, Pennsylvania, in April 1852 after graduating from Washington College and Jefferson Medical School. In 1863, he moved his practice to the Birmingham section of Pittsburgh. He held memberships in the American Medical Association and the Pennsylvania and South Side Medical Societies.

MINASSIAN, Simon G.

Military Service: Minassian served as acting assistant surgeon at U.S.A. General Hospital Pittsburgh from 24 March 1864 until 02 June 1865.

MOWRY, Robert Bruce

Military Service: Mowry served as a private volunteer surgeon. On one trip in early May 1864 at the request of Pennsylvania Surgeon General James King, he traveled to the battlefront with Drs. George L. McCook, H. T. Coffee of Pittsburgh, and several other physicians. The group served for ten days in the field and on steam transport ships assisting wounded soldiers at Belle Plain and Fredericksburg.[7] Mowry also participated as a volunteer surgeon after the Battle of Gettysburg. In a written testimonial included in the history of the Pennsylvania 155th Regiment, Dr. J. A. Reed from Lancaster, Pennsylvania, he described the service of Mowry and the group of other volunteer physicians as follows:

> While on the march to Gettysburg the writer was appointed Surgeon-in-Chief of the Second Brigade, First Division, Fifth Army Corps. It became his duty in less than ten days thereafter to take charge of the great field hospital on Little Round Top, Gettysburg. The enormous losses in that battle, the many operations on account of gun-shot wounds and from explosive shells, surpassed that of any previous engagement of the Civil War, because of the greater numbers engaged. The surgeons of the Army of the Potomac were greatly insufficient in number for this great emergency. The patriotic members of the medical profession appeared promptly from all parts of Pennsylvania and adjoining States for immediate duty. Pittsburg surgeons were among the first to report on Little Round Top, on July 3, 1863, before the cannonading had ceased to echo. The writer recalls the presence and active service of Doctors Thos. W. Shaw, John Dickson, A. G. Walter, G. L. McCook, Jr., Thos. J. Gallaher, Mowry, Jones, McCann, Childs, Cornman, and many more whose names cannot now be recalled, who came to alleviate and cheer the wounded. Many of the field hospitals and operating tables were under heavy artillery fire July 2nd and 3rd. The surgeon's duties were very much increased when the Confederates retreated, abandoning their badly wounded and sick.[8]

General Background: A graduate of the Western University of Pennsylvania, Mowry received his medical degree from Jefferson Medical College in Philadelphia in

1836. Following graduation, he established a practice in Pittsburgh and specialized in gynecology. He was a member of the American Medical Association and the Pennsylvania and Allegheny County Medical Societies. He was a founding member of the Allegheny County Medical Society in 1865. For several years, he served as president of the Pennsylvania Medical Society. Mowry was on the surgical staff of Western Pennsylvania Hospital for many years. He was also a founder of Allegheny General Hospital.

MURDOCH, Andrew C.

Military Service: Murdoch served as acting assistant surgeon at U.S.A. General Hospital Pittsburgh from 26 June 1863 until 26 August 1863.

General Background: Pittsburgh historian Sarah H. Killikelly described Murdoch's post-hospital work as follows:

> The appointment of a Draft Commissioner was followed by the appointment of a surgeon, Dr. A. C. Murdoch, to examine applicants for exemption on the ground of physical inability to bear arms. A room was assigned him in the Court House, and for several weeks his labors were most arduous. Private examinations were made in Dr. Murdoch's office, both before and after his office hours at the Court House, frequently protracting his labors far into the night.[9]

MURDOCH, James Bissett

Military Service: Murdoch served as a surgeon in the 24th Regiment New York Volunteers from 1862 until 1865.

General Background: Murdoch was born in Glasgow, Scotland, in October 1830. He graduated from the College of Physicians and Surgeons of New York City in 1854, and afterward served a one-year surgical residency at Bellevue Hospital. Upon completion of his residency, he took a position as Surgeon on the *North Star* steamer. Between 1855 and 1877, he practiced medicine in Oswego, New York, and then moved to Pittsburgh. After moving to Pittsburgh, he was a member of the American Medical Association as well as the Pennsylvania and Allegheny County Medical Societies. He was president of the Pennsylvania and Allegheny County Societies during his career. Murdoch was a surgeon on the staff of Western Pennsylvania Hospital, and when Western Pennsylvania Medical College opened in 1886, he served as its Dean and Clinical Professor of Surgery. Murdoch was married twice; his second wife was the youngest daughter of the Honorable J. K. Moorhead, president of the Monongahela Navigation Canal and the Atlantic & Ohio Telegraph Co., which later became Western Union Telegraph Company.

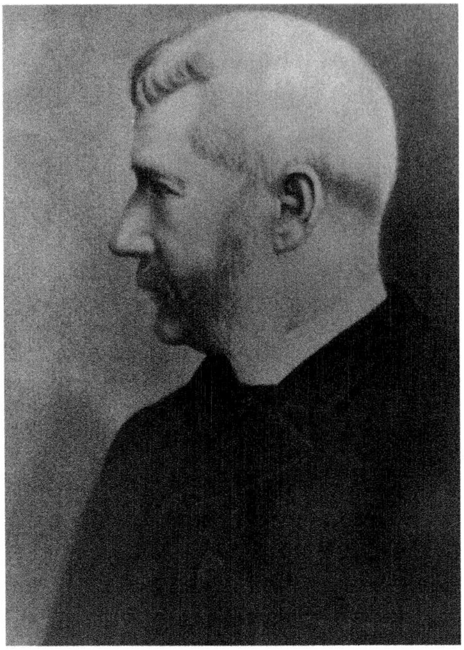

James B. Murdoch, M.D. (*Allegheny County Medical Society*)

PERCHMENT, P. D.

Military Service: Perchment served as a private in the 15th Pennsylvania Infantry and assistant surgeon in the 7th Missouri Calvary. He served for twenty-eight months and participated in the Battles of Antietam, Pittsburgh Landing, Second Bull Run, and others. After the war, he was a colonel in the Pennsylvania 14th Volunteer Infantry Regiment. Perchment participated in Pittsburgh's "Expedition to the Tennessee River" in April 1862.

General Background: Perchment attended Allegheny College in Meadville before enrolling at Jefferson Medical College in Philadelphia, Pennsylvania. He graduated with a medical degree in 1855. He was a long-term staff member of St. Francis Hospital and an examining surgeon for insurance companies.

PHILLIPS, Joseph A.

Military Service: Phillips served as assistant surgeon in the 9th Reserves Infantry (38th Volunteers) from July 1861 and mustered out on 12 May 1864.

General Background: Phillips was a member of the Allegheny County Medical Society from 1867 until 1897.

RANKIN, Andrew H.

Military Service: Rankin served as acting assistant surgeon at U.S.A. General Hospital Pittsburgh from 26 September 1864 until 03 February 1865.

RANKIN, D. N.

Military Service: Rankin served as assistant surgeon assigned to the U.S.A. Army of the Potomac. He was later transferred to U.S.A. General Hospital Pittsburgh where he served as acting assistant surgeon from 25 June 1864 until 24 April 1865. At the end of the war, Surgeon General James King appointed him a member of the Emergency Corps of Surgeons to look after Pennsylvania soldiers. From 1864 until 1866, he served as Pension Examiner for the 23rd District.

General Background: Rankin was born in October 1836 in Shippensburg, Pennsylvania. He studied medicine under his father, Dr. William Rankin. He subsequently graduated from Jefferson Medical College in Philadelphia. He returned home to practice medicine with his father until the outbreak of the Civil War. During his career, he was a prolific author of medical texts and articles and a member and officer of numerous professional medical organizations, including the American Medical Association and the Pennsylvania and Allegheny County Medical Societies. In 1884, he was chosen a delegate to the Eight International Medical Congress in Copenhagen, Denmark. In the same year, he was selected by the American Medical Association to serve as a delegate to the British Medical Association.

REA, John

Military Service: Rea served as acting assistant surgeon at U.S.A. General Hospital Pittsburgh from 08 December 1862 until 10 December 1864.

General Background: Rae served in both civilian and military capacities during the war. He was also civilian caretaker and physician-in-charge of Western Pennsylvania Hospital before and immediately after the hospital's transition to the federal government.

REDLICK, Charles A. W.

Military Service: Redlick served as surgeon in the 136th Pennsylvania Infantry for nine months, and later as an assistant surgeon in the 84th Pennsylvania Infantry (consolidated with 57th Infantry on 13 January 1865). In September 1862, he transferred to the 136th Pennsylvania Infantry. He mustered out of service on 29 May 1863.

REITER, William C.

Military Service: Reiter participated in the "Expedition to the Tennessee River." He also served as acting assistant surgeon at U.S.A. General Hospital Pittsburgh from 19 September 1862 until 19 June 1863.

General Background: Reiter joined the Allegheny County Medical Society in 1867 and remained a member until his death in 1882.

REX, Thomas A.

Military Service: Rex was appointed to the U.S Army Engineer Corps by Captain Montgomery C. Meigs and worked on the construction of the Washington Aqueduct. He also served as acting assistant surgeon at Finley Hospital from the winter of 1864 until the hospital closed in September 1865.

General Background: Rex was born in Philadelphia, Pennsylvania, in February 1838. He graduated Philadelphia College of Pharmacy in 1862. During the Civil War, Rex attended and graduated from Georgetown Medical College. After the war, he attended lectures at the University of Pennsylvania and graduated in 1866. He later moved to Pittsburgh to establish his practice. He was a member of the Allegheny County Medical Society and an examiner for the New York Life Insurance Company.

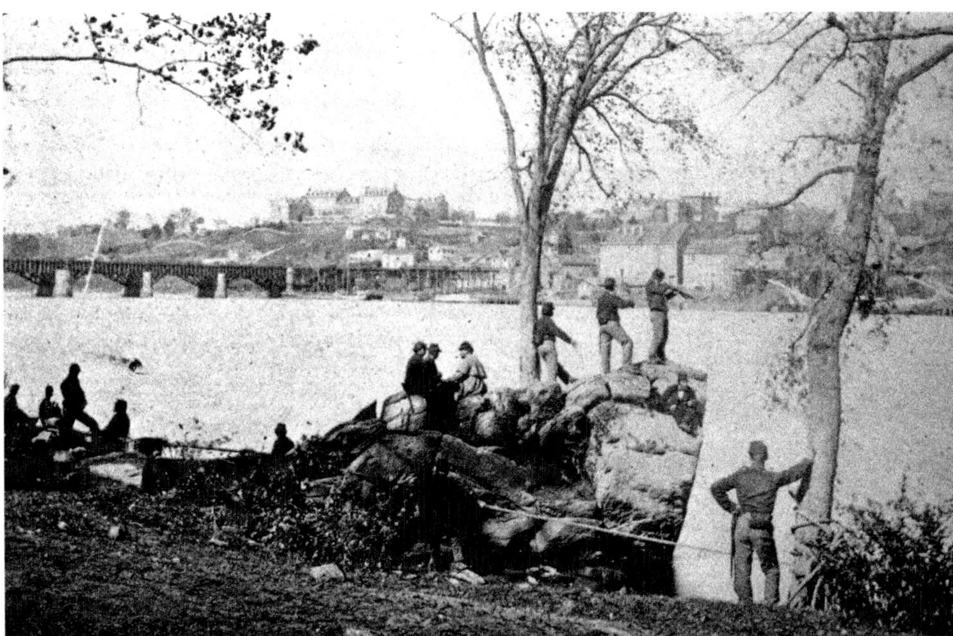

View of the Georgetown (Washington) Aqueduct connecting Georgetown, Washington, D.C., to Rosslyn, Virginia. (*National Library of Medicine*)

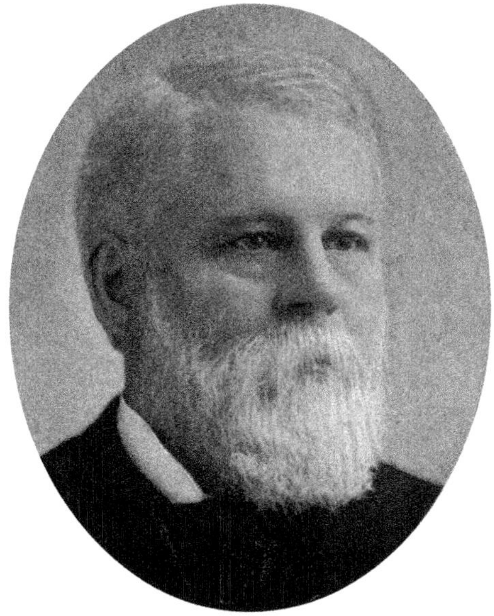

Thomas A. Rex, M.D. (*Carnegie Library of Pittsburgh. All rights reserved. Unauthorized reproduction or usage prohibited*)

RIGGS, David W.

Military Service: Riggs served as acting assistant surgeon at U.S.A. General Hospital Pittsburgh from 03 August 1864 until 14 January 1865.

ROBISON, George R. B.

Military Service: Robison served as assistant surgeon in the 71st Infantry (also known as Baker's 1st California Infantry) from May 1863 until he mustered out on 02 July 1864.

General Background: The youngest of twelve children, Robison, was born into a prominent farming family in Morgantown, West Virginia. In 1851, he enrolled in the College of Medicine and Surgery in Ohio. He graduated with his medical degree in 1853 and established a private practice in the Sharpsburg area.

SARGENT, Gorham P.

Military Service: Sargent served as acting assistant surgeon at U.S.A. General Hospital Pittsburgh from 26 April 1864 until 10 September 1864.

SARGENT, Rufus

Military Service: Sargent served as acting assistant surgeon at U.S.A. General Hospital Pittsburgh from 10 September 1864 until 09 March 1865.

SILLIMAN, Henry R.

Military Service: Silliman served as assistant surgeon at U.S.A. General Hospital Pittsburgh from 29 December 1864 until 08 December 1865.

SIMPSON, Robert B.

Military Service: Simpson was drafted and served as surgeon at U.S.A. General Hospital Pittsburgh from 18 April 1863 until 15 June 1865.

SMITH, Bascom B.

Military Service: Smith served as a private in Company "E" of the 123rd Pennsylvania Volunteer Infantry. He rose to the rank of sergeant major and participated in the Battles of Antietam, Fredericksburg, and Chancellorsville.

General Background: Smith was born in Allegheny City. Once he completed his early academic preparation, he enrolled at Allegheny College in Meadville, Pennsylvania. While at Allegheny College, he enlisted in the military and saw extensive action. After the war, he studied medicine with Dr. George N. McCook Sr. and later enrolled at the Bellevue Medical College in New York. He received his degree in 1869 and moved to Pittsburgh where he became associated with Allegheny General Hospital and the Allegheny Board of the Poor. Smith held membership in the Allegheny County Medical Society and served as visiting physician to the Allegheny City Home in Clermont for many years.

SMITH, Lee S.

Military Service: Smith first served as a private in the 1st Pennsylvania Artillery, and later as a sergeant in the 101st Pennsylvania Volunteer Infantry. After the war, he assisted in the reorganization of the Pennsylvania National Guard and served as assistant adjutant general of the Second Brigade. He was promoted to the rank of major in the 14th Pennsylvania Infantry.

General Background: After his service in the Civil War, Smith studied for the dental profession, but apparently, never obtained a degree. He opted instead to own and operate the Pittsburgh Dental Department located on Sixth Street for many years. His company provided dental supplies and appliances to dentists in the region.

SNIVELY, Whitmore

Military Service: Snively served as assistant surgeon with the 208th Pennsylvania Infantry Regiment from March 1865 until 01 June 1865, when he mustered out of service.

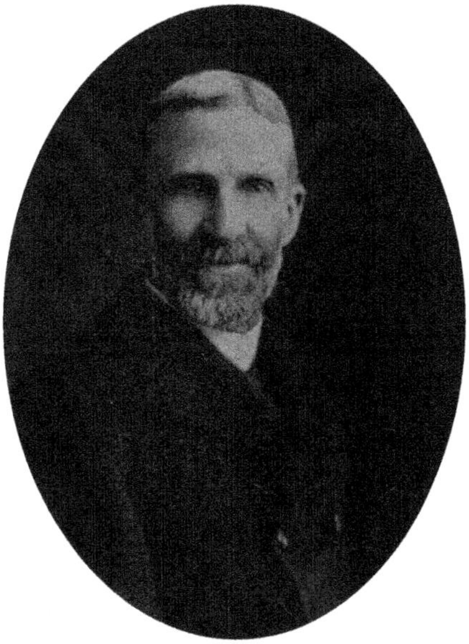

Whitmore Snively, M.D.

General Background: Snively was a member of the Medical Staff of Western Pennsylvania Hospital for many years, including the period when the Pittsburgh Subsistence Committee's Sanitary Soldiers' Home was officially transferred to West Penn in 1877. When Western Pennsylvania Medical College opened in 1886, he served as its first Professor of Practice of Medicine and Clinical Medicine.

SPEER, Alexander M.

Military Service: Speer served as surgeon and superintendent of U.S. Marine Hospital Pittsburgh from 1857 to the outbreak of the Civil War. He was appointed surgeon of the 12th Pennsylvania Volunteer Infantry from 25 April 1861 until 05 August 1861 and was then named surgeon of the 7th Pennsylvania Calvary (80th Volunteers), Army of the Cumberland. He later served as brigade surgeon and medical director of the Cavalry Corps of the Army of the Cumberland. In June 1863, he was assigned duty as surgeon in charge at U.S. Army Hospital at Covington, Kentucky, and later, took charge of the U.S. Army Eye and Ear Hospital at Cincinnati. He was brevetted lieutenant colonel for faithful and meritorious service before mustering out 14 October 1865.

General Background: Speer was the son of noted Pittsburgh physician, Dr. James R. Speer. He attended Pittsburgh's Western University and took up the study of medicine in 1849. He served as an apprentice under his father and house surgeon at Passavant and Mercy Hospitals. He was an 1853 graduate of Jefferson Medical College in Philadelphia. Shortly after graduation, he became a surgeon at Western Pennsylvania Hospital, a position he held until the outbreak of the Civil

War. Following his military service, he traveled to London and Paris to study ophthalmology. Upon his return, he made a specialty of treating diseases of the eyes and ears. He was a member of the Allegheny County Medical Society.

SPEER, J. S.

Military Service: Speer did not serve in the Civil War, but he was intimately involved in the Allegheny Arsenal incident in Pittsburgh three months before the firing on Fort Sumter. Speer was a cousin of President Buchanan and wrote to him regarding the planned transfer of weapons and munitions from the Arsenal to the South. His intervention helped in countermanding orders to ship the items. Boucher, in his book *A Century and a Half of Pittsburg and Her People*, recorded the matter as follows:

> Seeing the great danger approaching, realizing the baneful result of an open war between the national authorities and the citizens of Pittsburg, and perhaps deploring the bloodshed which might follow, he wrote to President Buchanan and laid the truth plainly before him. He told him of the feeling in Pittsburg and made him realize the needless danger the government was incurring. The very day that Dr. Speer's letter was due in Washington, Floyd was induced by some means, to countermand the order. The big guns were thereupon taken back to the arsenal amid shouts of joy and taunting epithets from the triumphant people of Pittsburg. Even if there is but little doubt that it was Dr. Speer's letter which directly brought about the countermand, it was the patriotic sentiment of Pittsburg as manifested by their threats of open resistance, that induced the thoughtful, unassuming physician, who was interested in the good name of the president, to lay the truth plainly before him.[10]

STILES, Richard C.

Military Service: Stiles served as acting assistant surgeon at U.S.A. General Hospital Pittsburgh from November 1862 until December 1862.

SUTTON, Rhodes S.

Military Service: Sutton was attached to the Medical Department of the U.S. Army from spring 1863 to the end of the Civil War. During his service, he was a surgeon in the Ninth Regiment of the 92nd Volunteers and Lochiel Cavalry. He mustered out of service on 18 July 1865.

General Background: Sutton was born in July 1841 to an affluent family in Indiana, Pennsylvania. His father was a successful businessman and banker. His mother was the daughter of a physician who served under General William Henry Harrison during the British Army's siege of Fort Meigs. Her grandfather was the State of Delaware's first surveyor-general and business partner of Revolutionary

War patriot, Robert Morris. Sutton's early academic education was above average. In 1856, he began to study at Elders Ridge Academy, where he spent one year. From there, he went to Tuscarora Academy in Juniata County for two and one-half years. He entered Jefferson College in Canonsburg in 1859 and graduated in June 1862. During his senior year, he began reading medicine with Dr. J. V. Herriott. The experience convinced him his future was in the medical profession. In 1862, he enrolled, as a private student of Professor D. Hayes Agnew, at Jefferson Medical College in Philadelphia. Under the tutelage of Dr. Agnew, who specialized in anatomy and physiology, he learned a great deal about the human body. He spent endless evenings in the dissection rooms. From early 1863 until spring of 1864, he served in the military. Upon discharge from the army, he returned to Philadelphia and his studies under Dr. Agnew, who by then had become affiliated with the University of Pennsylvania. In 1865, Sutton received his M.D. degree from that university. He then took a position as House Physician at Philadelphia's Blockley Hospital. Sutton moved to Pittsburgh in 1866 where he established a practice restricted to medical and surgical treatment of women. As his experience grew, so did his fame and recognition. He was a prolific writer of books on the diagnosis and treatment of diseases of women, and he regularly contributed to leading medical journals in America and Great Britain. Over the years, he was offered many prestigious positions at leading medical schools across the county, all of which he declined. In 1883, he opened a private hospital for the treatment of women. Sutton is credited with performing Pittsburgh's first laparotomy for removal of a cystic ovary.

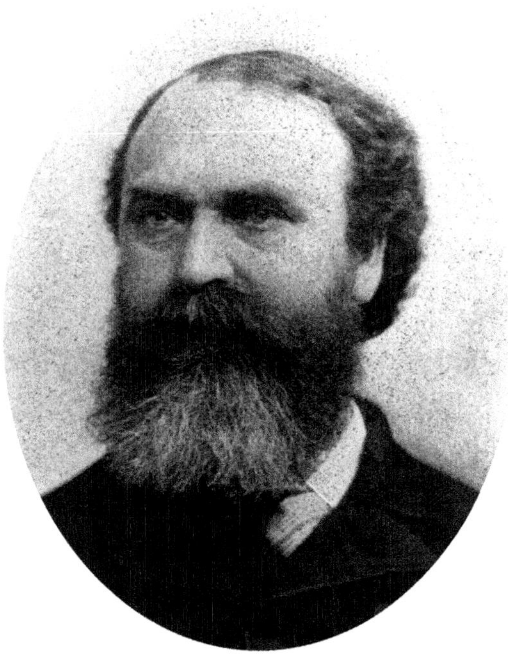

Rhodes S. Sutton, M.D. (Carnegie Library of Pittsburgh. All rights reserved. Unauthorized reproduction or usage prohibited)

THOMAS, Joseph Dio

Military Service: During the Civil War, Thomas served as a private in the Independent Battery "H" of the Pennsylvania Light Artillery.

General Background: Thomas served as apprenticeship under Dr. George McCook and graduated from Bellevue Medical College in New York City in 1869. After graduation, he established a private practice in Pittsburgh's South Side. He was a member of the Pennsylvania, Allegheny County, and South Side Medical Societies. He joined the Allegheny County Medical Society in 1871 and served one term as president. In 1886, upon the opening of the Western Pennsylvania Medical College, he served as a member of the board of trustees and as Professor of Genito-Urinary and Venereal Diseases. He was a proficient writer and contributed numerous articles to leading American medical journals. He also held a variety of public offices, including memberships on the city's 28th Ward council and the Board of Health, in which he served as an officer on several occasions.

TINDLE, R.M.

Military Service: Tindle served as surgeon in the Pennsylvania 61st Infantry. He mustered out of service on 28 June 1865.

TURDLE, Robert M.

Military Service: Turdle served as surgeon in the Pennsylvania Volunteers from April 1861 until August 1863.

UMBSTAETTER, Edwin S.

Military Service: Umbstaetter served as assistant surgeon in the 192nd Pennsylvania Infantry from May 1865 until being mustered out on 24 August 1865.

General Background: Umbstaetter joined the Allegheny County Medical Society in 1867 and resigned in 1871.

UPTON, George

Military Service: Upton was a member of the U.S. Veteran Volunteers and served as acting surgeon at U.S.A. General Hospital Pittsburgh from August 1865 until October 1865 when the hospital was returned to civilian control.

URE, Walter

Military Service: Ure served as private in the Pennsylvania Militia and fought at Antietam. After the Battle of Cold Harbor, he volunteered at White House Landing.

Later, at the request of Surgeon General Barnes, he passed the examining boards and was appointed assistant surgeon. In 1864, he served in the Ninth Army Field Hospital on the bank of the Appomattox. He later transferred to Shenandoah and served at the field hospital at Winchester, Virginia, until July 1865.

General Background: Along with his parents and seven siblings, Ure came to America from Scotland at the age of six. After initially settling in Springfield, Ohio, the family moved to Iowa. He received his basic academic education at schools in Cedar Rapids and Washington, Iowa. From 1855 to 1859, he attended Miami University Ohio, where he graduated with honors. Upon graduation, he moved to Allegheny City to study theology. He decided he preferred a career in medicine and entered an apprenticeship under Drs. Dickson and Hamilton. He subsequently entered medical school at the College of Physicians and Surgeons in New York City. In 1866, after his service in the Civil War, he returned to Pittsburgh to establish a general practice.

VAN DUYN, John

Military Service: Van Duyn served as acting surgeon at U.S.A. General Hospital Pittsburgh from 26 May 1865 until 01 July 1865.

WAGENSELLER, B.

Military Service: Wagenseller served as acting assistant surgeon at U.S.A. General Hospital Pittsburgh on 28 August 1861. He served until 28 October 1861.

WALKER, Mary E.

Military Service: Walker volunteered for medical service at the outbreak of the Civil War. Initially, her services as a doctor were disregarded. She was, however, permitted to work as a nurse at the temporary Patent Office Hospital in Washington, D.C. In 1862, Walker was appointed an assistant surgeon attached to an Ohio Regiment for a short period, and later in 1864, as acting assistant surgeon assigned to the 52nd Ohio Infantry Regiment. She provided medical services during or after many battles, including Chickamauga and the Battle of Atlanta. She was captured and was a prisoner of war from 10 April until 12 August 1864. In acknowledgment of her service as a surgeon, Dr. Walker was awarded a Congressional Medal of Honor in 1865. She is recognized as the very first woman to receive the award.

General Background: Mary Walker was born in Oswego, New York, in 1832. She graduated with a medical degree from Syracuse Medical College in 1855. She was among a handful of women who practiced medicine during the war. Her medical and surgical skills were soon recognized to be valuable early in the war as a Philadelphia newspaper commented: "She can amputate a limb with the skill of an old surgeon, and administer medicine equally well."[11]

Throughout her career, she championed women's rights and supported many causes seeking to increase opportunities for women to serve in professional roles. She was also recognized as somewhat of a maverick in dress, often wearing clothing associated with men. In 1863, she visited Pittsburgh, and her visit was recorded in a local newspaper:

> A Lady Creates an Excitement.—Dr. Mary E. Walker, a patriotic lady, who has conferred innumerable blessings upon sick and wounded soldiers in the Potomac army, arrived in this city on Sunday (25 October), in the noon train from the east, having in charge a sick soldier, who resides at Ravenna, Ohio. The soldier was given in charge of the Subsistence Committee, while the lady started out to obtain lodging at a hotel. Her dress being somewhat peculiar—in fact, unique—she attracted considerable curiosity, and soon found herself surrounded by a score of idle boys, while men and women stopped and stared at her as she passed. She had on a pair of pantaloons, and a military overcoat and cape, underneath which was a tunic reaching below the knees. Her headdress was a ladies hat, which had evidently been sometime in use, while her hair hung neatly behind in an ordinary net. She had on a white turn down collar, and a nock-tie neatly adjusted.
>
> In this eccentric garb, it is not strange that she became an object of much curiosity, in among the thousand and one surmises as to who and what she was, it was rumored that she was a rebel spy! It is said that she was positively refused admittance to two of our hotels, and not wishing to be subjected to the ill-mannered gaping of the populace, she asked to be conducted to the Mayor's office. She was escorted to that "excellent institution," where she made known her name and profession, and the object of her visit here. She is a regular graduate of a medical college at Cincinnati, and has been practicing medicine for eight years. She had her diploma with her. She adopted, her present style of

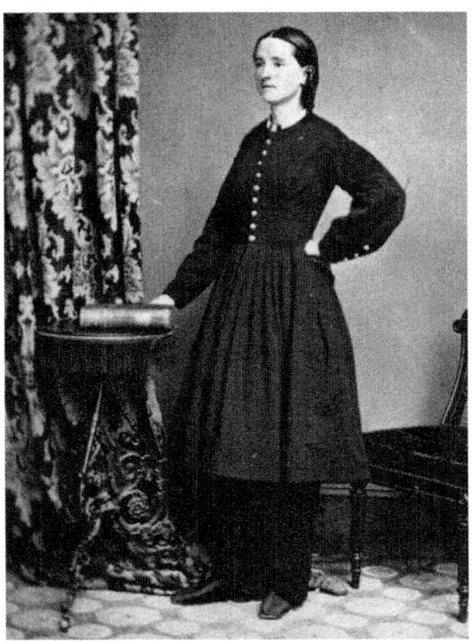

Mary E. Walker, M.D. (*Library of Congress*)

> dress, simply because it better suited the noble work in which she had been engaged—ministering to sick and wounded soldiers, in hospitals and on the field. She was introduced to one of our physicians, and became his guest during her stay in the city. She left in the midnight train for the West. She has promised to visit our city in two or three weeks, and deliver a lecture here for the benefit of sick and wounded soldiers.[12]

WALKER, Samuel

Military Service: Walker entered war service early as a "three-month" volunteer, serving as a private in the 13th Pennsylvania Infantry Regiment. He reportedly served as a hospital steward. Following this, he volunteered as a U.S. Sanitary Commission surgeon during the Union Army's Peninsula Campaign in 1862 and later reenlisted as assistant surgeon in Capt. Samuel C. Schoyer's 139th Pennsylvania Infantry Regiment. In the summer of 1863, he was ordered to Philadelphia to appear before the Army Medical Board.

General Background: Immediately following the Army Medical Board examination, Walker, for reasons unknown, returned to Pittsburgh to visit his wife and four-day-old infant. During his visit, military authorities arrested him for desertion. He reported he had lost the certificate he received from the Examining Board, which allowed him to return home on the condition he reports to local military officials each day. On the second day, Wednesday, 16 December 1863, he reported as required, but later visited a local drug store where he wrote the prescription: "Tincture of opium, two ounces; spirits of camphor, two drachms; simple syrup, one ounce. Directions—half a teaspoonful every two hours." The local newspaper reported that "The doctor took the drug home, and it is stated that he swallowed the contents of the phial in the presence of his mother, and in two or three hours afterward he was dead."[13]

WALTER, Albert G.

Military Service: Walter was a renowned orthopedic surgeon in Pittsburgh for many years. While he did not have traditional military service, he nevertheless volunteered his services treating wounded soldiers requiring orthopedic surgery, both in the field and at his clinic in Pittsburgh. He participated directly in the Pittsburgh "Tennessee River Expedition" and Gettysburg relief efforts.

General Background: Walter arrived in Pittsburgh from Germany in 1842. He established a surgical practice that grew in size and importance over the next decades. Born in 1811, he was orphaned early. He studied medicine, specializing in orthopedic surgery, at the University of Berlin. As his skill grew, he opened a clinic on Boyd's Hill above the Pittsburgh Courthouse. He frequently challenged the limits of surgery, often creating new techniques to repair deformed bodies. He became a prolific author of medical and surgical treatises, and he documented his surgical achievements in numerous books and journals. He is remembered for collecting specimens of his work and displaying them in a museum he created. The collection became part of the Western Pennsylvania Medical College. Walters married Frances Ann Butler, the daughter of Major John B. Butler, military storekeeper of the United States Arsenal in Lawrenceville in 1846.

WHITE, Charles B.

Military Service: White served as acting assistant surgeon at U.S.A. General Hospital Pittsburgh from 08 April 1863 until 18 July 1863. During this service period, he was in charge of the hospital.

WILLARD, Lewis H.

Military Service: Willard was appointed an army cadet and served at Satterlee Hospital in Philadelphia. In 1861, he transferred to Georgetown College Hospital, Washington, D.C., but later transferred to the U.S. Navy where he served as assistant surgeon. He remained in the Navy until November 1865.

General Background: Willard was born in Philadelphia in September 1838 and enjoyed a privileged childhood. He began his medical studies in 1860 at the Homeopathic Medical College. During his study, he worked in the office of Professor H. N. Guernsey and was placed in charge of the College Dispensary. He remained in that position until he received an appointment as an army cadet at Satterlee Hospital. While in the Navy, he returned for a short period to attend lectures at the University of Pennsylvania, after which he passed the military examination allowing him to serve as an assistant surgeon until the end of the war. After the war, he returned to Philadelphia and lectured at the Homeopathic College for one semester before leaving the city to accept a resident physician position at the Pittsburgh Homeopathic Medial and Surgical Hospital. In 1867, he established a private practice and joined the regular surgical staff of the hospital. Willard served as Dean of the faculty at the Pittsburgh Training School for Nurses. He was a member of the American Institute of Homeopathy, Pennsylvania Homeopathic Medical Society, and Allegheny County Homeopathic Medical Society.

WINNE, Charles K.

Military Service: Winne served as acting surgeon at U.S.A. General Hospital Pittsburgh from September 1863 until 06 October 1863.

WINSLOW, William Henry

Military Service: In 1858, Winslow was a Naval Academy midshipman. In 1862, he transitioned to active duty and became executive officer of the South Atlantic region. Dr. Winslow served on several U.S. Navy vessels, including the ironclads *Nahant* and *Monitor*, the sloop of war *Juniata*, and the gunboat *Ottawa*. He resigned his position and left the Navy with the rank of master in October 1865.

General Background: Winslow was born in August 1840 in Belfast, Maine. He could trace his ancestry back to Edward Winslow, Governor of Plymouth Colony in 1632. His naval military experiences were both distinguished and rewarding. After resigning from the Navy, he resumed his studies in academics and medicine. He went on to collect a number of degrees: a Ph.D. and M.D. from the University of Pennsylvania; an M.D. from the Long Island Hospital College in New York; an M.D. from Jefferson College in Philadelphia; and an M.D. degree from the Hahnemann Medical College in Philadelphia. After receiving his degrees, he traveled extensively to study with leading physicians in this country and Europe. For several years, he practiced in Philadelphia, but traveled to Pittsburgh in 1877 for unspecified "health reasons." In Pittsburgh, he specialized in diagnosing and treating diseases of the eye, ears, nose, and throat. For many years, he was the Pittsburgh Homeopathic Hospital's ophthalmic and aural surgeon. Winslow held memberships in many of the prominent national, state, and local homeopathic medical societies. He wrote extensively and contributed many works to leading medical publications. He also authored a naval history book and served as editor of several journals.

WISHART, *J. Wilson*

Military Service: Wishart served as surgeon in the 140th Pennsylvania Infantry from October 1862 until mustering out of the service on 31 May 1865.

General Background: Wishart joined the Allegheny County Medical Society in 1867. He died in 1902.

WOOD, *Charles*

Military Service: Wood served as acting assistant surgeon at U.S.A. General Hospital Pittsburgh from 28 August 1861 until 28 October 1861.

WOODS, *William S.*

Military Service: During the Civil War, Woods served as a surgeon. He was in charge of a hospital in Harrisburg, Pennsylvania, and of Benton Barracks in St. Louis. He died in military service while working among American Indians.

General Background: Woods practiced in the Birmingham section of Pittsburgh.

YOUNG, *Peter B.*

Military Service: Young served as acting assistant surgeon at U.S.A. General Hospital Pittsburgh from 14 January 1865 until 05 February 1865.

8

Early Hospitals and Medical Specialization

Considering the state of medicine up to the mid-nineteenth century, and the physician's inability to guarantee recovery from illness, it is not hard to imagine why permanent hospitals in Pittsburgh took so long to develop. The only recurring theme that supplied temporary hospitals was the frequent outbreaks of cholera, smallpox, and typhoid fever that periodically visited the city. Medicine had learned that quarantine at least offered some protection from contagious disease. The first temporary hospitals were by their nature established solely to protect the uninfected population from those afflicted with disease.

As noted earlier, the first temporary hospitals were those established by the military as shelters to quarantine smallpox victims. Capt. Simeon Ecuyer reported one such case at Fort Pitt during the summer of 1763. In his report, he stated he had prepared the fort for an anticipated Indian siege. He informed Colonel Bouquet:

> The fortifications having been badly damaged by floods, were with great labor repaired. The barracks were made shot-proof to protect the women and children, and as the buildings inside were all of wood, a rude fire-engine was constructed to extinguish any flames kindled by the fire-arrows of the Indians. All the houses and cabins outside the walls were leveled to the ground.[1]

The fort was so crowded by the families of the settlers that Ecuyer built a hospital under the nearby drawbridge.[2]

Fourteen years later in 1777–1778, Dr. (General) Edward Hand's hospital was established for similar reasons. In this case, however, it was constructed on a more permanent basis and became the first federally funded hospital and the only medical institution west of the Allegheny Mountains at the time. Since the hospital served soldiers, settlers, and American Indians, it can easily be argued it was the earliest structure that even remotely resembled Pittsburgh's first permanent public hospitals as they emerged in the late 1840s.

These temporary military hospitals survived only as long as did the epidemics. The first nuance of public hospitals also took the form of temporary shelters that served in a similar capacity of quarantining the afflicted after the settlement of Pittsburgh had been guaranteed by the military, and specifically only after most of the military had been removed from the confines of the Fort. As the civilian population became responsible for their healthcare during this transition, they relied heavily upon the military experience.

In general, the choices of structures used for these temporary hospitals were not good. A smallpox epidemic during the winter of 1845–1846 caused the city's old waterworks to be fitted out as a makeshift infirmary for the poor: "The building was originally used as a coal shed and was walled up into one room, in which were placed eight or nine beds, and in one corner stood a stove, table and utensils, etc."[3]

Between 1800 and 1860, countless news articles and public letters attest to the mounting frustration over the mentally ill wandering the streets, and the perceived growing criminal activities associated with these "lunatics." Public apprehension and increasingly vocal recriminations cajoled public officials into action.

Pittsburgh offered an amalgam of services through the provision of medical care for its poor and destitute in the city's almshouse and later its poor farm. The first almshouse was established in 1804. It was located in one of the city's oldest log houses at the foot of Coal Hill on the Monongahela River. The Allegheny City Almshouse replaced it in 1818. An 1844 newspaper article reports the annual salary for the period 01 April 1843–01 April 1844 for physician C. L. Armstrong was $100. During the same period, $38.04 was expended for medicines.[4] A year later, in April 1845, Drs. Fahnestock and George Watt were appointed "Physicians for the city and city Poor House."[5]

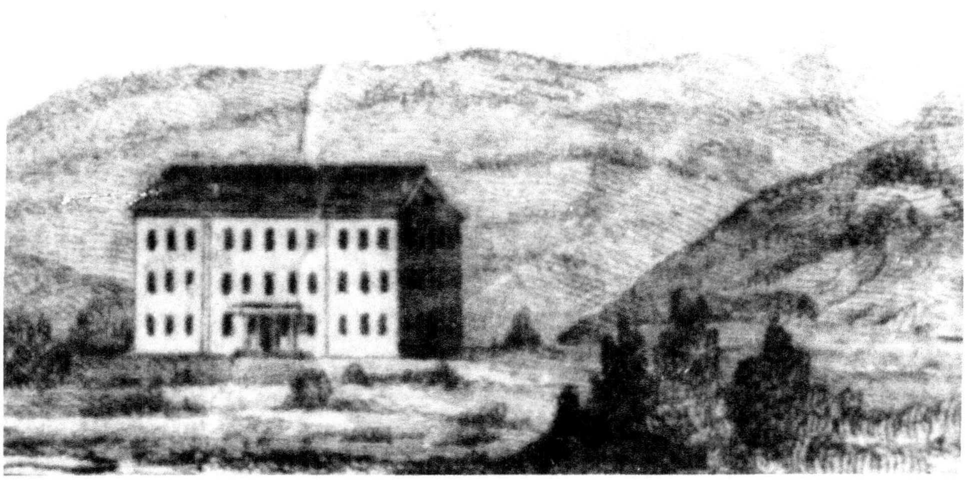

Allegheny City Poor House. (*Carnegie Library of Pittsburgh. All rights reserved. Unauthorized reproduction or usage prohibited*)

An editorial printed in the 23 July 1802 issue of the *Pittsburgh Gazette*, offers a graphic description of the health conditions in the city. It read:

> That the increase of diseases in this place has of late been greater in proportion than the increase of population, is a truth not to be disputed. From the opinion of a gentleman of the medical profession it is believed that many of the diseases which appear in this once healthy spot are produced from a vitiated state of the air, arising from causes obvious to the sense, narrow streets and alleys (to which too little attention has been paid by the officers of the police), filthy gutters, putrid vegetables and animal matter, the stench from foul slaughter-houses, and exhalations from ponds and stagnant water. Considering the activity, industry, sense of propriety and public spirit which the inhabitants of Pittsburgh generally possess, it is a matter of astonishment that nuisances so flagrant are suffered to exist.[6]

It was not that the citizens of Pittsburgh were opposed to the creation of a permanent public hospital. Many were, but just not enough to overcome the general skepticism about the benefits of institutional care. An editorial written on the 16 November 1842 offers this insight:

> Doctors
>
> Now that I am talking of doctors, what a strange set they are, and what a singular position they hold in society! Admitted to the fullest confidence of the world, yet by a strange perversion, they are the depositories of secrets that hold together the whole fabric of society, their influence is neither fully recognized, nor their power acknowledged. The doctor is now what a monk was once, with his additional advantage: that from the nature of his studies and the research of his art, he reads more deeply in the human heart. And penetrates into its inmost recesses. For him life has little romance. The grosser agency of the body, reacting ever on the operation of the mind, destroys many a poetic daydream, and many a high-wrought illusion. To him alone does a man speak "*son dernier mot*;" while to the lawyer the leanings of self-respect will make him always impart a favorable view of his case. To the physician he will be candid. Yet these are the men who, watching the secret workings of human passion, can trace progress of mankind in virtue and in vice. While ministering to the body, they are exploring the mind; and yet, scarcely is the hour of danger past, scarcely the shadow of fear dissipated, when they fall back on their humble position in life, bearing with them but little gratitude, and, strange to say, no fear![7]

The key issue preventing the establishment of a hospital in the 1830s and 1840s was the general ambivalence to medical practice. There were no sure cures. Government leaders were unwavering in their reluctance to expend public money for something viewed as only being needed intermittently during periods of an epidemic—or as a means to deal with insanity.

Even as the city's population, commerce, and influence grew, it took audacity and persistence for any of the city's leaders to counter negative public perception and will. A few did have the courage; with some using newspaper editorials and others direct action. The earliest recorded attempts to establish a permanent hospital began in the early 1830s, but the effort failed quickly. It took several more years, until 1837, for another attempt, which also failed.

Many things happened in Pittsburgh during the 1830s that seemed more worthy of the public's attention than the merits of a hospital. The city's population doubled between 1830 and 1835, business was booming, work was readily available, and progress was apparent everywhere. Most importantly, perhaps, was there was money to be made. With the exceptions of occasional epidemic diseases that visited the city, and a growing concern about insanity and mental illness, the state of any one person's health was not of immediate concern. Characterized as being written by "A historian whose life was spent in the atmosphere and in the influence of the nineteenth century" summarizes the accomplishments of the period:

> The decade of the thirties ended with the greatest advancement in all particulars Pittsburgh had ever witnessed. Among the many improvements, changes and advancements were the canal, the numerous turnpikes, the public school system, the orphan asylum, the first hospital, the increase in banking strength, the Board of Trade, the new bridges, increases in the number of newspapers, wonderful increase in population, great multiplication of schools, churches, the commencement of slackwater navigation, organization of insurance companies, promise of early completion of several railroads headed this way, organization of interests opposed to slavery, intemperance, the decadence of Jacksonism, the partisan warfare, the formation of the Whig party, the great industrial growth, city and suburban growth, and many other things inevitably tending towards local and neighborhood development.[8]

The "first hospital" referred to a temporary structure outfitted for use through conversion of an existing building. It was developed in response to the cholera epidemic that began in October 1832. Over a period of two months, thirty people died. A few months later, in May 1833, cholera returned to infect another 100 people and caused another seventy-five deaths. While the epidemics raged, city leaders, sanitary authority members, and city physicians quarreled among themselves and in public through letters to the local newspapers, with each camp claiming authority and ownership of the "facts" surrounding the cause, diagnoses, and remedy of the disease. Despite the deaths and unproductive dialog, construction of a permanent "public" hospital was defined by talk rather than productive action. The situation continued for years until March 1848 when Western Pennsylvania Hospital was chartered. The editor of the local newspaper called attention to the previous lack of resolve in the creation of the long-debated permanent public hospital when he noted through an editorial comment: "We observe that the contributors to the Western Pennsylvania Hospital are again at work. Will they do something this time?"[9]

While the debate over the benefit of establishing a permanent public hospital raged, a small congregation of Catholic nuns from Ireland took matters into their own hands. The Sisters of Mercy reached the city in December 1843. Six nuns and their leader, Mother Frances Warde, immediately began their work of teaching the ignorant, offering protection to young women of "good character," and ministering to the sick. Their convent and academy were located in an old building on Penn Avenue that had once been a hotel and concert hall.

They performed their benevolent work for several years before Roman Catholic Bishop Michael O'Connor challenged the group to accept more responsibility for ministering to those afflicted by epidemic diseases that recurrently visited the city. The Sisters accepted the Bishop's challenge, and in the latter part of 1846, they set about converting the concert hall into a small hospital. In December 1846, the *Daily Post* newspaper reported the proposed hospital development and noted the ongoing debate about the need for a "public" hospital:

> CITY HOSPITAL
> Yesterday we published a communication on the subject of a hospital proposed to be erected under the supervision of the "Brotherhood of St. Joseph," a Catholic Society of this city. So, then, Pittsburgh is to have a hospital at last, and one too, on the correct plan—free from sectarianism, and economical in its arrangements. The Protestants of this city, with their great wealth and numerical strength, should blush that the sick poor of their own people are to be protected and nursed by the Sisters of Mercy. The coal shed will soon be deserted in our city relieved from the expense of paying for keeping up that establishment.[10]

Their small "sectarian" hospital became known as Mercy Hospital, the city's first soon-to-be permanent hospital when it opened its doors on 01 January 1847. A newspaper announcement described the opening:

> PITTSBURGH HOSPITAL
> UNDER THE CHARGE OF THE SISTERS OF MERCY—Drs. Addison, Gazzam, Bruce and McMeal, General Attending Physicians; Dr. Werneburg, Physician for the Germans—The Institution is now open for the reception of patients.
> RECEIVING DAYS—Tuesdays and Fridays, from 8 to 10 o'clock, A.M. Cases of accidents can be received at any time.
> CHARGES—Three dollars a week in the general ward; five dollars with a private room. Medical attendance is included in these charges; payments to be made two weeks in advance.
>
> Any physician can send patients to the Hospital, and continue to attend them there, and any patient can engage any physician he chooses. In these cases the Institution will not be responsible for the physician's fees; each person will settle with such physicians. Leeching is an extra charge.

> As many free patients will be received as the means of the Institution will permit. Persons with contagious disease will not be received until accommodations can be prepared sufficiently ample to prevent any danger that the other inmates would incur.
>
> All the physicians will attend twice a week to visit the Hospital and will depute one of their number to attend the sick in the meantime. Advice will be given gratuitously to out-door patients on Thursdays and Fridays at 10:00, A.M.
>
> Pecuniary arrangements will be attended to by a committee of the Brotherhood of St. Josephs, which for the present consists of James Blakely, Esq., James May, John S. Cosgrove, John Coyle and Arthur Tiernan.[11]

The "concert hall" hospital, located at 638–640 Penn Avenue, operated for several months before it was determined a larger and more enduring structure would be needed for the growing numbers of patients seeking admission. Bishop O'Connor took the lead in gathering a charitably minded group of citizens to raise funds for a new structure. On 09 June 1847, the local newspaper reported:

> The present temporary Hospital affords ample evidence to the public of the necessity of such an institution, and we are much gratified to learn that the friends of the Mercy Hospital are fully organized and acting together in this charitable undertaking, in the most perfect union and harmony. We perceive by a notice from the Building Committee, that our citizens will be called upon for the purpose of aiding them in the erection of such suitable buildings as will be adequate to accommodate the increasing wants of suffering humanity; and we trust, indeed we have not the slightest doubt, that the liberality of the community will fully sustain the expectations of the very liberal and enterprising managers. The Mercy Hospital has been in operation four months. The number of patients so far amount to fifty-three, of which number four died, and there are at present sixteen in the institution.[12]

Amid concern patients with a contagious disease were a threat to the city, sufficient financial support was received to construct a new four-story hospital on Stevenson Street (on the Bluff in uptown Pittsburgh). It was noted in response to the fears of contagion, "This locality was then thinly inhabited, and was considered 'in the country.'"[13] At the cost of $15,000, a new facility was constructed. The new Mercy Hospital began operating in May 1848 with sixty beds and a small staff of physicians. Pittsburgh's first enduring hospital had finally arrived. The medical staff included Drs. Joseph Gazzam, George D. Bruce, William Addison, and Daniel McMeal. Dr. Thomas Shaw served as the hospital's first intern.

Despite the progress made in opening a larger and sufficiently remote sectarian hospital, the public continued to express concern about the need for a "public" hospital. Their sentiments expressed continued frustration over the lack of progress being made, and in particular, the lack of a facility to provide care for the insane. An opinion written in the newspaper stated:

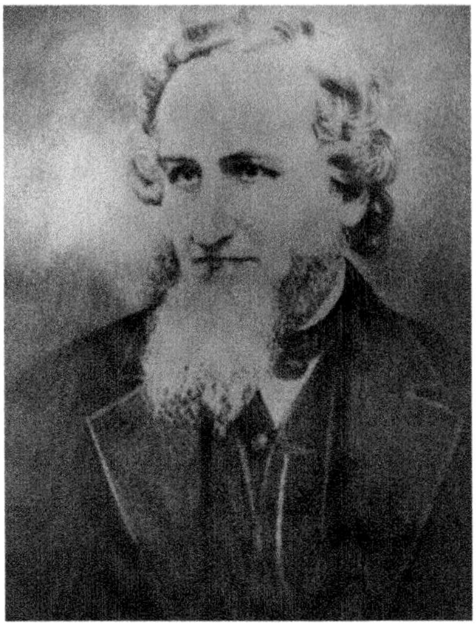

G. D. Bruce, M.D. (*Allegheny County Medical Society*)

> ... the hospital already instituted will be ample for those of our people who may be afflicted with disease. We ask, where is the use of another for the same purpose? Money has been subscribed, and a site donated, for the purpose of erecting a Hospital. Would it not be the part of wisdom to devote these means to providing a hospital for the insane? We have urged this matter heretofore, with what effect we cannot judge; but time only goes to convince us of the necessity of adopting our plan. Will those directly interested think of this?[14]

The "other hospital" was the proposed Western Pennsylvania Hospital. The author, whether aware of discussions taking place elsewhere in the city or not, would soon learn his pleas for an institution for the insane would take a positive turn with the opening of a new hospital in the early months of 1853. Before that, however, necessity again brought attention to the Sisters of Mercy and their hospital.

Mercy Hospital cared for "boatman" who became ill while working on the rivers for several years before the United States Marine Hospital was established in 1851. Upon opening of the Marine Hospital, those patients were no longer treated at Mercy. Besides losing patients, Mercy also lost the government income that paid well for their care. The remaining patients left were predominantly the poor who were unable to pay, which left the hospital with a challenging financial situation.

Over the last few years of the 1840s and the first few years of the 1850s, smallpox, typhoid, and cholera epidemics hit the city. Mercy Hospital provided the needed care since there was no municipal hospital. During the epidemics, it was noted:

> This hospital was filled to overflowing. The self-sacrificing Sisters even gave up their own beds and rooms that a few more might be cared for. They nursed the sick by day and night, seldom resting themselves during that awful period of distress. Only one

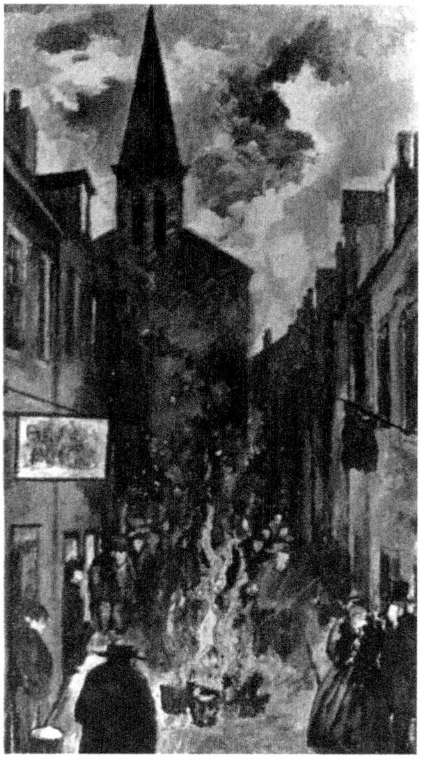

Coal fires and pitch pots burning on Pittsburgh streets to ward off cholera. (*Carnegie Library of Pittsburgh. All rights reserved. Unauthorized reproduction or usage prohibited*)

> man was left in the institution aside from the patients and he was there for the purpose of making rude coffins for those who died of the cholera.[15]

The hospital operated with cramped quarters and limited resources for several decades until a new 150-bed building was constructed in 1882. Upon opening the new building, the old hospital was converted into a "female ward" and dormitory for the sisters. In order to relieve continuing financial difficulties, it was determined the hospital would officially incorporate as a public institution, becoming eligible to receive State funding.

During the Civil War, the Sisters of Mercy Hospital took on added military-related responsibilities. In September 1862, in response to a request from the federal government, four nuns left Pittsburgh to serve as nurses at Stanton Military Hospital in Washington, D.C. On December 8, four others joined the group. In early 1863, the Sisters also began providing nursing assistance at Pittsburgh's Western Pennsylvania Hospital, which had recently been turned over to the army and converted into U.S. General Hospital Pittsburgh. A history of their service at the hospital was published in memoirs in 1918:

> In Pittsburgh the West Penn Hospital was used by the government for a Military Hospital, principally for Pennsylvania soldiers, and here such sick and disabled

> were sent as were sufficiently recovered to bear the fatigue of transportation from Washington or other places, to make room for cases direct from the field of battle. Our Sisters were invited to give their services here, which they cheerfully did early in 1863. In the Hospital the Sisters experienced the same courtesy from the officers as was extended to them elsewhere, every arrangement compatible with existing circumstances being made to lighten their duties. In both the hospitals a chapel was fitted up and Mass was celebrated daily when such convalescent patients as desired were at liberty to attend.[16]

The Sisters provided nursing services at the hospital until March 1865, just a short time before General Robert E. Lee's official surrender at Appomattox Court House on 09 April 1865. It was reported: "The Sisters remained at the West Penn Hospital until peace was restored, and all the patients discharged or cared for in other institutions."[17]

The Western Pennsylvania Hospital

Within ten weeks after Mercy Hospital's opening, a group of community leaders gathered to resurrect plans for the western "Pennsylvania Hospital." This hospital had been debated, planned, and partially funded in fits and starts since the early 1830s. On 09 March 1847, supporters of a new public hospital "for the reception and cure of the insane and afflicted, as well as the sick, helpless and infirm," met at the city's Odeon Building to form an association, under the corporate name of "Western Pennsylvania Hospital."[18] Dr. H. D. Sellers presided over the meeting with John Harper and Thomas M. Howe serving as secretaries.[19] Five days before the meeting, on March 4, a local newspaper offered notice of the planned meeting:

> The Pennsylvania Hospital
>
> We have one Hospital in successful operation under the superintendence of the Sisters of Mercy, who deserve all the credit of being the first to establish so excellent an institution in our city. It should be kept forever in remembrance that the ladies belonging to this benevolent Order were the pioneers in this good work, and crowned their efforts with success. But we shall soon have another Hospital. When those who always do the talking had exhausted to found "the Pennsylvania Hospital," George Breed, Esq., one of our most publically spirited and philanthropic citizens undertook the work, and we are credibly informed has succeeded beyond his most sanguine expectations. Mr. Breed is still receiving subscriptions and those citizens who intend to contribute, and have not been called on, had better now come forward. We understand that a gentleman residing in Manchester, has offered Mr. B. a lot of ground in the city of Allegheny, on condition that the hospital be erected thereon, which is said to be worth $4,500. This is a noble offer.[20]

Upon creation of the Association, a group of Pittsburgh's leading citizens were elected officers of the fledgling organization. They were Thomas Bakewell, president; George Breed and John Graham, vice-presidents; and M. Allen, John Harper, John Bissell, J. Carothers, William Ebbs, George Hogg, William Holmes, John Irwin, George W. Jackson, F. Lorenz, S. Lothrop, O. Metcalf, J. K. Moorhead, Jacob Painter, J. N. Shoenberger, Charles F. Spang, William J. Totten, William Wilkins, and W. W. Wallace as managers. Harmar Denny and David Shields became life managers.[21]

The meeting was successful in renewing enthusiasm for the project and garnering the donations and support that had previously been insufficient to launch a new hospital. With renewed vigor, the group prepared a charter for the hospital, which was approved nine days later on 18 March. A compelling reason for such quick action was the offer of numerous properties that might serve as the perfect site for the hospital. Of those offered, two pieces of property were considered: one parcel offered by James Anderson, Esq. was located in Manchester; the other was offered by J. S. Craft, Esq., and was located in Oakland. Since both sites were offered for sale at a discount, but neither was located in a manner thought conducive to easy access from the city in general, or to Allegheny City specifically. Under the circumstances, both offers were gratefully declined. Other subsequent offers, however, were thought

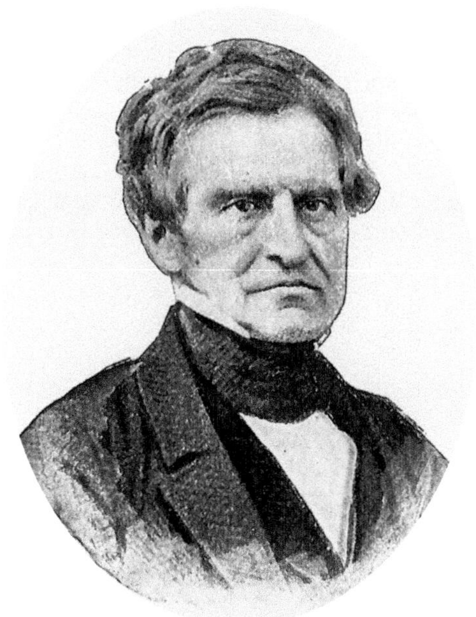

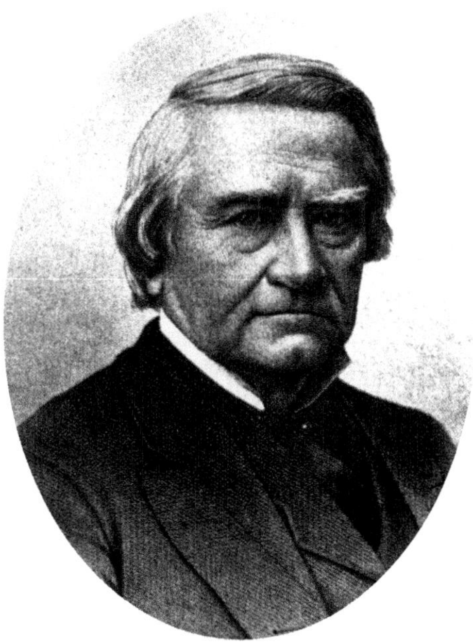

Above left: Thomas Bakewell, President of the Western Pennsylvania Hospital. (*Grand Army of the Republic 28th National Encampment program, Pittsburgh, 1894*)

Above right: John A. Harper, Manager of the Western Pennsylvania Hospital. (*Carnegie Library of Pittsburgh. All rights reserved. Unauthorized reproduction or usage prohibited*)

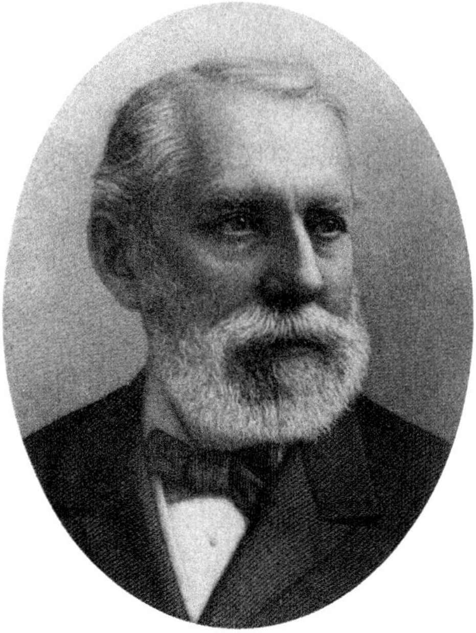

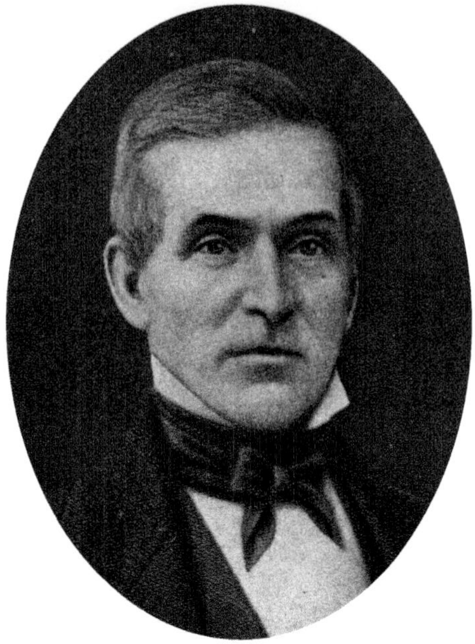

Above left: Charles F. Spang, Manager of the Western Pennsylvania Hospital Association. (*Carnegie Library of Pittsburgh. All rights reserved. Unauthorized reproduction or usage prohibited*)

Above right: Orlando Metcalf, Pittsburgh lawyer and Manager of the Western Pennsylvania Hospital. (*Carnegie Library of Pittsburgh. All rights reserved. Unauthorized reproduction or usage prohibited*)

Below left: James Kennedy Moorhead, Congressman and Manager of the Western Pennsylvania Hospital. (*Carnegie Library of Pittsburgh. All rights reserved. Unauthorized reproduction or usage prohibited*)

Below right: George Whitten Jackson, Pittsburgh banker, railroad builder, and Manager of the Western Pennsylvania Hospital. (*Carnegie Library of Pittsburgh. All rights reserved. Unauthorized reproduction or usage prohibited*)

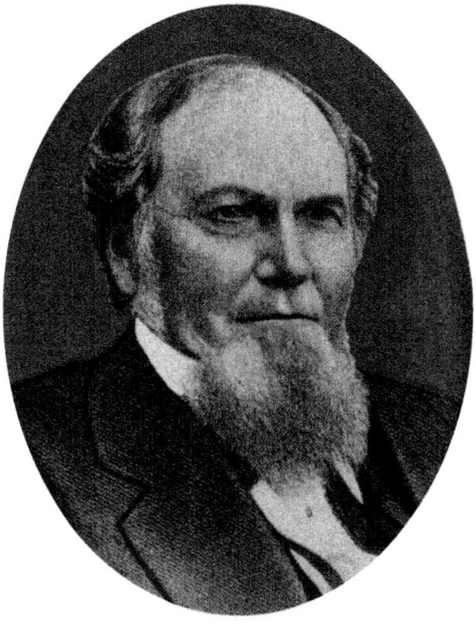

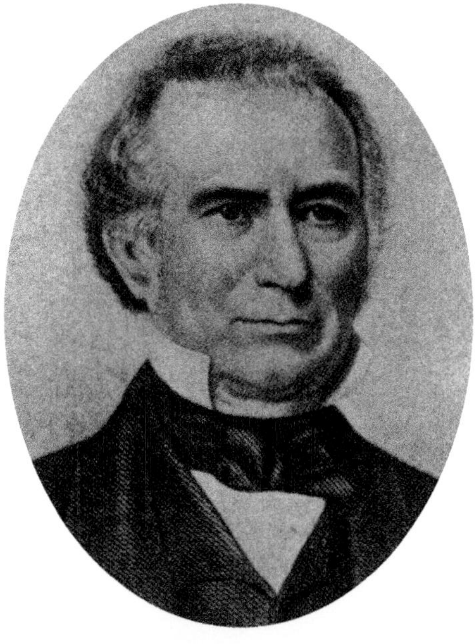

to be more strategically located, with two spectacularly well-suited parcels offered as outright donations. These two gifts included 24 acres located in the city's Ninth Ward owned by Mr. and Mrs. Harmar Denny and Mr. and Mrs. E. W. H. Schenley.[22] The board of managers considered the property's location and size advantageous, and they wanted to act quickly. Once again, the impact of the military on the development of medicine in Pittsburgh was exhibited through the philanthropic actions of the contributors.

Harmar Denny was born in Pittsburgh on 13 May 1794. He was the oldest son of Major Ebenezer Denny and Nancy (Wilkins) Denny. Major Denny was a celebrated Indian fighter and Revolutionary War officer who became Pittsburgh's first Mayor; Nancy Denny was the daughter of Captain John Wilkins, also of Revolutionary War fame, and the sister of William Wilkins who served in both the United States Senate and House of Representatives. Wilkins also served as the Secretary of War under President John Tyler from February 1844 until March 1845. Harmar Denny's wife, Elizabeth Febiger O'Hara, was the daughter of General James and Mary (Carson) O'Hara.

Captain Edward W. H. Schenley was born into a military family of the British Army. At a young age, he eloped from school to join the Army and served under the Duke of Wellington during the Peninsular War. In 1815, at the age of twenty, he saw service under General Edward Pakenham during the Battle of New Orleans. He was later awarded the rank of captain and served at the Battle of Waterloo where he was wounded. Ill health brought him to the United States for recovery where he met his future wife, Mary Elizabeth Croghan, a sixteen-year-old heiress from Pittsburgh.

Her mother, Mary Elizabeth (O'Hara) Croghan, and her father, William Croghan, Jr., both had military roots. Her mother's paternal grandfather was Major William Croghan who served under George Washington at Trenton, Princeton, Monmouth, Brandywine, Germantown, and Valley Forge. Her maternal grandfather, General James O'Hara, served at Fort Pitt and was extensively engaged in the Indian trade. At the outbreak of the Revolutionary War, he entered the service as a private and later became a captain in the 9th Virginia Regiment. He served under General George Rogers Clark at Vincennes and with General Greene at Guilford Court House. In 1792, he was appointed first Quartermaster General of the United States, an appointment that brought him the title of general. General O'Hara served in that capacity through the Whiskey Insurrection and Northwest Territory Indian campaigns.

Due to the generosity of the Denny and Schenley families, doubts that a new hospital could be built were effectively removed. The board of managers and the general public were excited about the prospects and thrilled that years of talk were now turning to action. On 25 June 1847, the editor of the *Pittsburgh Daily Post* went so far as to recommend the name of the hospital be changed from the Western Pennsylvania Hospital to "The Denny Hospital," the "O'Hara Hospital," or another such name as might better recognize the generosity of the property donors.[23]

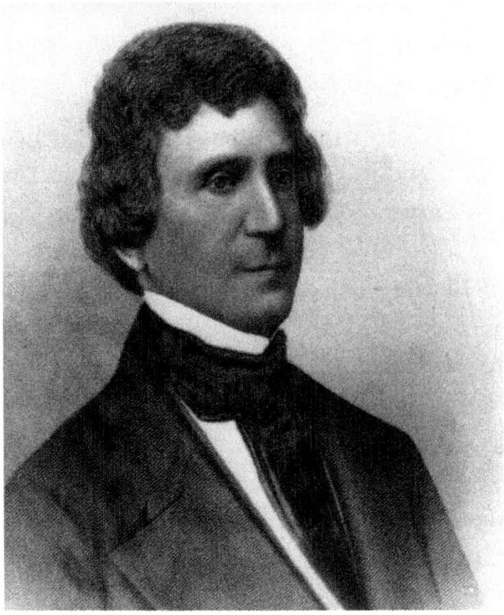
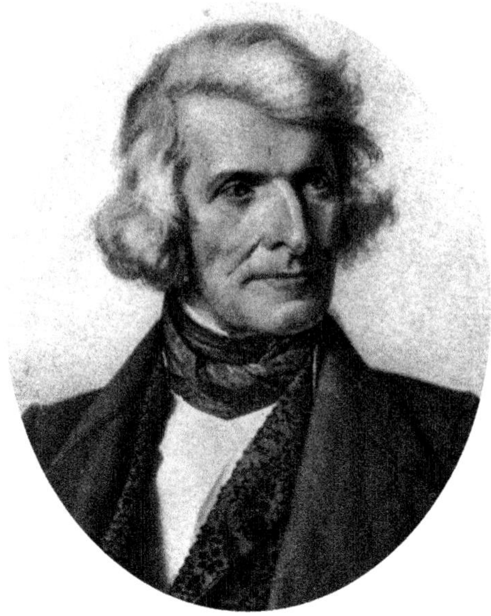

Above left: Harmar Denny. (*Heinz History Center*)

Above right: William Wilkins: Pittsburgh banker who served as a U.S. Senator and Representative, Secretary of War, and Minister to Russia. (*Carnegie Library of Pittsburgh. All rights reserved. Unauthorized reproduction or usage prohibited*)

Below left: Captain E. W. H. Schenley in his younger years. (*Carnegie Library of Pittsburgh. All rights reserved. Unauthorized reproduction or usage prohibited*)

Below right: Colonel William Croghan. (*Carnegie Library of Pittsburgh. All rights reserved. Unauthorized reproduction or usage prohibited*)

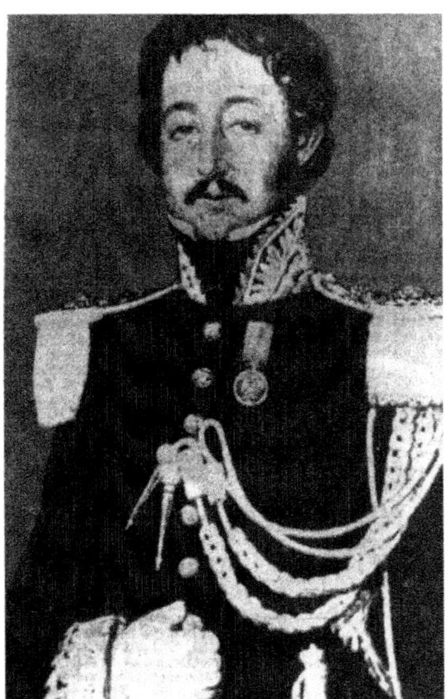
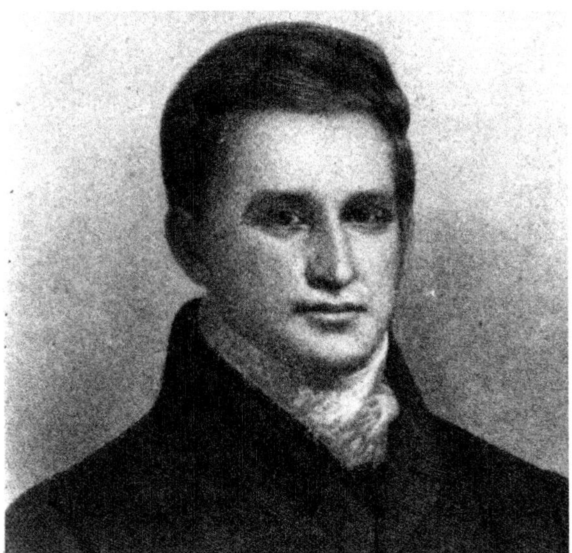

Before the land donation was settled, hospital managers faced two challenges. First, they needed to deal with how the original property donations adjoined each other. Initially, the properties were not sufficiently contiguous to promote efficient design. In their first annual report, the hospital's board of managers recounted the challenges and resolution to the final selection of a site for the hospital. They wrote:

> Among the other lots presented to the consideration of the Board, several portions of the well-known Springfield farm were offered upon liberal terms by H. Denny, Esq., and after learning the favorable opinion entertained by the Board of that location, Mr. and Mrs. Denny generously presented to the Institution a lot containing about eleven acres, adjoining the ninth ward of the city, and extending from Ferguson street along Smith, about 1100 feet to Fisk street. Shortly after the execution of the deed for this property, the Board were apprised by W. Croghan, Esq., of the benevolent intention of Captain and Mrs. Schenley to make a similar contribution, and of his determination to relinquish his individual interest therein to the Hospital.
>
> In consequence of this proposition, Mr. and Mrs. Denny proposed to exchange the lot which they had transferred, for an adjacent lot of somewhat larger extent and nearer to the city, which immediately adjoins the lot offered by Captain and Mrs. Schenley, from which it is separated by the old manor line. The Board gladly availed themselves of this proposal, under the conviction that it would prove highly beneficial, and now beg leave to congratulate the contributors on the possession of these munificent donations, which, together, contain more than twenty-four acres of ground, and present many advantages of position, admitting an extensive range of garden and pleasure grounds, and securing an ample supply of water from some of the most permanent springs in the vicinity, of sufficient elevation to be furnished on all the floors of the proposed building.[24]

Once the site decision was rendered, planning for the design and construction of the hospital began. However, another challenge presented itself. The issue was that after the donation was offered, Captain Schenley took exception to the possible use of his donated property for treatment of the insane. He was not thrilled by the prospect and threatened to withdraw his offer. In a letter dated 05 July 1848, Colonel Croghan wrote on behalf of Captain and Mrs. Schenley:

> No doubt you may have confidently believed the ground should be used at your discretion for an asylum for the insane as well as a hospital for the sick, indigent, the wounded, and otherwise afflicted. But you must believe me when I give you the assurance that the property should be used only for the latter purpose. It was my instruction it should be used as a "hospital" covering and embracing as many objects of charity as you might please, but in exclusion of the mad and insane.[25]

Upon receipt of the correspondence, the board was concerned that their plans for building a hospital would once again be thwarted. However, the public outcry was fierce and immediate. A notice in the newspaper of 06 July 1848 headlined "Backed Out," reported on the situation:

> We regret to learn that the gift of land to the Western Pennsylvania Hospital made by Colonel Croghan, on behalf of his daughter, and which he heralded some months since, is not likely to be realized. Captain Schenley has backed out, by coupling to the donation such a restriction as he knew the Board of managers would decline, or stultify themselves in accepting; which was, to exclude unfortunate lunatics from the benefits of the institution. Thank God! There is charity and philanthropy enough in this community to found and support the Hospital, without the aid of this English fortune-hunter or any of his daughters. We are unapprised of the course of the Managers in the matter.[26]

In essence, the question was whether or not the board of managers would comply with the donor's newly expressed wishes, or remain true to the organization's Act of Incorporation, which expressly stated the organization would "establish, maintain, and manage a hospital for the care of the insane and afflicted, as well as the sick, infirm and helpless."

A flurry of written communications flowed back and forth between Colonel Croghan (who initiated the donation in the name of Captain and Mrs. Schenley and was acting on their behalf) and Thomas Bakewell, president of the Western Pennsylvania Hospital board of managers. The issue was eventually favorably resolved and on 21 December 1848, the Pittsburgh Daily Post published a notice of an emergency meeting to be held that day in which the board of managers would consider a more favorable response they had received from the Schenley family. The newspaper reported:

> We are requested to call attention to the meeting to be held at Apollo Hall, this afternoon, at 2 o'clock, to consider important business connected with the Western Pennsylvania Hospital. We suppose this business will be the acception or rejection of the ground given by Capt. Schenley as a site for the institution. We do not know the terms of the donation; but if they are not of a character that will forever be favorable to the Hospital, they should be rejected. Unless the Deed is untrammeled, so that the Insane Asylum, a Hospital, or any other charitable Institution could be erected on the ground, what use is in it? For a sick Hospital only, so much ground is not wanted, particularly when the improvement will be enormously expensive. We do not understand the question at issue, but will endeavor to be present and apprise our readers of what will take place.[27]

At the meeting, the board was able to report the donor objection on including the insane had been removed, and all parties were now in agreement that construction of the new hospital could begin as quickly as possible. The hospital's next annual report in 1851 stated:

> In pursuance of the intimation given in the last annual report, all requisite legal documents have been executed by Mr. and Mrs. Harmar Denny, and by Mr. and Mrs. Schenley, conveying the munificent donation to the Hospital of more than 24 acres of ground, situated within and adjoining to the city, and forming the square bounded by Ferguson, Smith, Fisk, and Morton Sts.[28]

Once the matter was resolved, Harmar Denny and E. W. H. Schenley were duly named "life managers" as dictated by the hospital's by-laws and in recognition of their substantial donations of property. The hospital's charter provided:

> Any contributor who has already or shall hereafter subscribe the sum of $1000 as a single benefaction or who has already subscribed a less sum and shall increase the same to $1000, on payment of the same into the Treasury, shall be entitled to become a manager for life, and shall have the right to nominate and send in one patient to the hospital.

Denny and Schenley, by virtue of their property donations, were among the earliest major donors to join an illustrious list of Pittsburgh philanthropists supporting the new hospital.

The board of managers now took swift action. Over the following months additional financial donations were solicited and received, and the Building Committee studied and recommended architectural designs. Manager, and building committee member, Sylvanus Lothrop visited Philadelphia to consider how the design of the Pennsylvania Hospital and Pennsylvania Hospital for the Insane might serve the board's needs. Lothrop was particularly well suited for the job since he

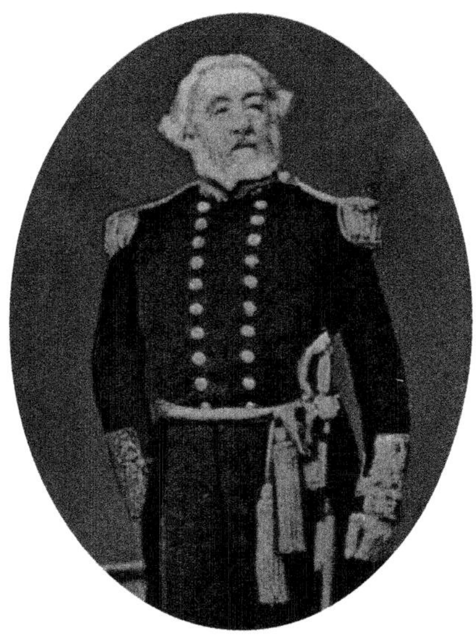

Captain Edward W. H. Schenley in his later years. (*Carnegie Library of Pittsburgh. All rights reserved. Unauthorized reproduction or usage prohibited*)

was one of Pittsburgh's most prominent businessmen and an engineer who helped design several of the city's bridges and the Allegheny Aqueduct. Lothrop was also chief engineer of the Monongahela Navigation Company, and he assisted in the development of the city's lock and dam system.

In Philadelphia, Lothrop met extensively with Dr. Thomas S. Kirkbride, superintendent of the Hospital for the Insane, and he became convinced a modified design of Kirkbride's hospital would best serve the needs of Western Pennsylvania. In the Board of Manager's annual report for 1848, Lothrop's recommendations were noted:

> This Institution is of greater extent than is at present required here, and it is applied exclusively to the relief of one class of patients, but as its general plan appears to embrace greater convenience than any other that has been met with, it has been adopted by the board as a basis for the Hospital, with such modifications in extent and detail as will render it more conformable to the particular objects of this Institution, and so arranged as to admit of a total separation of the various classes of patients, and of a gradual extension at a future time without impairing the general proportions of the building.[29]

Upon approval of the design concept, matters were turned over to the hospital's architect, Joseph W. Kerr. Soon, working plans were rendered, construction specifications developed, contractors engaged, and construction begun. The building was completed in November 1850 but remained empty due to the lack of funds to complete a water system, heating, bathing, and kitchen facilities. Upon receipt of a $10,000 grant from the State of Pennsylvania, and the generosity of the ladies of the "Helping Hand Society" and others in furnishing rooms and parlors, the facilities were completed and opened for the reception of patients on 13 January 1853.

After more than twenty years of discussions, planning, and intermittent fundraising, Pittsburgh's first chartered hospital built on a modern design finally emerged thanks to the donations of two families with a deep military heritage. Once opened, the operational and fiscal realities of operating a public hospital were soon understood. Thomas Bakewell in his 1853–54 Annual Report of the President noted that since the hospital's opening, 172 patients (ninety-two medical; eighty surgical; twenty-six insane) had been admitted with 139 being treated gratuitously. Of the total, nine patients had died. The numbers showed a slight improvement over the first few months of operation. During the first three months, only seven patients sought admission. The weekly rates charged for convicts was $2.50 to $3, while private patients were charged from $3 to $6, depending upon the difficulty of the case.[30] There were no paying patients recorded during its first nine months of operation.[31]

Reflecting on the challenging financial situation the hospital faced, Bakewell noted: "... the reception of pay patients is in no way injurious."[32] Bakewell also commented on the medical staff by reporting:

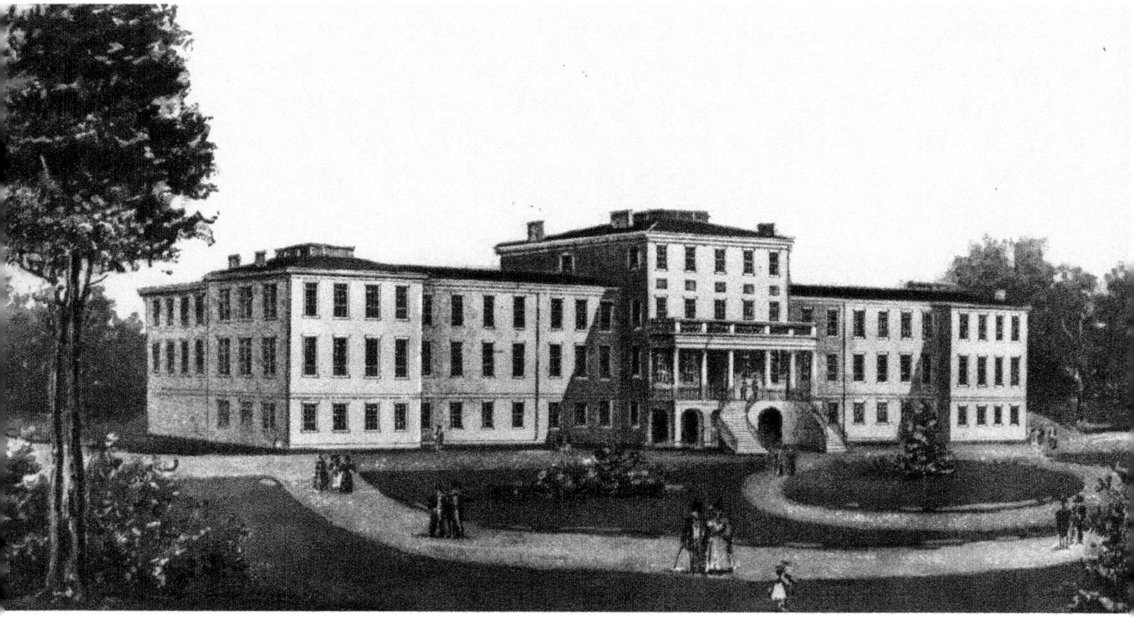

The Western Pennsylvania Hospital in 1853. (*Annual Report of the Managers of the Western Pennsylvania Hospital for 1851–1853*)

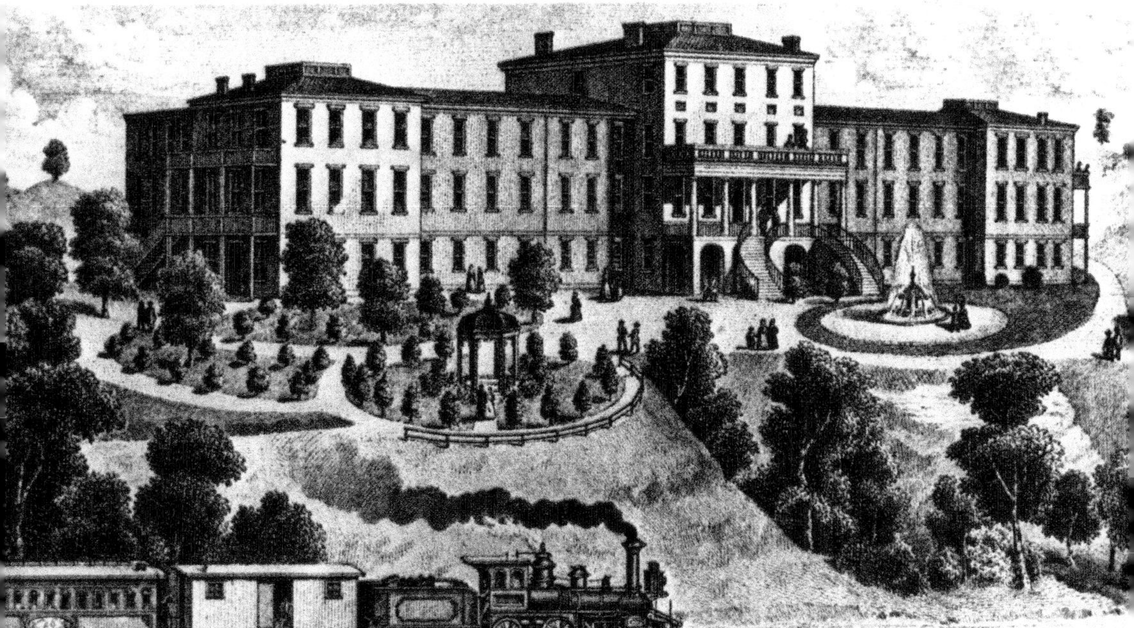

Architect's rendering of The Western Pennsylvania Hospital. (*Annual Report of the Managers of the Western Pennsylvania Hospital for 1883*)

> The Board entertains a grateful sense of the advantages which the Hospital has derived from the gratuitous services of the Physicians and Surgeons, who, by their frequent visits and kind attentions to the patients, have manifested their philanthropic dispositions, while the success of which has generally attended their ministrations, affords the strongest evidence of the skill and judgment displayed in the treatment of the various cases that came under their notice.[33]

Interestingly, out of a total of ninety-two medical admissions, 15 percent were admitted with intermittent fever and 28 percent with insanity.[34] Soon it became obvious the needs of the city's insane were becoming a major issue for the hospital. Bakewell reported: "A considerable portion of the patients, (mostly females), were afflicted with mania and other mental diseases."[35]

John Harper, who became the second president of the board of managers in 1867 after the passing of Thomas Bakewell, recounted the dilemma the hospital faced as it attempted to serve the insane: "The increasing demands upon the Hospital for the treatment of insane persons prompted the Managers to make additional provisions for them, and an outlay of money beyond the means of the institution became necessary."[36] Pittsburgh historian, Sarah H. Killikelly, also took note of the hospital's dilemma:

> There was an immediate demand upon this hospital for the admission of the insane, which continued to increase to such an extent that on May eighth, 1855, a supplement to the Act of incorporation was made by which the State appropriated ten thousand dollars towards securing accommodation for the mentally afflicted, and authorized the courts of Western Pennsylvania to commit to the hospital any person charged with punishable offense, who might be then insane, and a further supplement to the charter was made a year later, which carried with it a sum of twenty thousand dollars to further extend the department for the insane. It was then proposed and approved by the Governor to erect additional buildings for this particular class of patients, and the State to appoint annually three managers. This, however, after long and serious consideration, was deemed injudicious, and Miss Dorothy L. Dix was invited to a conference with the Board of Managers. Upon her advice, the managers sold the farm they had already purchased, on the left bank of the Monongahela river, and bought in place thereof one containing about three hundred acres on the right bank of the Ohio, seven miles below the city. This, with other tracts of land purchased subsequently through the aid of private funds, were all on the line of the Pittsburgh, Port Wayne and Chicago Railroad.[37]

Dixmont Hospital for the Insane

The decision to create a new hospital specifically for the insane was not without challenges. Managers of Western Pennsylvania Hospital were convinced many of the insane could be cured if treated early and with appropriate care. In contrast to other institutions in the country they felt were modeled as "Incurable Asylums," they posited the inscription from Dante's Inferno "Hope never enters here!" would not be emulated in western Pennsylvania.

With funding from the State guaranteed, the dilemma for the managers turned to the question of whether to expand the existing hospital in the Ninth Ward or to build an entirely new hospital. As Sarah Killikelly notes, it was Dorothea Dix's promotion of a separate hospital that convinced the managers. Indeed, she was a force that could not be taken lightly. The new hospital, bearing her name, specifically designed to care for the "mind diseased" attests to her considerable talents.

After months of debate and several real estate transactions, including the purchase and resale of property along the Monongahela River (now Homestead), a location on the right bank of the Ohio River (Kilbuck) was selected for the new hospital. The site offered approximately 300 acres of property, an ample fresh water supply, a stone quarry, and easy access to the railroad. Construction work began on 01 May 1860, with the hospital's cornerstone being laid on 19 July. By 11 November 1861, the Centre Building, Station House, Laundry Building, Water, and Gas Works were sufficiently complete to allow for the transfer of patients from the Ninth Ward hospital.

The Civil War brought major changes to the hospital's operation, and within ten years of its opening, Western Pennsylvania Hospital found itself directly connected to the military. In the hospital's annual report for 1862, the board of managers documented the circumstances:

> Several months ago an inquiry was made by the War Department with regard to the accommodation that could be obtained in this vicinity for sick and wounded soldiers, and after consultation with the State authorities, the Hospital in the Ninth Ward was offered for that purpose, so soon as the insane patients could be removed; and accordingly, about the middle of last month, the Hospital was transferred to the United States officers, who, after making the requisite repairs and alterations, have began to occupy the wards with their patients, assuming the whole expense of conducting it, except a small salary to be paid by the Board to Dr. Rea, who has been retained by the U.S. Surgeon, and who will attend to the preservation of the property and keeping it in order. By adopting this course, the Board trust that many valuable lives may be preserved, and much suffering spared to the valiant defenders of their country, at the same time that the sick, helpless and infirm among them may obtain the relief which their necessities require, while provision has been made for the reception of persons suffering from accidental wounds or casualties.[38]

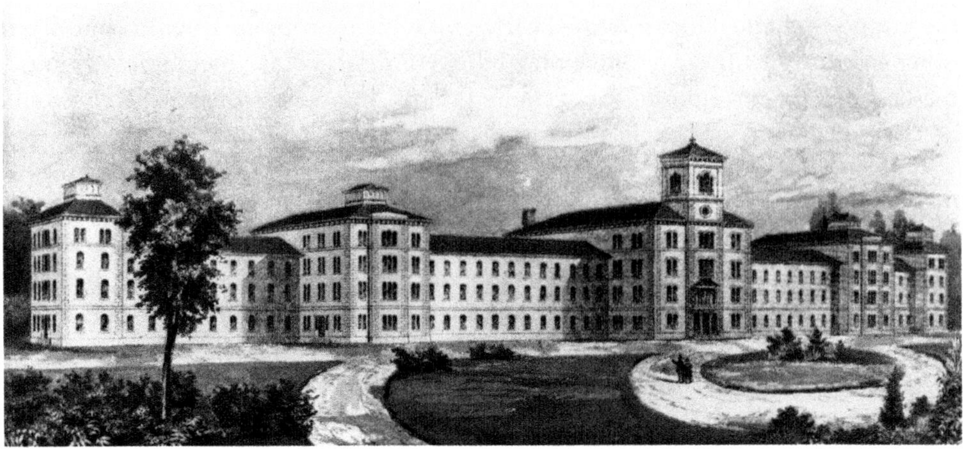

Dixmont Hospital for Insane, 1861. (*Annual Report of the Managers of the Western Pennsylvania Hospital for 1864*)

U.S.A. General Hospital Pittsburgh

Beginning in August 1861, a few months before Dixmont Hospital was sufficiently completed to accept the transfer of patients from the Ninth Ward facility, and before formal transfer of the facility to the federal government, the U.S. Army began assigning surgeons to the hospital. In December 1862, the hospital was officially transferred to the government and placed under the local control of the United States War Department's Department of the Monongahela. It would remain under federal jurisdiction until October 1865 when the hospital was officially returned to civilian administration. During the period of military occupancy, the hospital continued to accept general medical and surgical patients. Due to the hospital's location near railroads and heavy industry, arrangements were also made for the reception of cases of accidental injury.

Under military control, the army appointed thirty-seven surgeons to the hospital, engaged the Sisters of Mercy as nurses, and provided care for thousands of sick and wounded soldiers in the hospital proper and tents deployed on the hospital's property. During their time at the hospital, the Sisters of Mercy noted: "The horrors of combat were constantly increasing and plans were made by which, almost overnight, the hillsides of Pittsburgh were dotted with hundreds of tents, serving as emergency stations. These canvas hospitals dotted the hills as sheep dot the knolls while they graze."[39]

The Sisters went on to record that most of the soldiers treated wore Union uniforms and were from Pennsylvania, including many from Pittsburgh. However, Confederate soldiers in grey uniforms and those with different color skin were likewise cared for at the hospital: "Among these hundreds of soldier patients there were frightful emergency surgical cases. The Sisters never turned their heads away from any of these war-sick strangers within the gates because of the color of their uniform or face, or because his faith was not in accord with theirs."[40]

Sisters of Mercy Serving During the Civil War[41]

Stanton Hospital—Washington D.C.
Sister Mary Flavia Byrne
Sister Mary Estelle Curran
Sister Mary Vincent Delaney
Sister Mary Helen Devlin
Sister Mary Borgia Doherty
Sister Mary Bernard Duffy
Sister Mary Otillia Dusch
Sister Mary Anthony Gallagher
Sister Mary Berchmans Hostetter
Sister Mary Aloysius Ihmsen
Sister Mary Nolasco Kratzer
Sister Mary Joseph Laughran
Sister Mary Appollonia Leahy
Sister Mary Bernard Maher
Sister Mary Xavier Maher
Sister Mary Basil McGinn
Sister Mary Francis McCormick
Sister Mary Marcella McKeown
Sister Mary Remigius McQuade
Sister Mary Gonzaga Myers
Sister Mary Louis O'Conner
Sister Mary Celestine Rafferty
Sister Mary Johanna Rooney
Sister Mary Augustine Shuck
Sister Mary deRicci Tierney
Sister Mary Julia Ward

U.S.A. General Hospital—Pittsburgh, PA
Sister Mary Neri Bowen
Sister Mary Leo Driscoll
Sister Mary Benedict Duffy
Sister Mary Sebastian Gillespie
Sister Mary Berchmans Hostetter
Mother Mary Rose Hostetter
Sister Mary Basil McGinn
Sister Mary Madeliene O'Donnell
Sister Mary de Pazzi Russel

While under federal control, the army made alterations to the hospital and grounds including replacement of old small water pipes with larger pipes better suited for the dramatic increase in patients and the construction of two "frame" buildings. One of the structures was intended to serve as a "Protestant Chapel." After the Sisters of Mercy arrived, it was converted for use by the Catholic nuns. The chapel was designed so it could be quickly converted for emergency use as a hospital ward capable of holding fifty beds. A brief account of the hospital's work during this "military period" was presented in a newspaper article in August 1864:

The United States Military Hospital
The Philadelphia Ledger thus speaks of the Military Hospital in this city: One of the very best hospitals at present occupied by the United States is that located on one of the lots on the outskirts of Pittsburgh. This land was originally deeded to the State of Pennsylvania, in all about forty acres, on condition that it should be forever occupied for hospital purposes. The buildings erected upon it are three hundred and forty-five feet long, with a central portion about fifty feet square and three stories high. The rest is only two stories high, but with basement for offices. It was intended to hold about one hundred and fifty patients, and a considerable portion of the building was devoted to the insane of the western portion of the State. These, indeed, absorbed the whole building until the philanthropic Miss Dix succeeded in procuring the erection of the Dixmont establishment for this special purpose.

In September 1862, the buildings and grounds were tendered to the United States for a general hospital, and commenced with fifteen patients. Now there are eight hundred and thirty, among whom there have hardly been two deaths per month of late. Most of these patients are western Pennsylvanians, and they seem to recover wonderfully of their wounds. The location is eminently favorable for them, in the selection of the grounds is eminently favorable for the large number here located, most of them in tents.

Dr. Bryan, for twenty years a resident physician of the city, is the Surgeon in charge, and appears to be superintending the establishment with great success. The sickness prevalent at Vicksburg last season, has made him quite an invalid, but a gentleman of energy and great kindness of heart, everything connected with the hospital exhibits great attention to the comfort of his patients. New buildings have been erected, one of three a new dining hall being one hundred feet long by twenty-five feet wide. This is at present used as a place of worship on the Sabbath, where quite large congregations attend. The Chaplain, Rev., Mr. Bear, a liberal and pleasant gentleman, is pleasant and kind to all patients.

There are some forty-nine tents arranged in six rows, and this sort of outdoor life is found to contribute materially to the health of some of the patients at this season of the year, although so perfect are the arrangements, both of the buildings and the attendance, that the air is always fresh and pure for those who room in the buildings. In fact, except for the proverbial smoke at Pittsburgh, blackening all it comes in contact with, it is difficult to conceive how patients could possibly be in a better situation than is here provided. In consequence of the number of troops passing through from the west to the east, or the reverse, the hospital at Pittsburgh forms a most valuable point at which to deposit invalids whose wounds will not permit their traveling further. There are at present about six assistant surgeons in charge of the different wards, and fresh patients and surgeons are continually arriving, so that this is rapidly becoming a hospital of important, owing, no doubt, to the salubrity of the region and the ability with which it is managed. It would come however seem highly desirable that more and similar hospitals should be established along the line of the Pennsylvania Railroad and nearer to Harrisburg.[42]

A month earlier, one of the city's other newspapers reported:

> There are at present over seven hundred sick and wounded soldiers at the United States Hospital in the Ninth Ward, and there are arrangements made to accommodate as many more. The place presents a very clean and neat appearance, the wounds are dress carefully by surgeons of ability, the wants of the soldier supplied and well fed, and every attention bestowed to make the inmates happy and contented under the varied afflictions.[43]

Over the three-year span that the army occupied the hospital, there were periods when as many as 1,500 soldiers were cared for at the same time.

It should be noted that even though the General Hospital served as the city's primary military hospital, additional soldiers were treated at Mercy and Passavant Hospitals. At Mercy, it was recorded that the government paid ninety-four cents per day for each Union soldier treated.[44]

For the casual observer, the view of the Western Pennsylvania Hospital's grounds must have been amazing. Unfortunately, only written testimony like these newspaper accounts offers evidence of the sea of tents situated on hospital property. Until photographic evidence is discovered, the full visual extent of the army's use of hospital grounds must be left to the imagination.

The federal government returned the hospital to civilian control in October 1865. The hospital board of managers reported in their annual account for the year: "The Hospital buildings in the Ninth Ward were occupied by the United States authorities as a military hospital, until the 3d of October 1865, but some patients were admitted prior to that date."[45] The army stopped using the facility in July, but used the time between July and October to repair buildings and restore grounds. In July, the army began dismantling buildings they had constructed over the previous few years. A notice in the newspaper placed by the Deputy Quartermaster General's Office dated 17 July 1865 ran for several days offers a general description of the structures. The advertisement read:

> Sale of Public Buildings.—Will be sold Saturday, the 22nd instant at two o'clock P.M. at the General Hospital. FOUR WOODEN BUILDINGS, of the following dimensions, *viz*: Number one, 81 feet by 31 feet; Number two, 132 feet by 31 feet; Number three, 25 feet by 15 feet; Number four, 81 feet by 25 feet. A large quantity of old Lumber and iron at the fairgrounds. Payment cash, and in government funds. The buildings and lumber must be removed in 10 days after the sale. Signed O. Cross, Lt. Col. and D.Q.M.G.[46]

Another class of patients admitted during the military period and immediately afterward was veterans. If a soldier's medical circumstances were not pressing, they were often cared for at the Soldiers' Home. As noted earlier, the Home was located

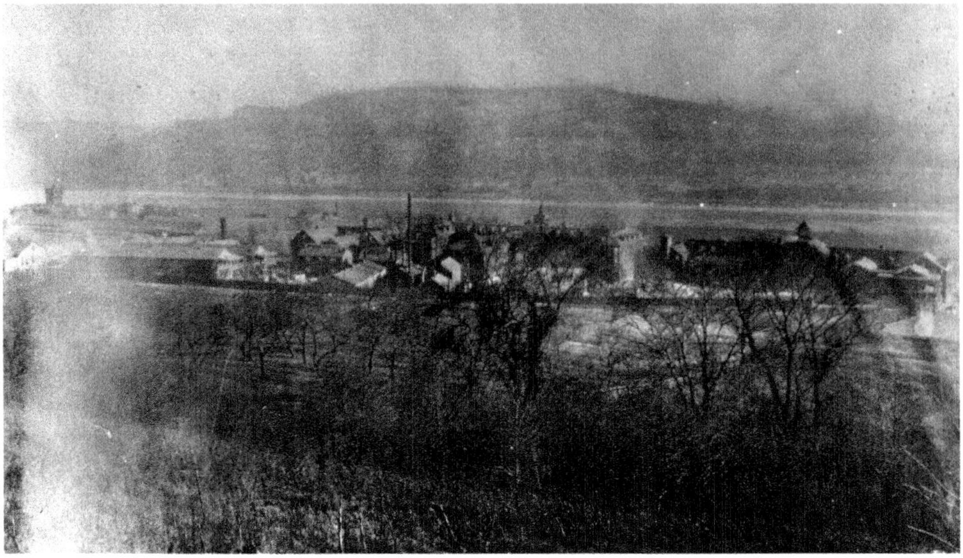

U.S. Army General Hospital, No. 22, Pittsburgh, Pennsylvania. This view is from the hospital building looking toward the Allegheny River. It is the only known image of hospital property during the Civil War period. (*National Library of Medicine*)

in the heart of the city and was operated by the Pittsburgh Subsistence Committee with medical direction by Dr. Andrew Fleming.

As military traffic increased through the city, the need for medical care grew exponentially. Frequently, the life-threatening nature of a soldier's illness or wounds was more than the group could handle in such a limited clinic-style setting, and they found it necessary to transfer the soldier to the hospital. In such instances, they were typically sent from the Soldiers' Home on Liberty Avenue to Western Pennsylvania Hospital a few miles away.

Once the institution was taken over by the federal government, it became known as U.S.A. General Hospital Pittsburgh or the "Ninth Ward" hospital. The arrangement with the hospital was fortuitous for the soldiers in meeting their immediate needs, and also for the city as it led to the formal establishment of the "Pittsburgh Sanitary Soldiers' Home" in 1866. This essentially became Pittsburgh's first veteran's hospital. At the time of the Home's incorporation in March 1866, the Soldiers' Home had already provided care for about 80,000 soldiers. Further details of the Home's continued evolution will be examined further in a later chapter.

Pittsburgh Infirmary—Passavant Hospital

During the spring of 1848, Rev. W. A. Passavant, pastor of the First Lutheran Church, decided to establish a hospital. He considered the time favorable since newspapers were filled with stories about proposed plans to organize and charter Western Pennsylvania Hospital. The Sisters of Mercy and the newspaper articles attesting to the initial success of their one-year-old hospital likewise served as a clarion call for action. If the Catholics and the Protestants were to have their hospitals, so too would the Lutherans. Thus, Passavant Hospital, first known as the Pittsburgh Infirmary, was born.

While the hospital was being contemplated and an initial site selected in Allegheny City's North Side, there was not an immediate rush to action. However, the return of three ill soldiers from the Mexican-American War and the arrival of cholera in the city provided the impetus needed for the hospital to open on 17 July 1849. The soldiers were ill from fever and had been stranded on boats on the river. Passavant, along with theological student Asa Waters, provided for their care in the new hospital.

Three companies of Mexican-American War soldiers had been raised in the city. During the war, more than 2,400 men from Pennsylvania had served:

> ... by the time both regiments returned home to be mustered out, after only a year and a half of service, their numbers had dwindled to mere 1,341 men. Death had claimed 477 Pennsylvanian souls, of which only fifty-two died as the direct result of combat. An additional 406 had to be discharged early, mainly due to sickness.[47]

On their return home, many arrived in Pittsburgh by boat: "The vessels began arriving at Pittsburgh on July 11, 1848, and continued to do so until the 18th. Companies A, I, and K of the First Pennsylvania Regiment and all of the Second Pennsylvania Regiment were mustered out at Pittsburgh between July 12, 1848 and July 25, 1848."[48] It is likely many other sick and wounded soldiers were treated at Mercy and Western Pennsylvania Hospital, however, that care was not documented. It was the admission of the three fevered soldiers that brought public attention to the Pittsburgh Infirmary.[49]

In 1849, the hospital accepted a number of cholera patients, which caused great alarm in the community. In a newspaper article published on 05 May 1849, it was reported: "A petition was presented on Thursday night to the Select and Common Councils of Allegheny City, praying that the introduction of cholera patients from steam boats into the Infirmary of Rev. Mr. Passavant, Allegheny City, might be stopped."[50] The petition stated:

> ... a painful anxiety and alarm now exists in the densely populated portion of the city, by the introduction from our sister city (Allegheny City), of foreign patients afflicted with the most fatal and dreadful of all diseases, the Cholera, into the infirmary but recently established in our midst, through the benevolence of a Reverend citizen of Pittsburgh. We feel constrained by a sense of duty to ourselves, our wives, and our children—by a proper concern for the purity, health, and happiness of our whole

> population, and by a sense of degradation of being made the common receptacle of the diseased of every infected port of our Western Waters...[51]

Upon receiving requests from the City's Mayor and Council, which was aroused by public threats of violence, it was subsequently decided it would be expedient—and much safer for all concerned—to remove the patients to another facility. Passavant loaded the patients in a wagon and transported them to the recently vacated Dr. Lacy's Female Seminary located in the Lacyville section of the city. The site was considered sufficiently distant from the general population to allay fears over the spread of contagion. The building and property were purchased for $5,000 and later expanded on adjacent property.

Later in the summer, Dr. Passavant successfully recruited four "Prussian" Deaconesses from the Lutheran Order of Deaconesses to serve as nurses. The Sisters were placed in the charge of a Pittsburgh resident, Sister Louisa Marthens. With the acquisition of the building and the arrival of nurses, the hospital was now able to accept up to forty patients. The new facility was dedicated on Sunday, 22 July 1849. In 1851, a new four-story building measuring 60 by 40 feet was constructed on the expanded property.[52] It would not be long before the hospital was filling a medical void in the city by providing care for growing numbers of contagious diseases victims. Between 1853 and 1854, the institution recorded 536 admissions, including thirty-eight typhoid patients, twenty-one smallpox victims, and sixty-four suffering from cholera.[53]

United States Marine Hospital

One other hospital that provided limited service to the military was the United States Marine Hospital. It opened between the time Mercy Hospital began operations in 1847 and the beginning of the Civil War. Originally intended for Wheeling, West Virginia, the federal government decided instead to establish a hospital in Pittsburgh. It took five years after congressional approval for the Secretary of War to select a site for the hospital. Moving slowly, it took three more years for building to begin. Construction stopped and restarted over the years, as appropriations would allow. Fourteen years after approval, the Pittsburgh Marine Hospital was completed in 1851.

While the hospital was designed to treat ill seamen, it also served soldiers for a short period early in the Civil War. As noted earlier, it was after the Battle of Shiloh in early April 1862 a contingent of volunteers left Pittsburgh on the "Expedition to the Tennessee River" to retrieve sick and wounded soldiers. Most of the sixty-eight soldiers they returned with were taken to the Marine Hospital. A newspaper article in May 1862 offered a brief update on their recovery by reporting:

> The Wounded Soldiers—The brave heroes of the battle of Shiloh, now in the Marine Hospital in the care of the City Committee are rapidly recovering from their wounds

> and diseases. It is hoped by the physicians and nurses that all those now under treatment will recover, although the nature of the wounds of several would seem to preclude the possibility of a reasonable hope.[54]

The remainder of the wounded was placed at Mercy Hospital and Western Pennsylvania Hospital.

As the soldiers recovered at the Marine Hospital, the federal government was finishing work at nearby Western Pennsylvania Hospital converting the institution into the new U.S.A. General Hospital Pittsburgh. From that point forward, sick and wounded soldiers were treated there, except during times of overflow or emergency when some were cared for on a *per diem* basis at Mercy Hospital.

Other Hospitals

Following the opening of Dixmont Hospital in 1861, a number of other hospitals were founded in Pittsburgh. In fact, between the close of the Civil War and the turn of the century, thirteen hospitals opened. Compared to how long it took for the city's first three hospitals to get started, it was almost as if a spigot had now been opened.

Medical care had dramatically improved since the firing on Fort Sumter. In four short years, the odds of recovery from wounds or disease—whether on the battlefield or in a hospital—were remarkably higher than before the war. Surgery, medical care, nursing, and better use of drugs now offered real chances for successful treatment and full recovery. Old public prejudices about hospitals being viewed as places to die faded fast. They were quickly replaced by an era of receptive patients, enlightened medicine, and a renewed focus on improving public health.

FAITH-BASED HOSPITALS

1865 **St. Francis Hospital** (originally known as German Franciscus Hospital) was the first post-war hospital to begin operations. Opened only six months after General Lee's surrender, the fifty-bed hospital began accepting patients on 30 October 1865. The institution was sponsored by Roman Catholics and was located on Thirty-fourth Street in the Lawrenceville section of the city. Further development of the hospital was driven by the arrival of a group of three Sisters from Buffalo, New York, who were associated with the order of St. Francis. The hospital was officially incorporated on 20 June 1868. Within a few short years, patient demand had outgrown the hospital's physical space, and it was decided a new building would be required to meet the growing demand. In 1872 a new four-story building was opened. In 1885 the hospital added a separate department for treatment of insane women.

1890 **Columbia Hospital** (originally known as Little Memorial Hospital) was founded through the efforts and support of the Presbyterian Church. It was originally located in the North Side section of Allegheny City and later moved to Wilkinsburg.

1893 **Presbyterian Hospital** began operating in 1893 and officially incorporated on 04 May 1895. The original hospital was located on Montgomery and Sherman Avenues in the North Side section of Allegheny City. The hospital later moved into a new building in the Oakland section of the city.

1895 **Pittsburgh Hospital** (originally known as Charity Hospital) began operating in May 1895 under the direction of the Catholic Sisters of Charity. The hospital was opened in a small dwelling house on Stanton Avenue in East Liberty. A new expanded facility was built and opened in December 1905.

1896 **St. John's General Hospital** was founded by Protestant Deaconesses from the Mary J. Drexel Home of Philadelphia, but was later taken over by the Sisters of Divine Providence, a sisterhood of the Roman Catholic Church. It was originally developed as a Lutheran institution located on McClure Avenue in the Woods Run section of Allegheny City, primarily to provide care for accident cases coming from the many mills located in the area.

1898 **St. Margaret's Memorial Hospital** was created by members of the Protestant Episcopal Church on the corner of Forty-sixth and Davison streets in the city's Lawrenceville district. The hospital was made possible through a bequest of John H. Shoenberger, Esq. in honor of his wife, Margaret Cust Shoenberger.

The demand—or desire—for hospitals also grew because of competition. Religious preference, nationality, and neighborhood now became critical factors in determining where each new hospital would emerge. A consistent backdrop to the development of all these hospitals was the region's rapid population growth beginning in the mid to late 1840s. This was particularly true initially for the Irish and Germans immediately before and after the Civil War, but also for Italians and all the eastern Europeans who flooded the city later in the nineteenth century.

Another compelling reason for the creation of new hospitals after the war was the return of physicians who were now better educated and battle-tested. An influx of new doctors seeking professional or economic benefit from Pittsburgh's booming economy also helped fuel growth.

Before the war, the city's only specialty medical service was for mental disease. That class of patients was now well cared for at Dixmont Hospital. At the end of the war and immediately afterward, specialized services for veterans were in high demand and would remain so for several decades.

The other specialties that grew rapidly post-war were orthopedic surgery and treatment of diseases of the eyes, ears, nose, and throat. While vestiges of these specialties were evident before the war, there were now many more physicians—some with skills honed in battle and others recently graduated from medical schools—arriving in the city eager to establish a practice. Brief descriptions of the other hospitals created between 1865 and 1900 include:

SPECIALTY-BASED HOSPITALS

1866 **Homeopathic Medical and Surgical Hospital** (also known as the Pittsburgh Homeopathic Hospital and later as Shadyside Hospital) opened on 01 August 1866 in an old mansion on Second Avenue near Smithfield Street. Its charter was awarded 04 April 1866. The hospital was created to fill the needs of those who practiced homeopathy and those who sought such treatment. The hospital expanded on the original site in April 1884. In 1910 it moved to Shadyside. Related to the hospital was the Pittsburgh Training School for Nurses, which was opened in 1884. In 1892, the hospital expanded its services by adding an eye and ear dispensary.

1891 **Pittsburgh Hospital for Children** was opened on 04 June 1891on Forbes street in the city's Oakland area. Its construction was principally funded through the generosity of Miss Jane Holmes. The hospital was officially incorporated on 18 March 1887. Its initial purpose was to treat children with orthopedic disorders.

1895 **Eye and Ear Hospital** was initiated on 20 May 1895. It was located at the corner of Fifth Avenue and Jumonville Street in the Oakland area of the city. Pittsburgh writer and historian, Sarah H. Killikelly, was a primary benefactor. On 22 June 1895, the hospital was chartered and a new location was obtained on Penn Avenue. Its first board of managers was composed of thirteen women and two physicians who were eye specialists engaged in the medical and surgical treatment of diseases of the eye, ear, nose, and throat.

1891 **Rosalie Foundling Asylum and Maternity Hospital** was opened on 26 November 1891 under the auspices of the Catholic Sisters of Charity. Initially, the hospital operated in a small house on Forbes Street in Oakland but later moved to larger premises located on the corner of Cliff and Manila streets in the city's Hill District. The move was necessitated by public outrage over the hospital's caring for supposedly "immoral" women. The hospital's maternity department served two distinct classes of patients: 1) unmarried women seeking to restore character and reputation, and 2) married women whose financial circumstances precluded care at other institutions. The hospital's foundling department operated as a distinct unit with independent staff.

1893 **Reineman Maternity Hospital** opened in 1893. It was the first institution of its kind in Western Pennsylvania. Created by Adam Reineman, it was deeded to the Western University in 1894, but its title was held by the Western Pennsylvania Medical College. Due to the high cost of operating the hospital, the University agreed to transfer the hospital to the College. An arrangement between the University and the Medical College was subsequently made with the College becoming a department of the University. In exchange, the University acquired stock in the Medical School, albeit without voting privileges. The building was subsequently remodeled and enlarged. It was located on Polish Hill adjacent to Western Pennsylvania Medical College, and not far from Western Pennsylvania Hospital. While under the control of the Medical College it was used as a teaching facility for educating students in obstetrics and gynecology. In 1895 after receiving a large donation from Isaac Kaufmann, a prominent Pittsburgh merchant, the hospital site was expanded and a new building was added. The Emma Kaufmann Clinic was officially opened in 1897. It included an amphitheater and several treatment rooms. The donation was accompanied by a ten thousand dollar gift to create a chair of medicine.

COMMUNITY-BASED HOSPITALS

1880 **Allegheny General Hospital** was chartered on 18 October 1882. The one hundred-bed hospital was located on the corner of East Stockton Avenue and Weiser Street on the North Side of Allegheny City. It was not long before the hospital became too cramped to handle a growing patient load. An annex was added in 1887, creating room for the addition of twenty-five beds. The hospital operated on the original location until just after the turn of the century when continued growth required the building of a new structure on a new site. The new building holding four hundred and fifty beds was completed in 1904.

1893 **South Side Hospital** opened for the reception of patients in 1893 on South Twentieth and Carson Streets in the city's South Side area. It had taken almost four years, and two failed attempts to establish the hospital, but Drs. John Milton Duff, J. D. Thomas, M. A. Arnholt, and their associate members of the South Side Medical Society persevered. With improved public interest and funding from a "Ladies' Aid Society" and other donors, a cornerstone was laid in 1893 and the hospital opened shortly afterward.

The dramatic growth of Pittsburgh and the early development of its first permanent hospitals took many decades to accomplish, but once the Sisters of Mercy ignited the flame of competition by opening Mercy Hospital in 1847, the city's healthcare engines were stoked, primed, and ready for rapid advancement. From the opening date of Mercy Hospital, Pittsburgh's first hospital to accept patients, to the opening of St. Margaret's Hospital in 1898, sixteen hospitals were opened before the turn of the century.

The Civil War provided a new lens through which the rest of the country—and the world—could see the manufacturing might of the city and the interminable energy and industriousness of Pittsburgh's people. The city's rivers provided access to seemingly unlimited amounts of food and manufactured goods. Arms and munitions used in battle, including cannons of a size the world had never before seen, were routinely shipped by river and rail. Thousands of soldiers and sailors from the city and its suburbs added critical mass to the country's army and navy. The city delivered hundreds of doctors, nurses, and other medical volunteers, to the battlefront to support and heal the wounded. If Pittsburgh was indeed the "domain of Vulcan," with its "great furnace of Pandemonium with all its lids lifted," as Glazier noted in his book, *Peculiarities of American Cities*, the city's industries certainly found their impetus in war and reconstruction, so too did the cities medical establishment.[55]

The expansion of industry and the creation of hospitals was not the only beneficial outcome of the war. Medical care, in general, had made major strides. Physicians learned new methods of diagnoses and treatment; nurses transitioned from unpaid volunteers offering basic comfort to ill and wounded soldiers, to trained professionals proficient in delivering care under the most challenging circumstances. In tandem with those offering medical care, thousands of ordinary citizens found ways to complement the work of both groups by banding together to provide food, clothing, hospital materials, transportation, and sundry other beneficial products and services to support the war effort and its wounded warriors. In four years, ordinary people proved capable of extraordinary deeds of healing and compassion. Collectively, their philanthropic work created a launch pad from which future generations would benefit in unimaginable ways.

9

Post-Civil War Medical Advances

Comparing the state of medicine in Pittsburgh and around the country before and after the Civil War is like seeing the hands of a clock move abruptly from midnight to six o'clock in the morning. The transition from medical care delivered on the frontier to that now developed in response to the Civil War was astonishing. In Pittsburgh specifically, a new day in healthcare had dawned, and once again, it was the city's physician-soldiers who forged the way.

The Care of Veterans

One of the first and longest lasting changes came about as the result of Dr. Andrew Fleming's work with the Pittsburgh Subsistence Committee. As noted earlier, Fleming was among a small group of people in July 1861 who formed the Pittsburgh Subsistence Committee. Offering food, drink, comfort, and medical care to soldiers traveling through the city proved to be a daunting but rewarding task—one that would affect medical care for veterans for decades.

Fleming was a very busy doctor in 1861. After graduating from medical school in 1855, he served an eighteen-month residency at the Pennsylvania Hospital in Philadelphia. He returned to Pittsburgh in early 1857 to join the practice of his preceptor, Dr. Joseph P. Gazzam. Gazzam had a leading medical practice in the city, and Fleming quickly established himself as an eminent physician and prodigious medical writer.

An early paper, *Blood Stains in Clinical Trials*, was published in a leading national journal in October 1858. In 1861, in book form, it would become nationally recognized as the definitive work on the subject. In its introduction, Fleming remarked:

> In the trial of criminal cases, especially where the evidence is of a circumstantial character, it is frequently of the greatest importance to determine of what certain spots are composed, in order to fix the guilt or attest the innocence of the accused. To this end science has been employed, and frequently, by the weight of her testimony alone, has acquitted the innocent or condemned the guilty.[1]

The monograph was crafted in response to a special request from Edwin M. Stanton, a personal friend, leading Pittsburgh attorney, and soon to be Cabinet member under presidents, James Buchanan and Abraham Lincoln. Fleming dedicated the work to Stanton by stating: "In obedience to whose suggestion, this effort was undertaken to remove a difficulty long felt in criminal trials, this small tribute to his personal and professional excellence, is respectfully dedicated."[2]

Fleming was active in research, writing, and practice. His work with the Subsistence Committee was establishing and managing its medical service. A local newspaper described the work of the department by writing: "Some time ago it was

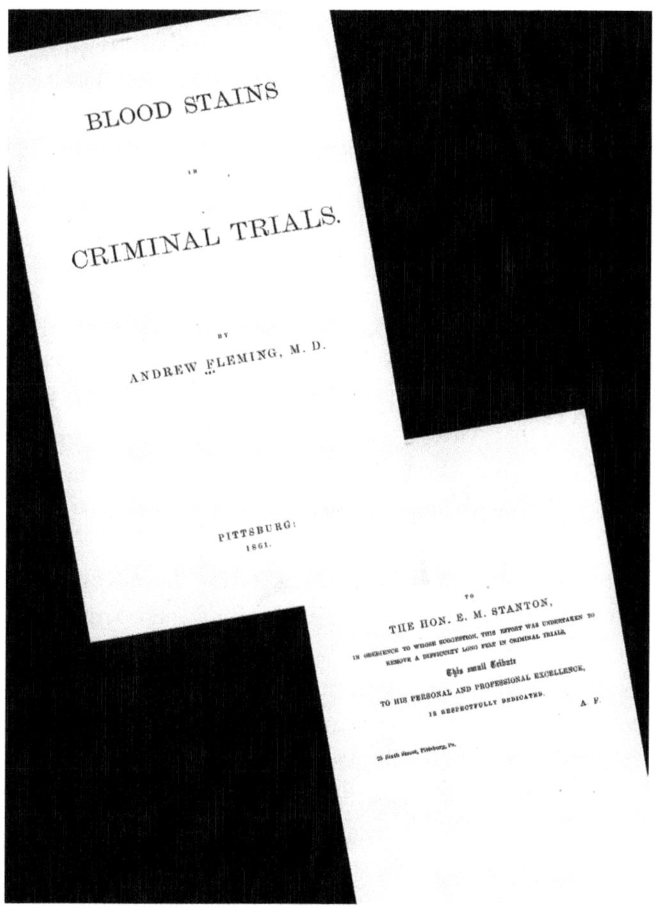

Dr. Andrew Fleming's *Blood Stains in Clinical Trials* title page and dedication. (*National Library of Medicine*)

found necessary to provide temporary lodging for sick and wounded soldiers unable to pursue their journey, and also for those destitute of means and without proper papers for securing transportation. Great relief and much aid have been given to many in this way."[3] A biographical account of Fleming's work during this time explained his efforts:

> Early in the war, in 1861, a Soldiers' Home was opened near the Union Station in Pittsburgh, by the Subsistence Committee, to care especially for the multitudes of sick and wounded soldiers on their homeward journey. Dr. Fleming was at this home, on the arrival of the trains, every noon and every midnight, dressing the wounds of the sufferers and prescribing medicine for the sick. As the number of soldiers needing attention was from twenty-five to one hundred each noon and midnight, these merciful ministrations took from one to three hours of his valuable time, but during the four years of the war, he rarely failed to make the two daily visits.[4]

As the war progressed, so too did the demand for medical services. In May 1864, space limitations of the original medical department were resolved by expansion into new and larger quarters on Liberty Avenue. One city newspaper announced the pending opening of the new quarters as "Opening of the Soldiers' Home—The ceremonies connected with the opening of the Soldiers' Home of the Pittsburgh Subsistence Committee, will take place at the Home, No. 347 Liberty street, on Thursday evening, May 5th."[5] One week after the opening of the Soldiers' Home, another newspaper provided additional background:

> ... last week, larger and more commodious rooms were completed, which were opened last Thursday evening.... The rooms appropriated to this laudable purpose are in the second, third and fourth stories of one of the large buildings on Liberty Street, opposite the Central depot. They are neatly and tastefully fitted up, with every convenience for sick soldiers. There are a dining room, kitchen, sitting rooms and sleeping apartments. Here soldiers—sick and weary—can at all times, when passing through the city, find a quiet resting place—in a word, A Home.[6]

In cases where soldiers were too ill or their wounds too severe for adequate care in the small medical department, they were transferred to Western Pennsylvania Hospital. Transfers took place before, during, and after the hospital transitioned from civilian care to Army military service between late 1862 and mid-1865. The Subsistence Committee's medical department and the hospital also served those mustering out of military service throughout the war.

Once the Civil War had concluded, the Soldiers' Home continued providing care for "honorably discharged" sick and wounded veterans, but slowly transitioned all of its services to Western Pennsylvania Hospital. The Subsistence Committee officially disbanded in January 1866. Admirably, under Dr. Fleming's care, the

Home provided medical attention for almost 80,000 soldiers during its short four and one-half years of existence. When the Subsistence Committee disbanded, the Soldiers' Home ceased operating under the Committee's charter. It was re-chartered by the Pennsylvania State Assembly in March 1866, with all of its services now fully transitioned to Western Pennsylvania Hospital.

Under terms of the transfer, residual funds from the Pittsburgh Sanitary Fair were used to pay for care rendered at Western Pennsylvania Hospital. The agreement lasted until September 1877 when the remaining funds, in the amount of $198,383.71, were used to establish an endowment sufficient to guarantee veterans "of the Volunteer Armies of Western Pennsylvania," would continue to receive free medical care. A joint committee of the region's Grand Army of the Republic and hospital managers would administer the fund. The endowment lasted well into the twentieth century.

Medical and Scientific Advances

While the provision of medical care for veterans was an early post-war priority, many other changes in medicine and medical care delivery were taking place at the same time. The Allegheny County Medical Society was formed within weeks of the war's end. Within a year, Allegheny General Hospital, the city's newest hospital opened. Nursing care was likewise changing dramatically as professional nurses, both males and females, with war experience, were returning to take positions in the hospitals.

Physicians were similarly affected by four years of war. Before the war, it was common to find physicians who served an apprenticeship but had never gone to medical school practicing next to one who attended a university or medical college. There were many times more of the former than the latter. It would have been highly unusual to find a physician, particularly in the eastern and southern states, with extensive trauma training before the war. That changed immediately after the war's earliest battles, where amputations, once an anomaly, now became frequent. Similarly, injuries from gunshot, saber, or bayonet were wounds almost never seen in cities and towns—except, perhaps, in the western territories—for several generations before the war were now routine.

Patient transportation was now highly effective and by war's end had become a specialized branch of medical service; triage was now a routine practice, and sanitation and quarantine practices were greatly improved. In surgery, the safe use of anesthetics was now commonplace and newly developed specialty procedures, including plastic surgery, neurosurgery, eye surgery, and others were embraced by individual physicians and adopted for singular focus in hospitals around the country. Bonnie Brice Dorwart, in her *Essential Civil War Curriculum—Civil War Hospitals*, describes several specialty hospitals that emerged during the war: "Eye injuries—

Desmarres Hospital, Washington, D.C.; Eye injuries—Athens, Georgia; Spinal cord, brain, nerve injuries and epilepsy—Turner's Lane Hospital, Philadelphia; Gangrene—Memphis; Eye and Ear—St. Louis; Erysipelas—Nashville; Feet and toes lost to frostbite—Wilmington, Delaware; Mutilated soldiers—New York City; Female venereal diseases—Hospital Number eleven—Nashville Tennessee; Soldiers' syphilitic diseases—Hospital Number fifteen—Nashville Tennessee; Serious venereal diseases—Kingston, Georgia."[7]

With the end of hostilities, a majority of the volunteer surgeons returned to their home cities. Others enrolled in medical school before returning. The opportunity was ripe to obtain a medical degree. For some, the prospects of specialization offered new ways of differentiating their practices and increasing prospects for higher incomes. These decisions were especially important since there were now significantly more physicians and surgeons competing for patients than had been the case just four years before. Due to the influx of these more recently educated and now battlefield-trained physicians, competition in the civilian market dramatically increased.

There were also the physicians who came from Europe during the war. They were typically better educated, and most were well accustomed to using diagnostic instruments like stethoscopes, microscopes, and thermometers. Particularly early in the war, such equipment and skillsets gave them an edge over their American counterparts. They did not shy away from using such knowledge and expertise for competitive advantage.

In the two decades following the war's end, new scientific discoveries continued to energize the entire field of medicine. Antiseptic surgery, germ theory, experimental medicine, and other scientific and therapeutic advances essentially brought positive changes for both physician and patient. Doctors and hospitals were now better equipped to diagnose and cure disease and perform life-saving surgery.

The battle between allopathic physicians and those practicing alternative medicine was fundamentally settled since the allopaths had been successful in excluding most "irregular" medical practitioners from war service. Except for homeopathy, alternative treatments did not survive the test of war. To endure, the homeopaths found it necessary to create proprietary medical colleges, nursing schools, hospitals, and professional societies.

Pittsburgh's First Medical School

Prospects for establishing a medical school in Pittsburgh were presented by Western University professor Robert Bruce in 1822. The concept of adding a professional school to complement the University's academic program was theoretically a good idea, but in practice, a stretch too far and too soon. Originally founded as Pittsburgh Academy in 1787, the school had only recently, in 1819, achieved university status.

From its beginning, the school struggled financially, and even though it faced mounting pressure from the public and State to add professional training to its traditional liberal educational programming, its leaders could not generate the resources, or common agreements, needed to launch such a venture.

Efforts to create a medical school were not demonstrated again until 1848. Like the discussion in 1822, this attempt met with failure. Dr. Andrew Fleming made another effort in 1864, as did the officers of Western University in 1880, but they also proved ineffective.[8] It took a group of frustrated, but determined physicians from Western Pennsylvania Hospital to break the stalemate. Civil War surgeon Dr. Cyrus B. King organized the effort to establish a medical school in Pittsburgh. King was chief physician and curator of Western Pennsylvania Hospital as it transitioned from military to civilian control in 1865. He also served as the first superintendent of the Pittsburgh Soldiers' Home as it transitioned from Pittsburgh Subsistence Committee oversight to Western Pennsylvania Hospital's. He continued to be a leading figure at the hospital and in the general medical community for decades. His success in organizing the medical college was realized in June 1883, when the Western Pennsylvania Medical College was formally chartered.

Together with a group of leading city physicians, who each purchased stock in the new organization, they collectively funded the school. A total of 250 shares of stock valued at $100 per share were sold. With the sale of the stock, funding was sufficient to construct a new building to house the college. The facility was built near Western Pennsylvania Hospital on property located at Thirtieth and Brereton Streets in the Polish Hill area of the city. Standing four-stories high and containing classrooms, a dissection room, laboratories, a medical museum, and a large two-story amphitheater, the building took a little more than two years to complete. The Medical College officially opened in September 1886 with an initial class of fifty-seven students.

Another compelling reason for a medical school in Pittsburgh resulted from an act passed by the State Legislature in 1881, "requiring medical graduates who wanted to practice in Pennsylvania, but who had received their training elsewhere, to be endorsed by a Pennsylvania medical college."[9] With no medical college in Pittsburgh, physicians in the city were at a considerable geographic disadvantage compared to their peers in the eastern part of the state who benefitted from the four colleges located in Philadelphia at the time.

A majority of the college's stockholders were medical staff members at the Western Pennsylvania Hospital. However, the hospital's board of managers determined there would be no formal affiliation with the college. Nevertheless, college faculty used the hospital for clinical training, which was made accessible by way of an underground connecting tunnel. The first faculty included twenty-two of Pittsburgh's leading physicians, one Ph.D., and an attorney. Among the physicians, at least one-third had served in the Civil War. The faculty included:

First Faculty of the Western Pennsylvania Medical College[10]

James Bissett Murdoch, M.D.	Dean
Samuel Ayres, M.D.	Professor of Mental and Nervous Diseases
William J. Asdale, M.D.	Professor of Diseases of Women and Secretary of the Faculty
N. W. Brown, M.D.	Professor of Diseases of Children
Hugo Blanck, M.D.	Professor of Chemistry
Austin G. Case, M.D.	Professor of the Diseases of Children
J. G. Connell, M.D.	Professor of Botany, Materia Medica, and Therapeutics
James Creaer Dunn, M.D.	Professor of Diseases of the Skin
John Milton Duff, M.D.	Professor of Obstetrics
William T. English, M.D.	Professor of Physical Diagnosis
Herman W. Hechelman, M.D.	Professor of Diseases of the Eye and Ear
Thomas L. Hazzard, M.D.	Professor of Physiology
Cyrus B. King, M.D.	Professor of Orthopedic Surgery
J. Chris Lange, M.D.	Professor of Principles and Practice of Medicine
James B. Murdoch, M.D.	Professor of Practical and Operative Surgery
John S. Mabon, M.D.	Professor of Diseases of Nose and Throat
Eugene G. Maston, M.D.	Professor of Pathology and Histology
James McCann, M.D.	Professor of Principles and Practice of Surgery
Edgar A. Mundorf, M.D.	Professor of Pathology and Histology
T. M. T. McKennan, M.D.	Professor of Anatomy
Whitmore Snively, M.D.	Professor of Practice of Medicine and Clinical Medicine
Jeremiah Tingley, Ph.D., LL.D.	Professor of Chemistry
J. F. Slagle, Honorable	Professor of Legal Medicine
J. D. Thomas, M.D.	Professor of Genitourinary and Venereal Diseases
E.A. Wood, M.D.	Professor of Dietetics and Hygiene

The composition of the faculty was similar to the stockholder group, with a majority of the physicians being members of Western Pennsylvania Hospital staff. All of the involved physicians were also members of the Allegheny County Medical Society.[11] Civil War veteran James B. Murdoch, M.D., was appointed Dean. Dr. John Milton Duff, another veteran, served as professor of obstetrics and as the college's very first lecturer.

In 1887, the curriculum was expanded to two years, in 1891 to three years, and in 1895 to four years. Over that period, other changes occurred, including formal affiliation with the University of Pittsburgh in 1892 and the sale of the college to the University in 1908 for the sum of $100,000. At the time of the sale, "there were three brick buildings, the original enlarged to five stories, with three lecture rooms, a dissection room, seven laboratories and sundry assembly and reception rooms; the Kaufman Outpatient clinic next door; and the Reineman Maternity Hospital on Millwood Avenue."[12]

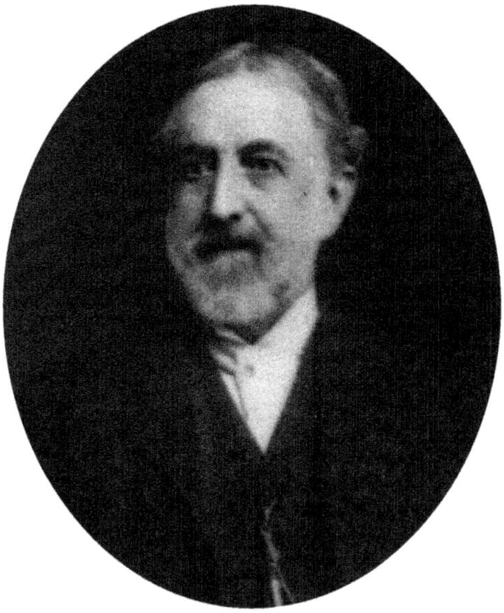

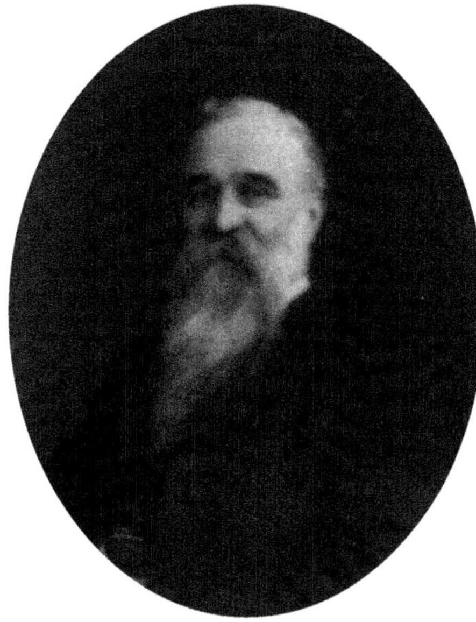

Above left: Cyrus B. King, M.D., original organizer of the Western Pennsylvania Medical College and Professor of Orthopedic Surgery.

Above right: William J. Asdale, M.D., Professor of Diseases of Women and Secretary of the Faculty of the Western Pennsylvania Medical College.

Below left: J. C. Lange, M.D., Professor of Principles and Practice of Medicine at the Western Pennsylvania Medical College.

Below right: John S. Mabon, M.D., Professor of Diseases of Nose and Throat at the Western Pennsylvania Medical College.

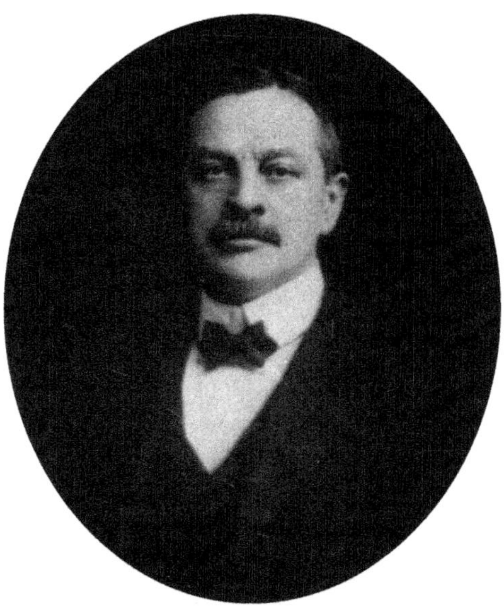

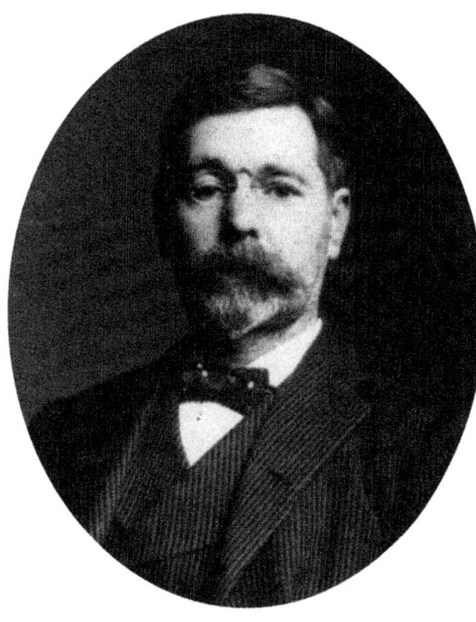

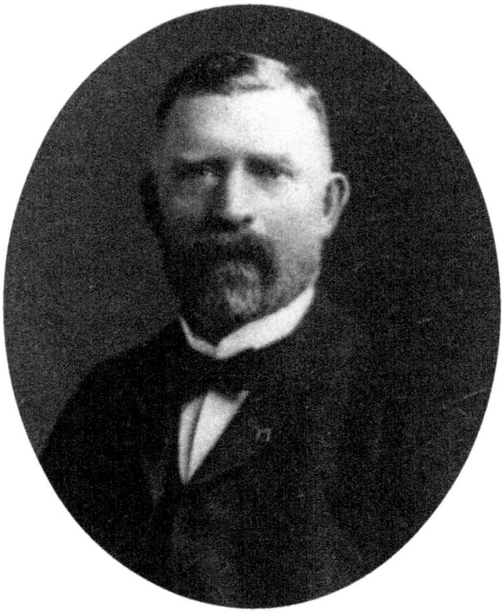

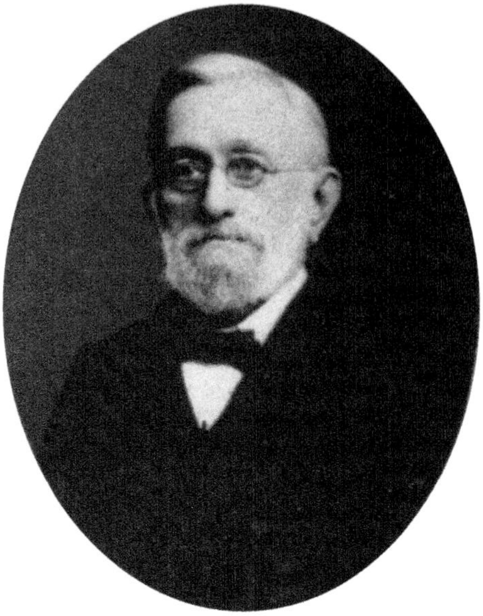

Above left: John M. Duff, M.D., Professor of Obstetrics at the Western Pennsylvania Medical College.

Above right: J. Tingley, Ph.D, Professor of Chemistry at the Western Pennsylvania Medical College.

Below left: E. G. Matson, M.D., Professor of Pathology and Histology at the Western Pennsylvania Medical College.

Below right: E. A. Wood, M.D., Professor of Dietetics and Hygiene at the Western Pennsylvania Medical College.

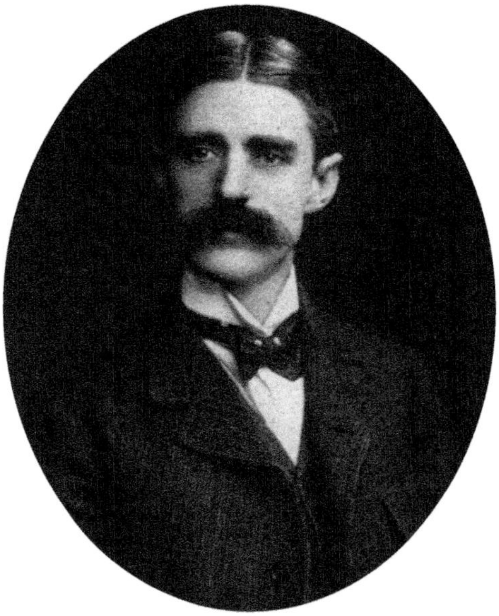

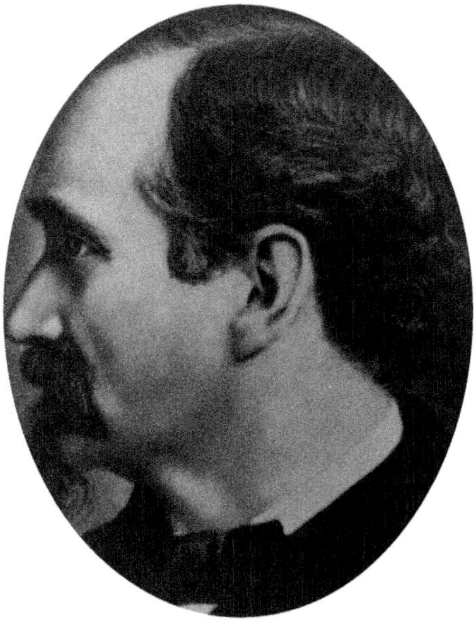

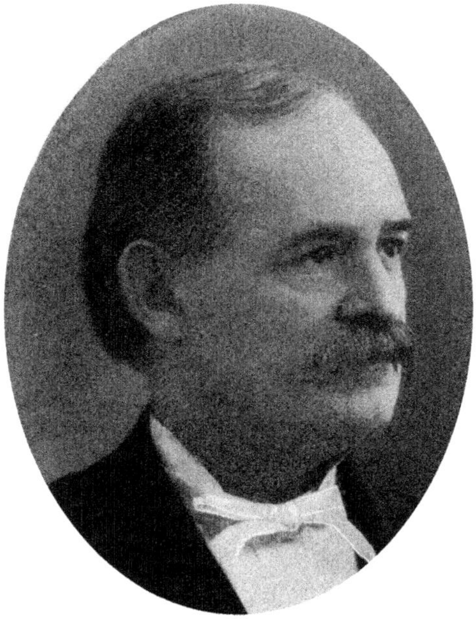

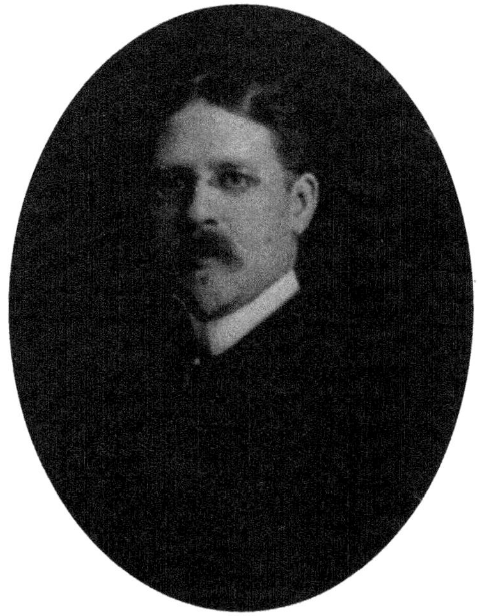

Above left: J. D. Thomas, M.D., Professor of Genitourinary and Venereal Diseases. (*Carnegie Library of Pittsburgh*)

Above right: T. M. T. McKennan, M.D., Professor of Anatomy at the Western Pennsylvania Medical College.

Right: Western Pennsylvania Medical College Announcement 1890–1891. (*The Western Pennsylvania Hospital*)

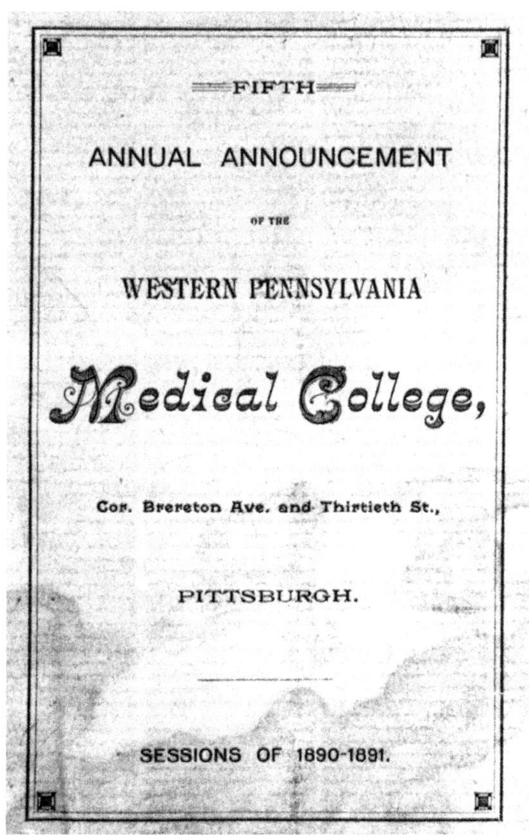

FIFTH

ANNUAL ANNOUNCEMENT

OF THE

WESTERN PENNSYLVANIA

Medical College,

Cor. Brereton Ave. and Thirtieth St.,

PITTSBURGH.

SESSIONS OF 1890-1891.

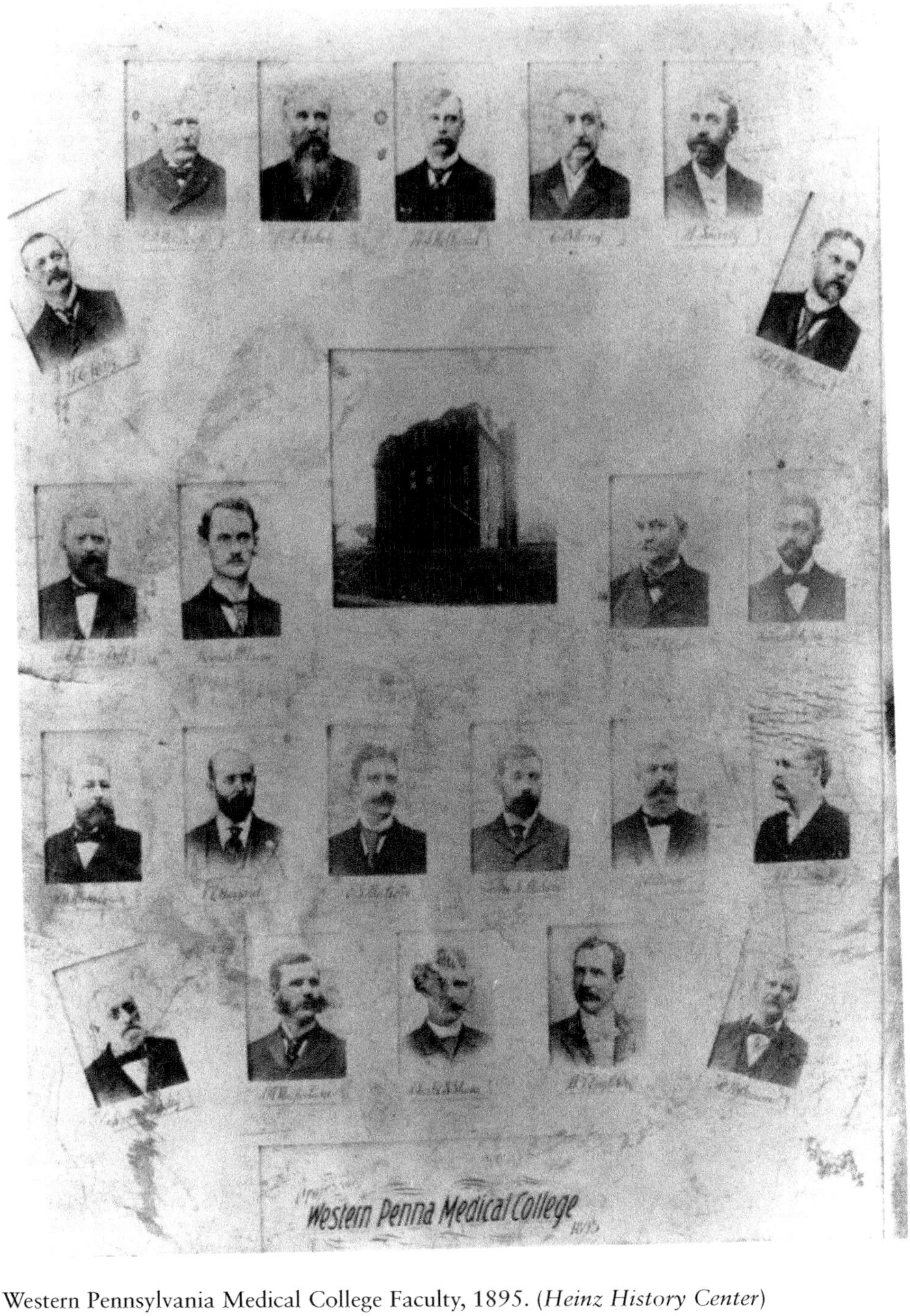

Western Pennsylvania Medical College Faculty, 1895. (*Heinz History Center*)

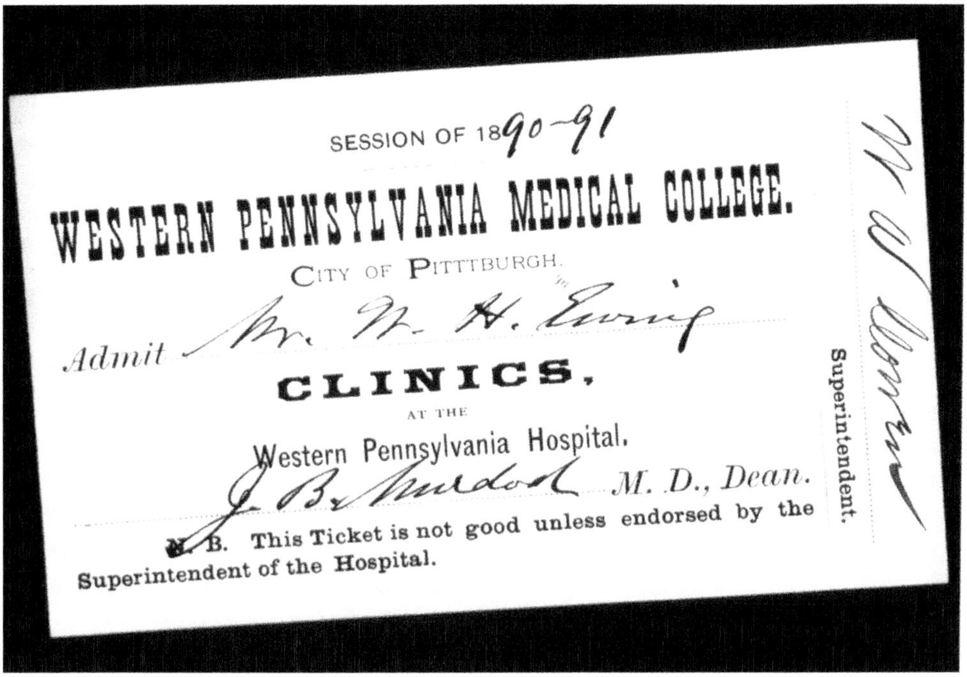

SESSION OF 1890-91

WESTERN PENNSYLVANIA MEDICAL COLLEGE.

CITY OF PITTTBURGH.

Admit Mr. W. H. Ewing

CLINICS,

AT THE

Western Pennsylvania Hospital.

M. D., Dean.

N. B. This Ticket is not good unless endorsed by the Superintendent of the Hospital.

Superintendent.

Western Pennsylvania Medical College clinic ticket for 1890–1891 session. (*The Western Pennsylvania Hospital*)

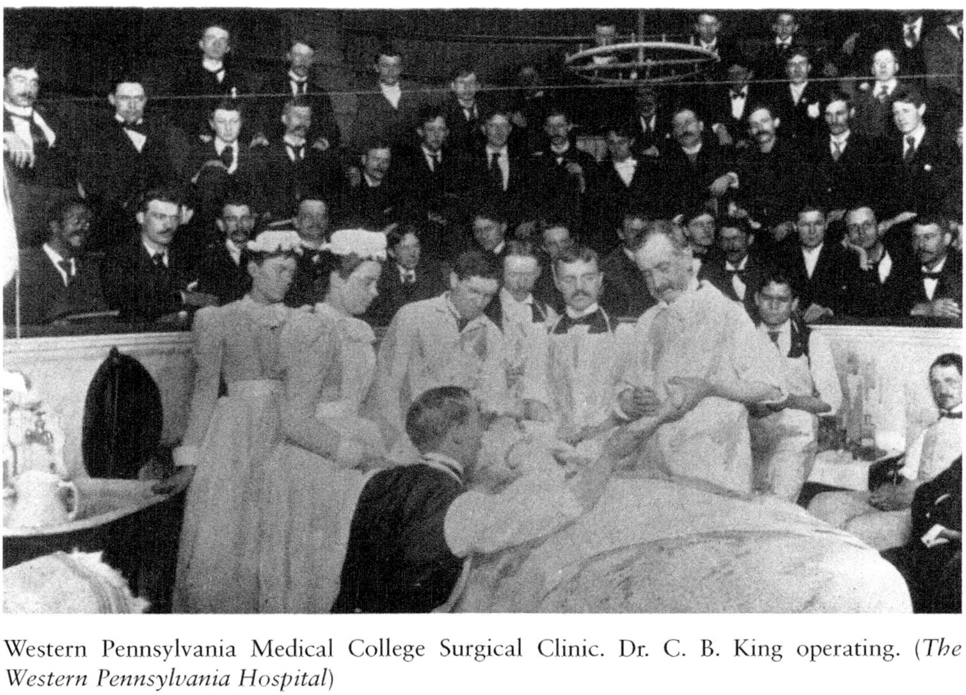

Western Pennsylvania Medical College Surgical Clinic. Dr. C. B. King operating. (*The Western Pennsylvania Hospital*)

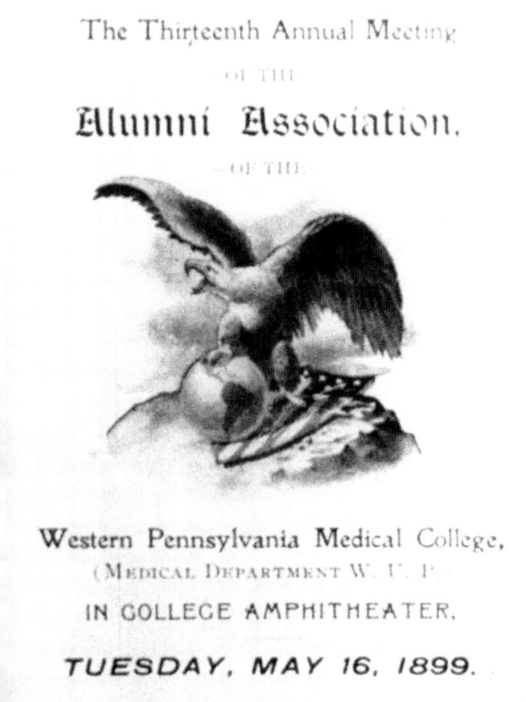

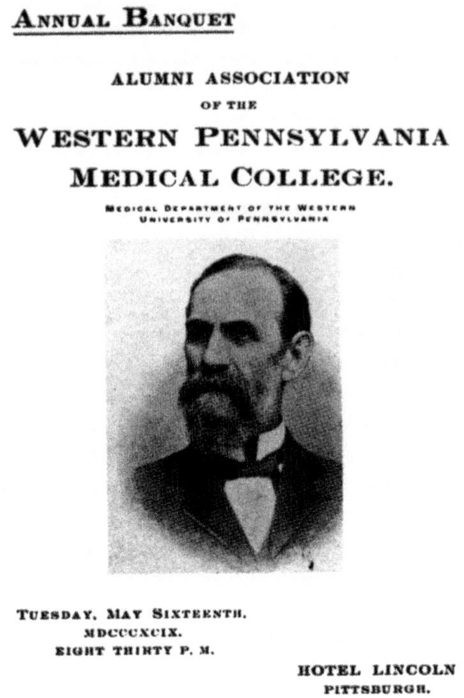

Above left: Western Pennsylvania Medical College Alumni Association program cover, 1899. (*The Western Pennsylvania Hospital*)

Above right: Western Pennsylvania Medical College Alumni Banquet program 1899. (*The Western Pennsylvania Hospital*)

Below: Western Pennsylvania Medical College medical fraternity letterhead masthead. (*The Western Pennsylvania Hospital*)

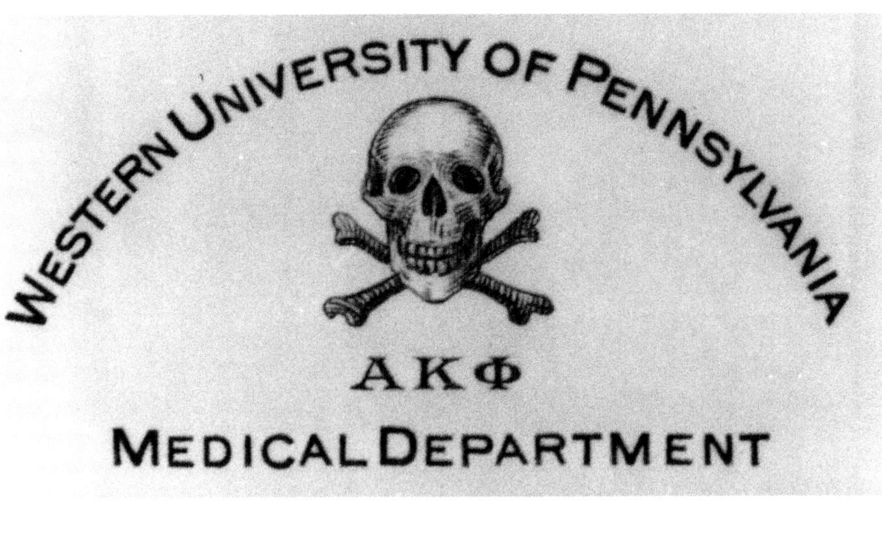

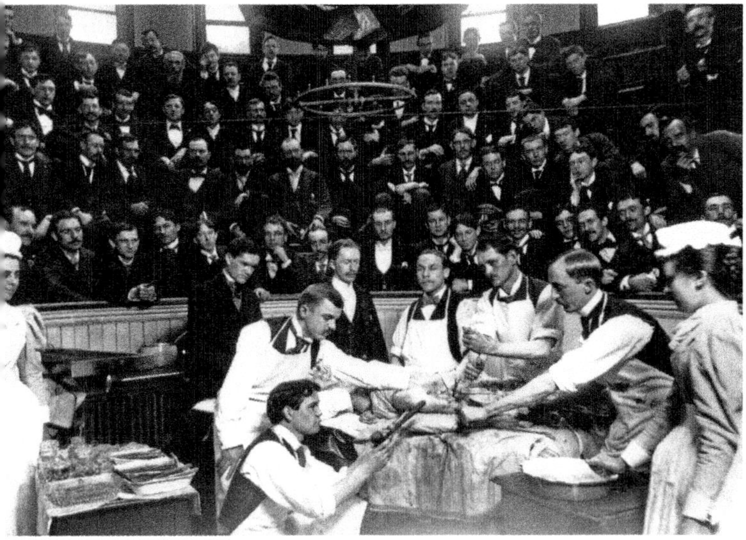

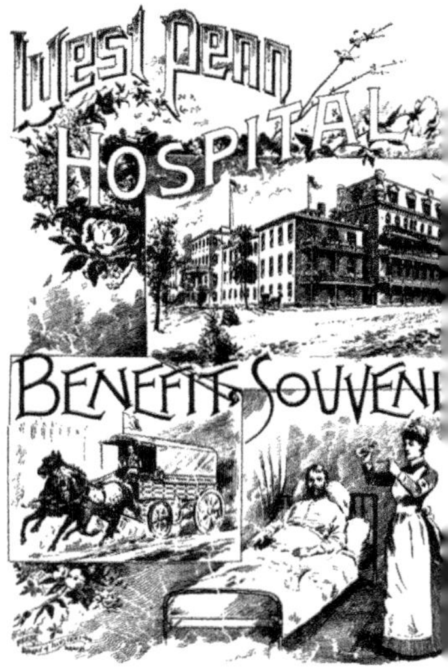

Above left: Western Pennsylvania Medical College amphitheater with Dr. Thomas McCann operating with surgical drill. (*The Western Pennsylvania Hospital*)

Above right: Western Pennsylvania Hospital Benefit Souvenir program cover 1888. (*The Western Pennsylvania Hospital*)

Below: Western Pennsylvania Hospital Medical Department in the late 1880s. (*The Western Pennsylvania Hospital*)

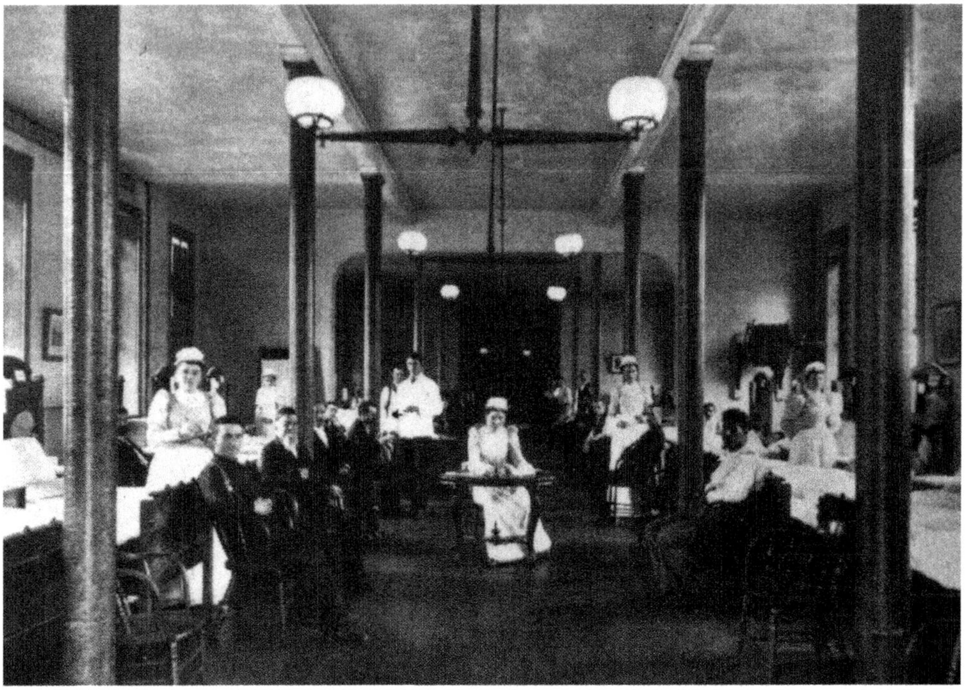

Specialty Care: Hospitals and Practices

Rapid change in medicine had indeed become routine. It was almost as though everything established as normal and traditional before the war was now ripe for disruption. A degree from a medical college or university became a prerequisite for acceptance into community practice and for professional recognition among peers. New medical and surgical specialties were created that required skilled practitioners and dedicated facilities. Innovative treatments and surgical techniques now offered hope where there was little before. New instruments and diagnostic tools were developed, and their use quickly adopted. Treatment for mental illness was now recognized as an integral part of medical care. The conditions for delivery of care were compassionate and effective. Public health measures were now forethought rather than a reaction to an episodic epidemic.

While the evolution of medicine in Pittsburgh was dynamic during the last half of the nineteenth century, its trajectory was not always straightforward. There was much to accomplish as newly adopted practices were demonstrated, tested, contested, and refined. A brief review of some of the highlights include:

Care for the Insane

With the founding of the Western Pennsylvania Hospital for the Insane at Dixmont in 1861, progress was made in how individuals with mental illness were treated and in the environments in which their care was delivered. The buildings and grounds were state of the art, and progressive treatment practices were adopted immediately. Hospital leadership continued to receive counsel and advocacy support from Dorothea Dix for several decades after the hospital's opening. For more than a quarter century, her activism on behalf of the city's mentally ill, and her attention to the hospital and its patients helped influence public opinion, state and local government officials, policy makers, and philanthropists.

After developing, testing, and perfecting new strategies for improving nursing care during the Civil War, she shared her experiences with many, including Dixmont's administrative leadership. Many of her practices and routines were readily adopted. In 1870, Dix established a library for patients, and in 1876, she spent an entire six-week period at Dixmont as a guest of superintendent Dr. Joseph A. Reed. In 1887, a formal course of nursing instruction for mental health patients was incorporated. In 1895, Dixmont opened a training school for nurses and graduated its first class of thirteen female and three male nurses in early May 1897. Dix's impact on the hospital left a legacy that would survive for generations.

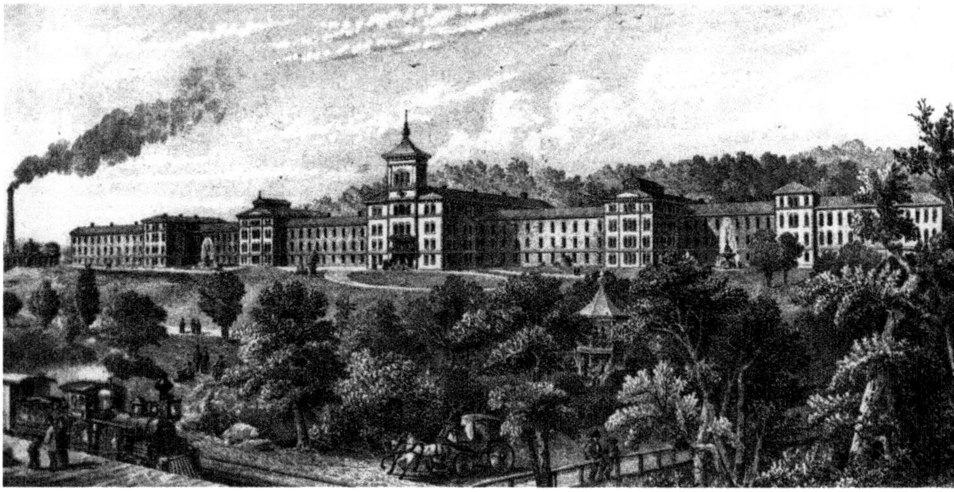

Western Pennsylvania Hospital for the Insane at Dixmont 1880. (*Report of the Managers of the Western Pennsylvania Hospital 1880*)

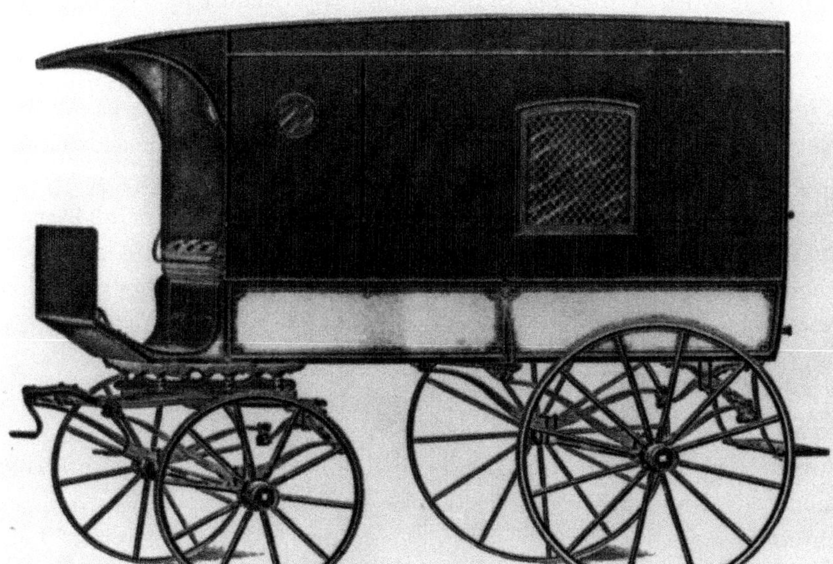

Asylum van used for transporting inmates, *c.* 1890. (*National Library of Medicine*)

Specialty Hospitals Large and Small

August 1866

The Pittsburgh Homeopathic Medical and Surgical Hospital provided a site for homeopathic care that eliminated competitive pressure from the city's allopathic mainstream physicians. The allopaths had become adept at developing exclusionary measures that prohibited homeopaths and other alternative medical practitioners from practicing in the city's hospitals and professional societies. In 1892, the hospital added a clinic for specialized treatment of diseases of the eyes and ears.

September 1883

The Terrace Bank Sanitarium for Women was opened as a private hospital on Ridge Avenue in Allegheny City. The institution was owned and managed by Dr. Rhodes S. Sutton, a Civil War surgeon and one of the city's most prominent physicians. The hospital was founded as a place where invalid women could be restored to good health. In 1889, Dr. Sutton served as president of the Pittsburgh Obstetrical and Gynecological Society. At the end of his term, he offered a detailed background on his trailblazing work performing an ovariotomy, a procedure he developed in 1875. He described the rationale for opening his private hospital:

> The advantages to the patient and operator, are great. The nursing is, as a rule, better. The hygienic surroundings are more under control, the precautions looking to the avoidance of sepsis, are more thoroughly understood by the attendants, and are more successfully carried out. An audience is more critically selected, or avoided. Everything for an emergency is at hand, the patient is kept more secluded, and faults in her diet are less likely to occur. The encouragement afforded those to be operated by those already operated and convalescent, has been a very marked feature in favor of the private hospital.[13]

June 1891

Pittsburgh Hospital for Children was initially opened to treat children with orthopedic disorders. Services were quickly expanded to include a full range of medical and surgical services. Civil War veteran Dr. Francis "Frank" Lemoyne promoted the development of a specialized hospital for children after years of dealing with childhood illnesses and injuries. Just a few years before the hospital's opening, in 1886, Lemoyne reported that 59 percent of all deaths in the city were those of children. He was frustrated by the lack of resources devoted to their care, so he engaged other leading doctors and philanthropists to intervene. The hospital proved successful in reducing deaths from injury and debilitating disease from its beginning.

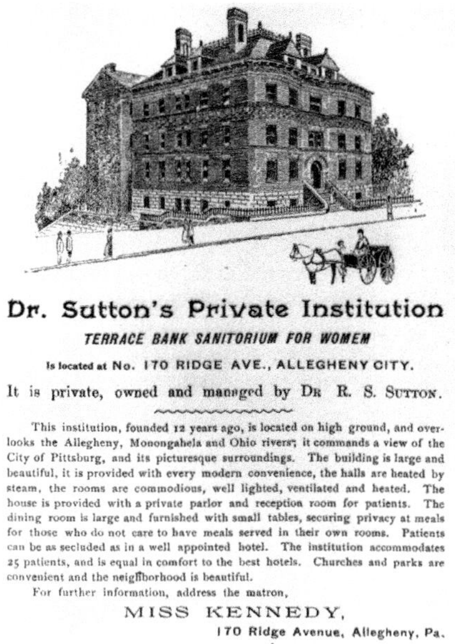

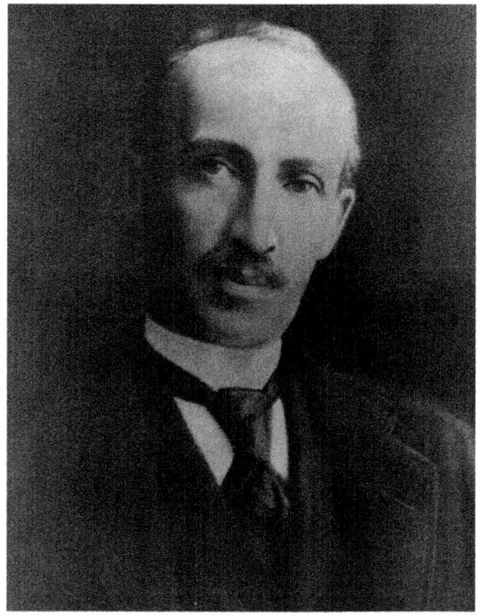

Above left: Dr. Sutton's Terrace Bank Sanitorium for Women 1895. (*J. M. Kelly's Handbook of Greater Pittsburg, 1895*)

Above right: Francis "Frank" Lemoyne, Civil War veteran and surgeon at the Western Pennsylvania Hospital. Founders of the Pittsburgh Children's Hospital. (*Allegheny County Medical Society*)

July 1891

The Keeley Institute opened its doors as the city's first institution to specialize in the treatment of alcohol and drug addiction. In 1895, the Institute had treated more than one thousand patients since opening.

1893

Reineman Maternity Hospital was founded as the city's first specialty maternity hospital. The institution holds a unique place in the city's medical history, as it is arguably the bridge that formally connected Western University to Western Pennsylvania Medical College. This resulted in the creation of the University of Pittsburgh School of Medicine and Elizabeth Steel Magee Hospital. While university and college leaders had long considered such an arrangement, it was Adam Reineman's gifts of the hospital structure to the University, and the title to the property to the college, that provided the functional and financial framework for affiliation.[14]

Spring 1894

Dr. Golwitzer's Hospital was another private hospital that opened in the Schenley Park area of the city for treatment of diseases by use of hydropathy, steam treatment,

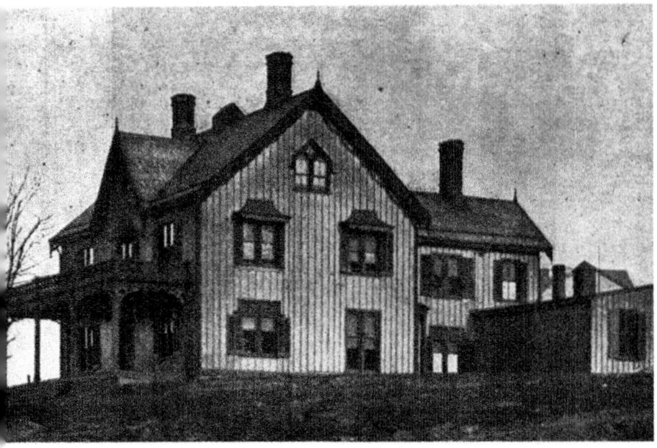

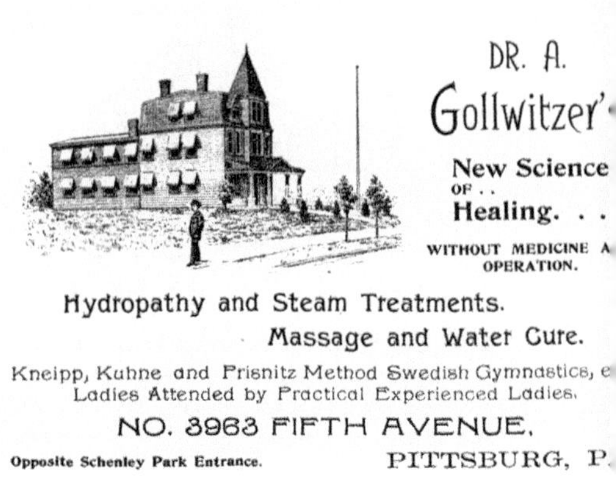

Above left: Reineman Maternity Hospital. (*The Western Pennsylvania Hospital*)

Above right: Dr. Golwitzer's Hospital. (*J. M. Kelly's Handbook of Greater Pittsburg, 1895*)

and massage. The treatments were marketed as being useful for "nervousness, rheumatism, general debility, neuralgia, sleeplessness, epilepsy, indigestion, lung troubles and typhoid fever." Like homeopathy, the city's mainstream physicians viewed such practices with skepticism.

July 1894

The Oakland Private Hospital was located on the corner of Fifth Avenue and Bouquet Streets in the city's Oakland area. Dr. D. E. Wiles developed the hospital as a hybrid healthcare facility offering a list of services, including treatment of diseases of women, nervous diseases, lying-in (bed rest before and after delivery), and addiction treatment.

May 1895

Eye and Ear Hospital was chartered to minister to all those who suffered from any disease of the eye and ear and were unable to pay. The hospital offered medical and surgical treatment of diseases of the eye, ear, nose, and throat.[15]

Specialty Practices Evolve

The Civil War provided an opportunity for physicians and surgeons to treat large numbers of patients with similar diseases and injuries. Baptism by fire in war proved cathartic, as the sheer volume of patients and the intensity of their wounds and illnesses proved to be a remarkable laboratory in which physicians became experts in specialized treatments or procedures. Those who became specialists, either in the field or as surgeons in the Army specialty hospitals, returned home to apply their newfound skills. Pittsburgh benefitted from their experiences. Some of the earliest specialists in the city included:

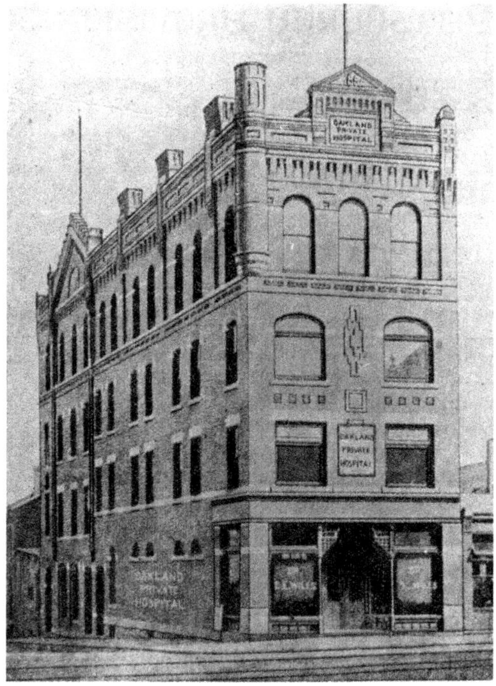

The Oakland Private Hospital. (*J. M. Kelly's Handbook of Greater Pittsburg, 1895*)

John J. Buchanan

The son of a Civil War surgeon, J. J. Buchanan was born in Wellsville, Ohio, in 1855. His family moved to Allegheny City after the war. In 1873, Buchanan enrolled at Western University of Pennsylvania and graduated four years later. He attended medical school at the University of Pennsylvania and received his medical degree in 1881. Buchanan served an internship at Western Pennsylvania Hospital, where he studied surgery under Dr. James McCann and others. At West Penn, his surgical skills were perfected during a period when the hospital was treating more industrial accident victims than any other institution in the country. Following the internship, his father helped him obtain a position as a surgeon to the Pennsylvania Railroad. He also served as a surgeon at the Pittsburgh Free Dispensary. In 1884, along with Drs. Koenig, Werder, and Shaw, he was one of the creators of the *Allegheny County Medical Bulletin*, the city's first permanent medical journal. The year 1892 was particularly rewarding for Buchanan. He was named to the new permanent medical staff of Mercy Hospital, and in July, he performed life-saving surgery on noted Pittsburgh industrialist, Henry Clay Frick, after a failed assassination attempt by anarchist Alexander Berkman. The extensive training he had received in surgically treating traumatic injuries was put to good use that day. For the next several decades, Buchanan was one of the city's most prominent surgeons. In 1919, upon Frick's death, a donation of $1.4 million was given to Mercy Hospital. The gift was the largest given to a Pittsburgh charitable organization up until that time.

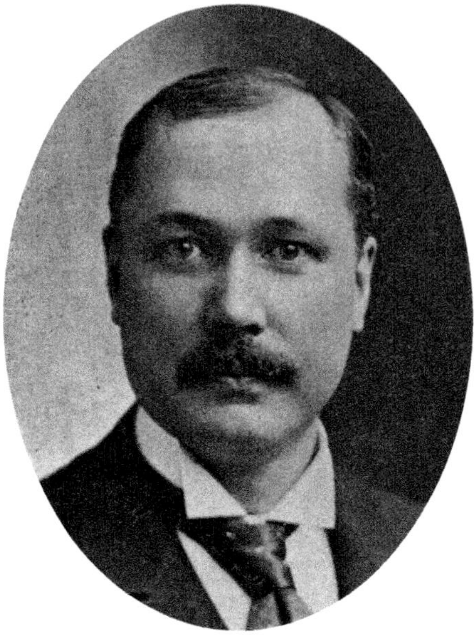

John J. Buchanan, M.D. (*Carnegie Library of Pittsburgh. All rights reserved. Unauthorized reproduction or usage prohibited*)

William Hudson Daly

Daly, a Civil War veteran who took advantage of the lessons of war, became the first physician in the city to specialize in laryngology. He arrived in the city after graduating from the University of Michigan in 1866. He began his specialty practice late in the 1870s after spending time studying in England and continental Europe. Daly was an accomplished writer who published more than fifty articles. He wrote on topics ranging from gunshot wounds, tonsils, burns, leprosy, and malaria, to his most famous treatise on asthma-related respiratory disorders. This paper drew the attention of the dean of British laryngologists, Sir Morrell Mackenzie, who wrote in the *London Journal of Laryngology and Rhinology*: "There can be no doubt that Dr. Daly may justly be regarded as the founder of the surgical school of rhinology in the United States."[16] Throughout his time in Pittsburgh, he was associated longest with Western Pennsylvania Hospital and the Allegheny County Medical Society. In 1894, he was elected president of the American Laryngological Association, and in 1897 he served as president of the American Laryngological, Rhinological, and Otological Society.

John Milton Duff

A Civil War veteran, Duff was among Pittsburgh's earliest physicians specializing in obstetrics and gynecology. His practice was long associated with South Side Hospital and Western Pennsylvania Medical College. At the College, he was the first Professor of Obstetrics.

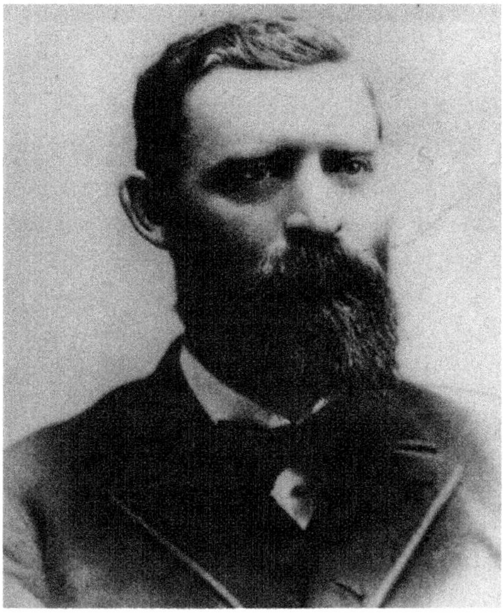

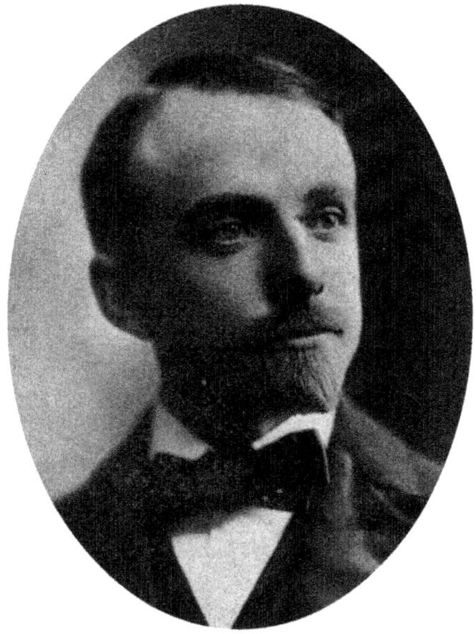

Above left: John Milton Duff, M.D. (*Allegheny County Medical Society*)

Above right: Chevalier Jackson, M.D. (*Carnegie Library of Pittsburgh. All rights reserved. Unauthorized reproduction or usage prohibited*)

Chevalier Jackson

Considered the inventor of the modern bronchoscope and esophagoscope, Jackson was recognized around the world for his expertise in the field of laryngology. Born in Pittsburgh on November 4, 1865, Jackson attended the Western University of Pennsylvania from 1878 until 1882. Following graduation, he apprenticed with Dr. Gilmore Foster, and in 1884, he entered Jefferson Medical School in Philadelphia. He later studied under Sir Morell Mackenzie in England. Mackenzie was one of the world's earliest pioneers of laryngology. In 1887, Jackson returned to Pittsburgh and established an office on Sixth Street near Penn Avenue, which was then considered Pittsburgh's specialist row. With the assistance of Dr. William H. Daly and others, he quickly developed a large practice. In 1890, he invented the esophagoscope, and in 1899, the bronchoscope. In 1900, he became chief of Laryngology at Western Pennsylvania Hospital. In 1902, he decided to improve his esophagoscope by adding light to the instrument. This small enhancement proved to be a remarkable achievement, and the practice of laryngology was changed forever.

James McCann

After serving as assistant surgeon during the Civil War, McCann returned to Pittsburgh, established a private practice, and became a staff surgeon at Western Pennsylvania Hospital and surgeon with Pennsylvania and Lake Erie Railroad. His experiences in the army, hospital, and railroad afforded him the opportunity to become one of the city's preeminent surgeons. Like Dr. Albert G. Walter, McCann was recognized for adoption and advocacy of a "conservative" approach to surgery and antiseptic treatment of wounds and surgical incisions. At Western Pennsylvania Hospital, he associated himself with three other Civil War veterans: Drs. Frank Lemoyne, C. B. King, and J. B. Murdoch. Together, they had an impressive surgical record. Charles R. Wilson, Jr., M.D., noted in 1977: "By 1884, West Penn surgeons had performed more amputations than any hospital in the Country, primarily as a result of railroad and machinery injuries. At the time, the Hospital's average daily census of 177 surpassed that of Pennsylvania Hospital (164), Massachusetts General (168), and St. Luke's, N.Y. (155)."[17] A statistical analysis of the amputations performed at West Penn between January 1877 and January 1884 was published in the October 4, 1884 issue of *The Medical News*. The article reported resident physicians William H. Mercur and Ellwood B. Haworth had documented more amputations were performed at Western Pennsylvania Hospital in 1883 alone than in any other institution in the United States. A majority were the result of railroad injuries.[18]

Alexander M. Speer

Along with Dr. Albert G. Walter, Speer was one of the city's first physicians to specialize in treating diseases of the eyes. Speer had extensive military service during the Civil War, including running one of the country's first specialty hospitals, the U.S. Army Eye and Ear Hospital at Cincinnati. It was this experience that led Dr. Speer to embrace the specialty upon discharge from military service. After leaving the army in 1865, Speer traveled to London and Paris to study ophthalmology. Upon his return, he began his specialty practice.

Rhodes S. Sutton

Dr. Sutton's interest in medicine came early. He was born in 1841 in Indiana, PA, and enjoyed the benefits of good schooling and private tutoring. His mother was the daughter of a Revolutionary War surgeon. Sutton graduated from Jefferson College at Canonsburg in 1862 and enrolled at Jefferson Medical College in Philadelphia. Between early 1863 and the spring of 1864, he served in the military. After discharge, he enrolled at the University of Pennsylvania where he received his medical degree in 1865. In 1866, Sutton moved to Pittsburgh and established a specialty practice focused on the medical and surgical treatment of women. In 1883, he opened The Terrace Bank Sanitarium for Women. At the time, it was one of the largest private hospitals of the kind in the United States.

C. Jane Vincent

Dr. Vincent was Pittsburgh's first resident female physician, as well as one of the area's earliest pediatric specialists. After graduating from Franklin College in Ohio, she studied medicine with Dr. R. S. Hunt in Brookville, PA. She later received a medical degree from Women's Medical College of Pennsylvania. She then spent one year at Nursery and Childs Hospital on Staten Island, New York. She arrived in Pittsburgh in 1883 and became affiliated with United Presbyterian Hospital for Children, the Orphans' Home of the Presbyterian Church, and the Day Nursery. In 1891, Dr. Robert Bruce Mowry reported on her work by writing: "Since Dr. Vincent's arrival in this city she has been conspicuous for her successful practice and her able demonstration of the fact that women not only make thorough physicians, but are perhaps superior to men among their own sex, in their clearer and more delicate apprehension in diagnosing diseases."[19]

Albert G. Walter

Walter was the father of "conservative surgery" in Pittsburgh. In fact, in 1867, he published a book on the topic. He received his education at the University of Konigsberg and spent a year at the University of Berlin where he received additional training in anatomy and orthopedics. He later enrolled at the Royal College of Surgeons in England where he received surgical training from some of the country's leading experts. He moved to Pittsburgh in 1842. The city was the perfect location for him to establish a practice as the city's railroads, mills, and factories produced a significant number of workforce injuries. He developed a thriving practice focusing on industrial accidents. At the time, these injuries typically resulted in amputation—a procedure he felt unnecessary in many cases. With a growing patient base, he refined his skills and saved many limbs that would otherwise have been lost. He became very proficient in preserving mangled limbs and restoring function to the extent that found favor with his patients, his peers, and the community at large. In 1859, Walter reported he successfully treated a traumatic ruptured bladder by laparotomy. It was the first operation of its kind in the city. As his work became better recognized, he expanded his practice to include surgical repair of congenital deformities of the body and the eyes. In the introduction to his 1867 book on conservative surgery, he wrote:

> Having been ardently, and almost exclusively engaged in the profession of Surgery, to which more than thirty years of faithful labor, in public and private practice, have been devoted, in a locality, too, where accidents and injuries caused by machinery were unusually frequent, the author, in treating these cases, soon became convinced that the efforts of Nature at salvation and restoration, in injuries, especially in those of a grave character, and her conservative aims, on which the surgeon, alike as the physician, has mainly to rely, in order to lead the case to recovery, had, alas been too often either entirely overlooked, or plainly misunderstood.
>
> A radical change, therefore, in the surgeon's duty and responsibility in the attendance of these cases, forced itself upon his mind, namely: First—To discard the common routine of practice, sanctioned by age, of sacrificing every limb, with soft and bony

> tissues lacerated and crushed; and Second—To act merely as an intelligent assistant to Nature's wise, bounteous, and marvelously omnipotent vis medicatrix [the healing power of nature]—inherent in the whole of her animal and vegetable creation. With this resolve, he broke the path which he eventually followed, and that he has been well repaid for his exertions, the subjoined treatise will bear ample witness.
>
> The gratification of having rescued, by a conservative practice, hitherto not promulgated, a vast number of persons suffering from the varied catalogue of fearful traumatic injuries, from mutilation, danger, and death, prompts the author to lay his views and experience before his brethren of the profession, thus adding to Surgery another branch of conservative treatment, equal, if not superior, to any other which the genius, learning, and skill of modern surgeons have so much enriched already.[20]

It should be noted by the time he published his book, Walter had performed surgery on a great number of wounded soldiers on the battlefield as well as a significant number of maimed veterans at home.

A few years after he had arrived in the city, he opened a clinic on Boyd's Hill near the city's Courthouse. In 1844, and for several years afterward, he advertised the clinic's services in local newspapers:

> Pittsburgh Infirmary. For the Restoration of Deformities of the Human Frame. The subscriber has returned to the city and intends to establish an Infirmary for the reception of deformed members, such as Club or Reeled feet, contracted joints, wry-neck, and Straubism or Squinting. There is no institution of this kind as yet in the

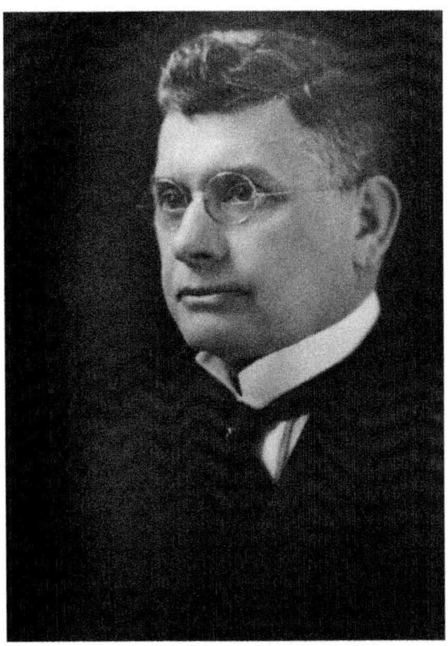

Markley C. Cameron, M.D., specialist in diseases of women. (*Allegheny County Medical Society*)

> country, though much needed. Patients from a distance would find the establishment exclusively devoted to the restoration of the above named deformities. The easy access to Pittsburgh, by river and canal almost at any season of the year, one of the healthiest spots in the country, would offer great facilities for those desirous of being relieved. His ample experience and well know success gives sufficient guaranty that the welfare of those entrusted to his care will be greatly promoted. Albert G. Walter, M.D.[21]

A year later, he refined his advertisements and added details about some of his other specialty work. An advertisement appearing in January 1845 noted he had expanded his services to include "Diseases of the Eye, such as Cataract, etc."[22]

Some other Pittsburgh physicians created specialty practices by the late 1880s. These included Drs. C. B. King, Orthopedic Surgery; W. J. Asdale, Diseases of Women; J. D. Thomas, Genito-Urinary and Venereal Diseases; J. D. Dunn, Diseases of the Skin; A. G. Case, Diseases of Children; Herman W. Hechelman, Diseases of the Nose and Throat; John S. Mabon, Diseases of the Nose and Throat; Charles W. Wilkin, Obstetrics; M. C. Cameron, Diseases of Women; H. R. O'Connor, Genito-Urinary and Venereal Diseases; W. T. Burleigh, Diseases of the Skin; and, W. C. Bane, Diseases of the Eye and Ear.

Advancing Medical Education: Pittsburgh's Early Medical Journals

Once specialty practices and institutions began to emerge, there was renewed interest in publishing medical reports and case studies. While some of Pittsburgh's leading practitioners had written books and submitted articles to national journals over the past several decades, there was a noticeable void in the publication of local professional journals. To promote these new specialty practices and institutions, it was increasingly important for physicians in the region to become aware of these new services and potential advantages. Without the benefit of awareness, opportunities for referrals and admissions would suffer.

The first documented attempt was made in 1819 with the publication of the *Western Eclectic Repertory, and Analytical Review, Medical and Philosophical*. Created by two physicians, Drs. J. Lewis and D. M. Kirkpatrick the project was short-lived.[23] The next publication that had wide distribution in the city—at least among those practicing homeopathy—was *The Hahnemannian Monthly*, which was published in Philadelphia but distributed widely in Pittsburgh. The publication was initiated in August 1865. The introduction to the first volume illustrated the tension that existed between the homeopaths and those practicing traditional, or allopathic, medicine.

> While we are strongly impressed with the great responsibility of the position we have been persuaded to assume, we earnestly appeal to the forbearance, charity, and support

> of our colleagues; by their assistance we hope to make this periodical a useful and instructive organ, worthy of receiving an equal share of patronage with our respected elder cotemporary, the Review; both aiming to accomplish the same end, both holding the same guiding principles in the practice of our school, both devoted to the further development of the medical sciences founded on the immutable natural laws first applied to the healing art by Samuel Hahnemann. We will endeavor to disarm our common adversaries and opponents of the Alloeopathic school, by showing them the errors of their proceedings, the means by which they may adopt a better and safer method of cure than they have done hitherto; and for that purpose we will present the readers of the Journal, from time to time, with incontrovertible arguments, especially in the shape of those stubborn facts, "statistics," without which no argument, how ever clearly it may be presented, can successfully be sustained or be of much avail; but arguments sustained and supported by statistics will lead the inquiring mind, in and out of the profession, to investigate; and investigation once honestly undertaken must, as it always does, lead to a full conviction of the truth of Homoeopathy.[24]

Homeopaths were deeply entrenched in the fight for survival, and despite repeated attempts by the allopaths to dismiss their practices as bunkum, these practitioners and their institutions and journal managed to survive into the 1930s. In the last decade of the twentieth century, it was estimated only 1,500 to 2,000 homeopathic physicians were practicing in the United States. The number in Pittsburgh had dwindled to a mere handful. Even though no medical schools existed to replenish the ranks, homeopathic practices were at the time enjoying a renewed interest among naturopaths, acupuncturists, and research institutions, and their appeal remained strong to a small segment of the general population.[25]

Dr. Robert Gallagher launched another mainstream medical periodical, the *Pittsburgh Medical Journal*, in 1880. It too was transitory, lasting only three years. In 1886, the *Pittsburgh Medical Review* was yet another attempt. This periodical, initiated by Dr. X. O. Werder survived and later became the *Pennsylvania Medical Journal*, the first official organ of a State Medical Society in the United States.[26] In January 1890, the *Journal* reflected on the ongoing battle against homeopathy. In that issue, the editor, Dr. Adolph Koenig, with commentary, reproduced an address published in the *Journal of the American Medical Association* that read:

> HOMOEOPATHY AND MEDICAL PROGRESS.—
> The address of Dr. Nathan Jacobson before the Syracuse Medical Association, published in the Journal of the American Medical Association for March 15, should be read by every member of the profession. It is entitled "Homoeopathy and Medical Progress During the Present Century," and is a historical and critical review of what we believe to be an expiring sect. Its perusal is particularly recommended to those gentlemen, who while deriding the absurdities of Hahnemannism, believe that it has had a good influence on medicine. Such a belief can exist only with ignorance of the precepts of homoeopathy.

> The advances of medicine have been in the lines of rationalism, not mysticism; they are due to work in the laboratory and by the bedside, assisted by chemistry, physiology, pathology, by the microscope and the thermometer; they have not been, and can never be, aided by the speculative fancies of dogmatists or the partial and inaccurate observations of hare brained sectaries. Whatever of indirect benefit has accrued to medical science from other schisms and sects, homoeopathy has had no such influence. Hahnemannism is the Boeotia of medicine, out of which can come no good thing.[27]

From its beginning in 1886 until transitioning into the *Pennsylvania Medical Journal*, the *Pittsburgh Medical Review* carried the latest news of medical advances in the city as well as around the country and the world. While a majority of the local articles highlighted the work of the city's specialty practitioners, numerous other articles routinely condemned quackery. The primary target was most often homeopathy. However, purveyors of patent medicines were held in even lower esteem. In the January 1890 edition of the *Review*, Dr. Koenig wrote the following editorial:

> DRUGGISTS AS AGENTS FOR QUACK MEDICINES.—Under the present method of medical practice, and in the absence of sufficient legal enactments governing the sale of drugs, the relationship existing between the physician and the pharmacist is both necessary and intimate. That their intercourse may be satisfactory a feeling of mutual esteem and confidence is essential. From the physician's standpoint faith in the honesty, as well as in the skill, of the pharmacist is emphatically necessary, for it is the only guarantee he can have that his prescriptions are properly compounded and that he and his patient are not abused. As a rule this confidence in the integrity and uprightness of the druggist is not withheld, but it is at the price of much charitable forbearance on the doctor's part, and in spite of the ocular evidence presented in every drug store of patent-medicine placards, wrapping papers in which the doctor's prescriptions are enclosed, advertising some nostrum to his patient, almanacs for gratuitous distribution, and all the other man-traps known to quackery, for which the druggist is the cheerful and energetic agent.
>
> This offense is of universal prevalence and of great antiquity, and in justification of it the druggist is accustomed to say to the physician that the people demand these patent medicines, and that if he does not supply them his neighbor will, and so the press of competition forces him into the business, in which he is but a passive agent. These are conspicuous instances of the evil that exists in high places, and they certainly indicate the urgent need of a more wholesome business code in the drug trade.[28]

Dr. Koenig and the *Review* were on target in expressing rage over quacks and the sale of patent medicines. Their anger, and that of other physicians around the country, would continue until the passage of The Pure Food and Drug Act in 1906. The Act prohibited interstate transportation of impure and contaminated food and drugs and required labeling that identified the composition and quantity of a large range of drugs, including opium, morphine, heroin, cannabis, and alcohol.

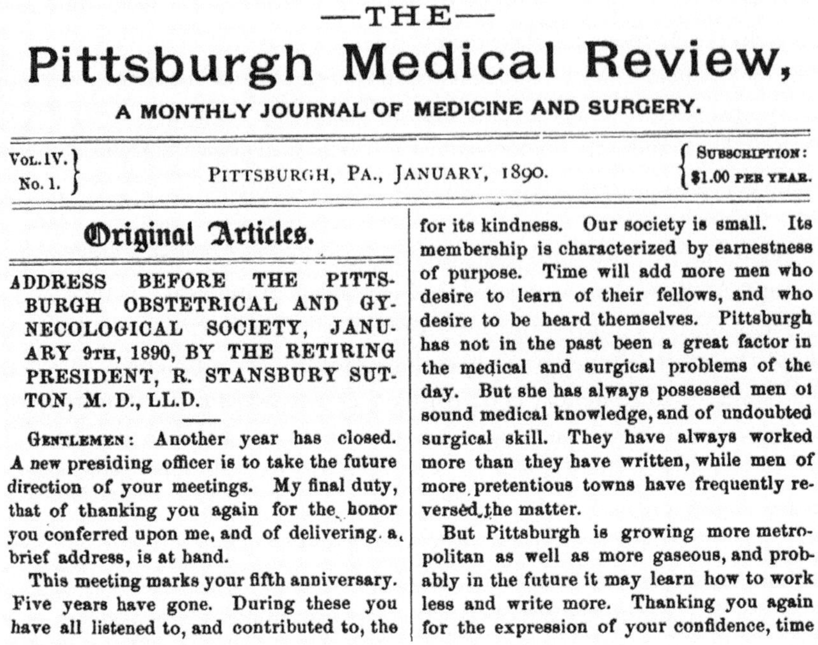

—THE—

Pittsburgh Medical Review,

A MONTHLY JOURNAL OF MEDICINE AND SURGERY.

VOL. IV. No. 1. PITTSBURGH, PA., JANUARY, 1890. SUBSCRIPTION: $1.00 PER YEAR.

Original Articles.

ADDRESS BEFORE THE PITTSBURGH OBSTETRICAL AND GYNECOLOGICAL SOCIETY, JANUARY 9TH, 1890, BY THE RETIRING PRESIDENT, R. STANSBURY SUTTON, M. D., LL.D.

GENTLEMEN: Another year has closed. A new presiding officer is to take the future direction of your meetings. My final duty, that of thanking you again for the honor you conferred upon me, and of delivering a brief address, is at hand.

This meeting marks your fifth anniversary. Five years have gone. During these you have all listened to, and contributed to, the for its kindness. Our society is small. Its membership is characterized by earnestness of purpose. Time will add more men who desire to learn of their fellows, and who desire to be heard themselves. Pittsburgh has not in the past been a great factor in the medical and surgical problems of the day. But she has always possessed men of sound medical knowledge, and of undoubted surgical skill. They have always worked more than they have written, while men of more pretentious towns have frequently reversed the matter.

But Pittsburgh is growing more metropolitan as well as more gaseous, and probably in the future it may learn how to work less and write more. Thanking you again for the expression of your confidence, time

Above: Pittsburgh Medical Review masthead 1890. (*HathiTrust*)

Below left: X. O. Werder, M.D., creator of the *Pittsburgh Medical Review*.

Below right: Adolph Koenig, M.D., editor of the *Pittsburgh Medical Review*. (*Allegheny County Medical Society*

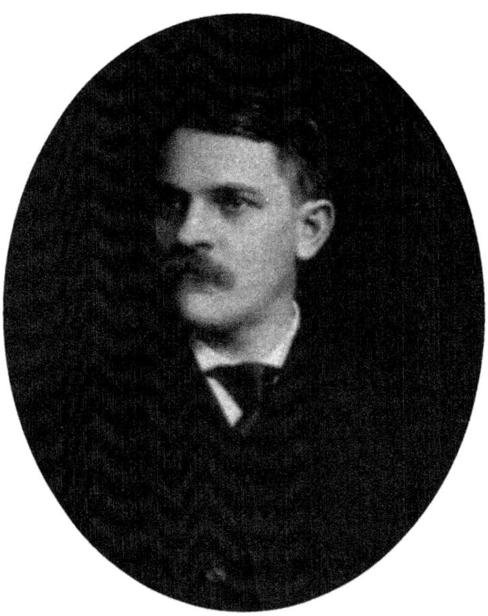

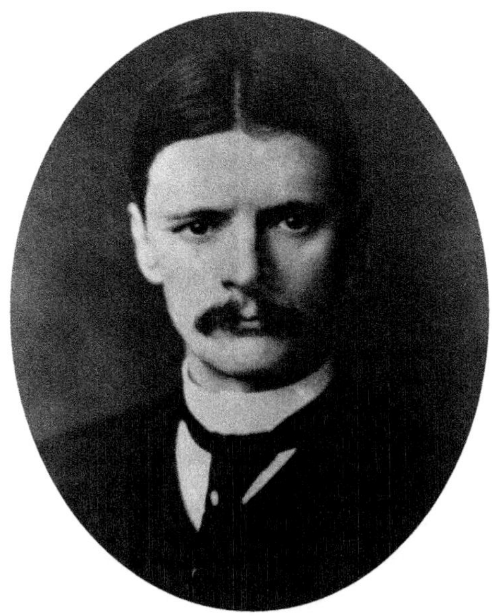

Conclusion

The changes that took place in the practice of medicine and the delivery of healthcare in Pittsburgh before, during and immediately following the Civil War were dramatic. Rip Van Winkle may have slept through the American Revolution, but the city's doctors did not sleep through the Civil War. In four years, they were transformed, as were the city's hospitals and health service organizations. The changes over the last decades of the nineteenth century were similarly profound, and much of the transformation that took place was directly attributable to the city's physician-soldiers and the experiences they gained during the war.

While the United States was at war with itself, clinicians and researchers across the world were busy advancing scientific medicine. New diagnostic tools and procedures were being developed and deployed with increasing regularity. Private and university-based scientific and clinical laboratories were established, and their discoveries were readily adopted. Many physicians began utilizing a robust experimental design. Germ theory was slowly but surely displacing the old miasmatic model.

Before the Civil War, it would take decades for European advances to influence medical practice in the United States. Now, such improvements became routine. Upon their post-war return to Pittsburgh, the city's physicians immediately applied what they had learned from their war experiences. A new era in medicine had dawned. The city now had a cadre of highly trained and experienced doctors who were eager to embrace and apply these discoveries. Expectations for professionalism and self-regulation were now the rule rather than the exception. Modern medicine in Pittsburgh had indeed arrived.

Specialty medical practices and hospitals emerged; professional societies and scientific journals communicated discoveries and informed clinicians on best practices; and, public health standards were drafted and regulations adopted. A new medical college assured the city of an ample supply of better-trained physicians than ever before.

Competitive maneuvering between the hospitals was ongoing. Generally, the contest was between homeopaths and allopaths, with each group seeking dominance in the local market. Confrontations occurred regularly in professional settings and newspaper editorials. Their debates raged for decades with little effect. The battle over prominence and technology, however, was a different matter. Technology was an area where one institution could easily outdo the other.

By the 1880s, nursing was an area ripe for competition. Professional nursing improved greatly during and immediately after the Civil War. The roles that Dorothea Dix and the Sisters of Mercy played in elevating nursing to a profession have already been described. There were many other individual men and women, and religious orders, who provided critical nursing services during the war. While Dix and the Sisters of Mercy had a more direct impact on healthcare in Pittsburgh, all those who served as nurses during the war played a role in advancing nursing as a career choice nationally. Without the benefit of battlefield training, other methods for educating nurses had to be developed.

The first school of nursing to develop in Pittsburgh was located at the Homeopathic Medical and Surgical Hospital. The Shadyside School of Nursing was opened in 1884. It was founded by three of the hospital's physicians. The gauntlet was thrown, and it would only be a matter of time before other hospitals followed. In 1892, the Western Pennsylvania Hospital opened the Western Pennsylvania Hospital Training School for Nurses. In 1894, it took a dramatic step forward by becoming the first to admit male students. Mercy Hospital opened its nursing school in 1893. Dixmont and South Side Hospitals opened theirs in 1895.

Considering that industrial accidents were routine during this period, emergency surgical services were a large part of the business for all of the city's hospitals. Western Pennsylvania Hospital's location near the railroad was advantageous in this regard, as was its ambulance service, which was considered one of the best in the city.

In the battle over technology, West Penn leaped ahead in 1886 to become the first institution in the city to install a telephone switchboard. With the switchboard and celebrated ambulance service, the hospital was now a logical first choice for emergency care. The same year, West Penn also became the first and only hospital in the city to become affiliated with the Western Pennsylvania Medical College. The battle for prestige and dominance was in full bloom.

In the last fifteen years of the nineteenth century, other major medical advances took place in the city. The most noteworthy was recognition of the value of Wilhelm Roentgen's discovery of X-rays. Physicians reading the latest medical journals learned of the discovery; those associated with the military found an immediate application. Six months after its discovery, on 10 June 1896, Roentgen's tube was used by the U.S. Army to locate a bullet in a victim who had been accidentally shot.[1] A cascade of other reports on the successful use of X-rays followed, and by the next year, Adolph Koenig, editor of the *Pittsburgh Medical Review* was reporting

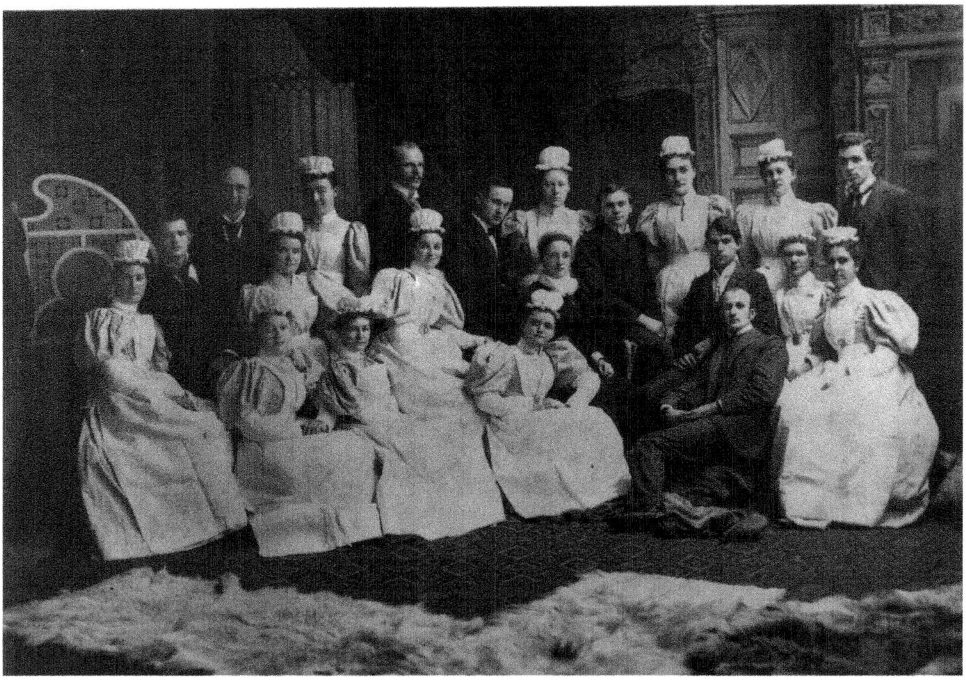

The Western Pennsylvania Hospital Training School for Nurses, student class, *c.* 1895. (*The Western Pennsylvania Hospital*)

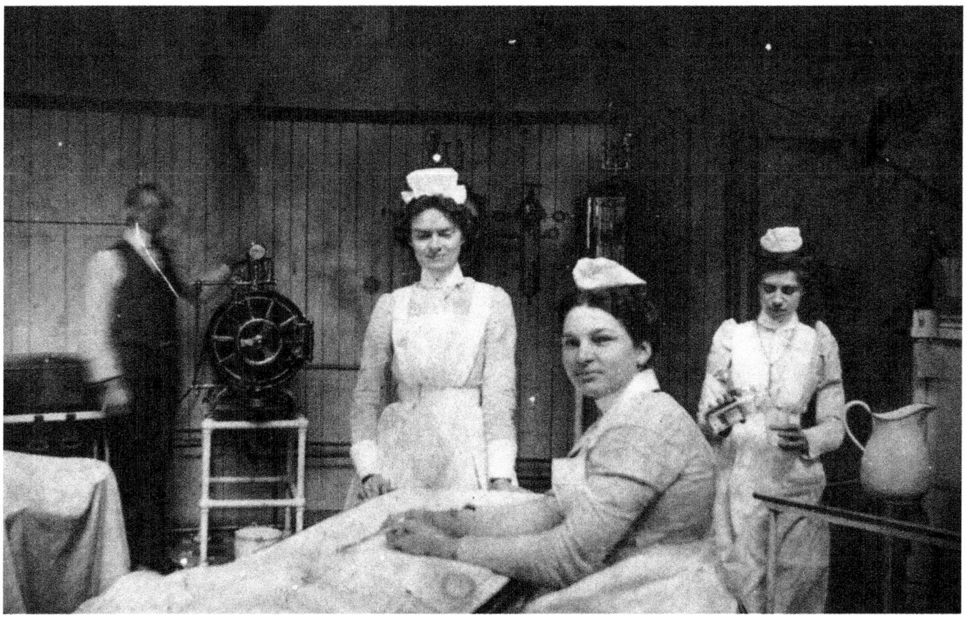

Western Pennsylvania Hospital operating room nurses, *c.* 1895. (*The Western Pennsylvania Hospital*)

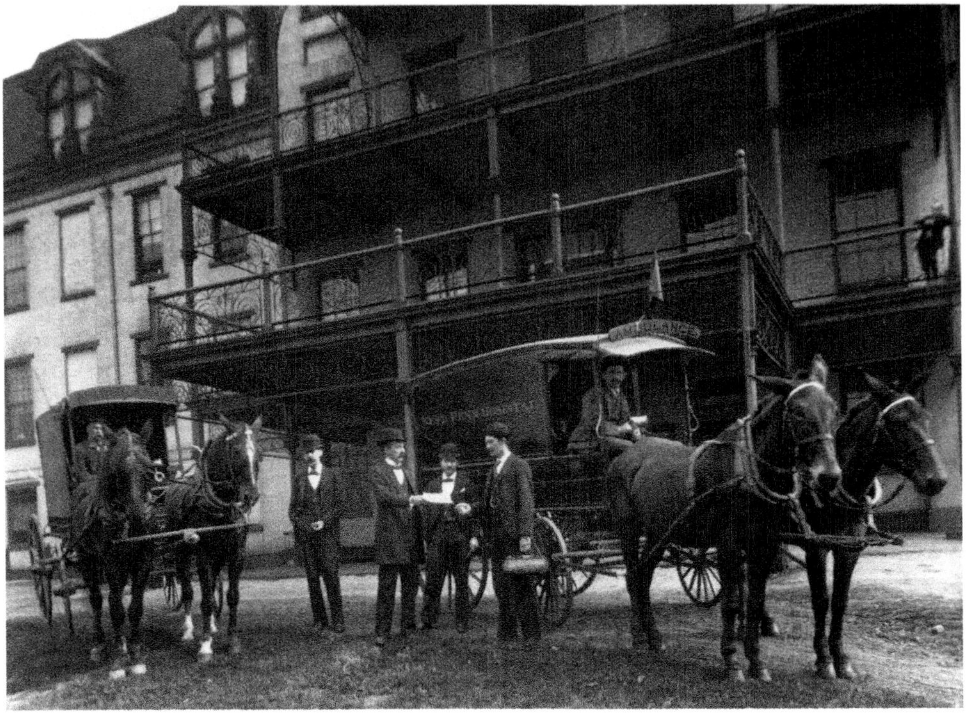

Western Pennsylvania Hospital ambulances, *c.* 1895. (*The Western Pennsylvania Hospital*)

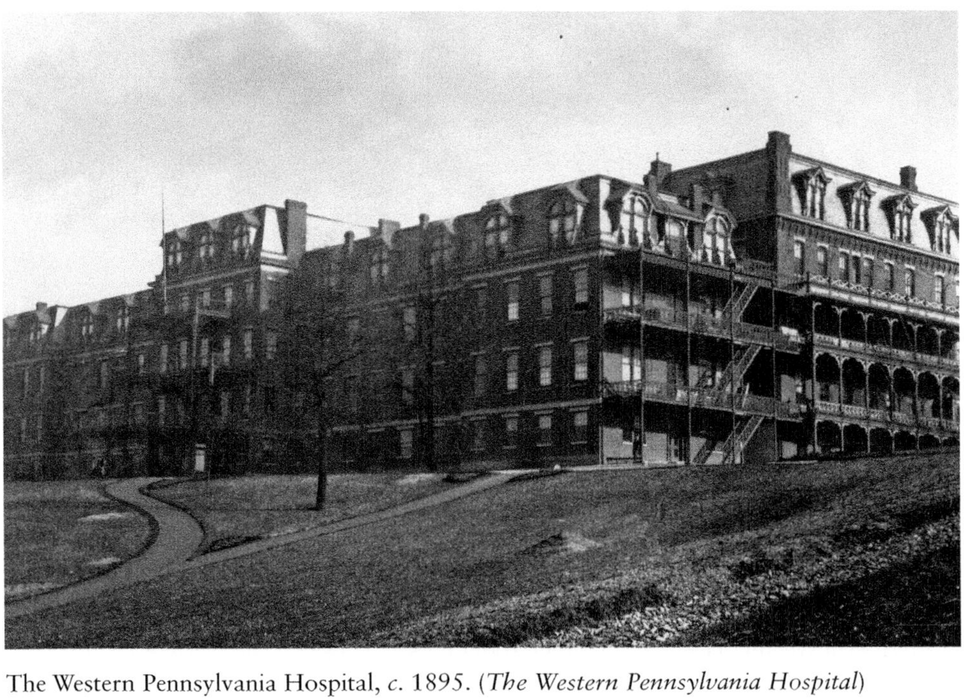

The Western Pennsylvania Hospital, *c.* 1895. (*The Western Pennsylvania Hospital*)

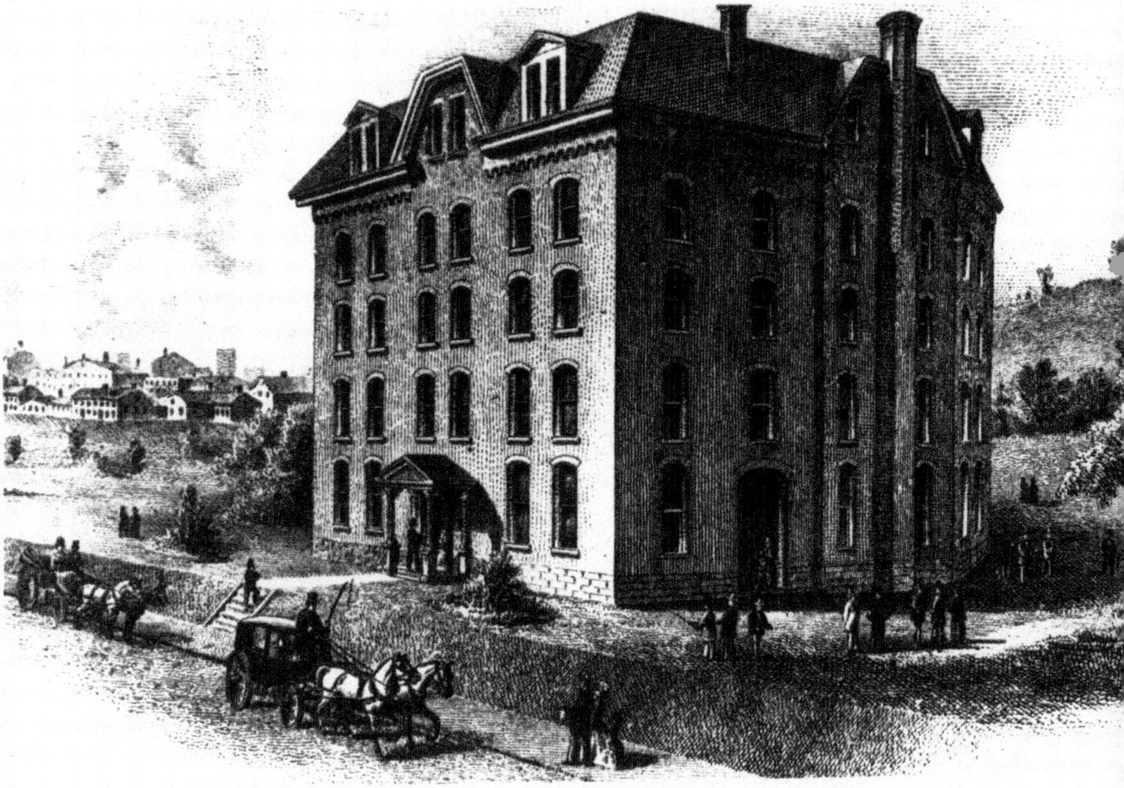

Western Pennsylvania Medical College. (*The Western Pennsylvania Hospital*)

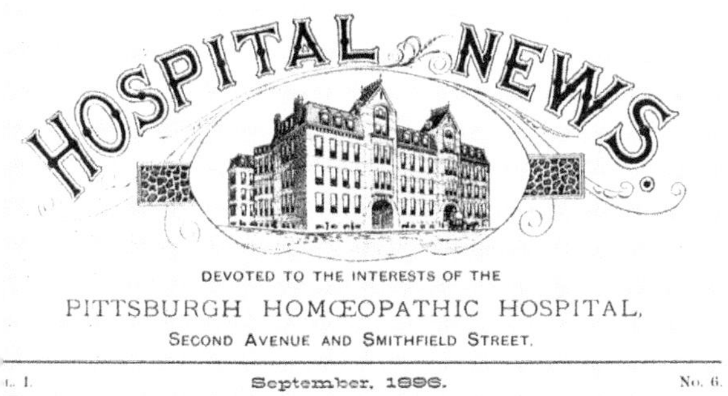

HOSPITAL NEWS

DEVOTED TO THE INTERESTS OF THE
PITTSBURGH HOMŒOPATHIC HOSPITAL,
SECOND AVENUE AND SMITHFIELD STREET.

September, 1896. No. 6.

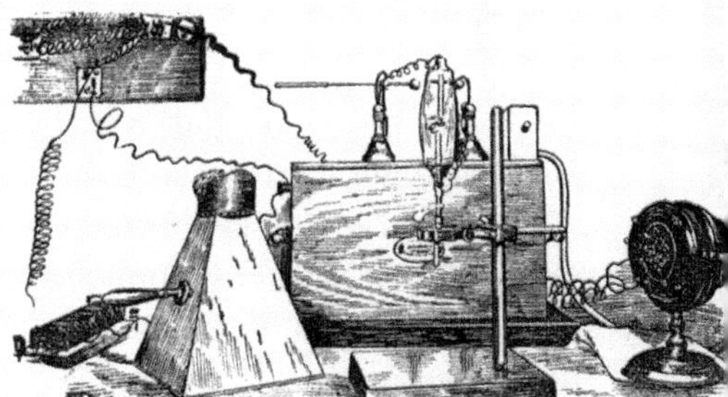

OUR X-RAY APPARATUS.

Above left: Pittsburgh Homeopathic Hospital "Hospital News" masthead 1896. (*Hospital News: September 1896*)

Above right: Pittsburgh Homeopathic Hospital X-Ray Apparatus. (*Hospital News: "Our X-Ray Apparatus," September 1896*)

on its clinical value. Shortly afterward, the Pennsylvania Medical Society met in Pittsburgh, and the Allegheny County Medical Society read a paper titled "The X-ray and its Use in Medicine and Surgery."[2]

Within a few short years, the X-ray had become a critical diagnostic tool. The Homeopathic Medical and Surgical Hospital was the first hospital to install an X-ray apparatus during the summer of 1896. The homeopaths were greatly amused to see a steady stream of allopathic physicians from West Penn and Mercy request invitations to view this modern diagnostic marvel.[3]

As the nineteenth century came to a close, it was clear medicine in Pittsburgh had evolved spectacularly. Within one generation, public perception of the value of doctors and hospitals was markedly improved.

During the last few years of the decade, medical advancements in Pittsburgh continued. Dr. Chevalier Jackson forever changed the field of laryngology by improving on his inventions of the bronchoscope and esophagoscope. Jackson's mentor, Dr. William Hudson Daly, likewise challenged the status quo by provoking a national debate over the safety and wholesomeness of feeding soldiers preserved beef during the Spanish-American War.

At the outbreak of war, Daly was quick to volunteer, as did the Managers of the Western Pennsylvania Hospital. West Penn was the first Pennsylvania Hospital to respond to Gov. Daniel H. Hasting's appeal for assistance in caring for sick and wounded returning from the Spanish-American War. As noted in the hospital's annual report for 1898:

> The management was the first to anticipate the Governor's application for extension of hospital care to soldiers of the army then and now on active duty in the Spanish War. Shortly after the breaking out of hostilities, it instructed the Superintendent to receive such soldiers on the same terms and as freely as he is required to do for veterans of the War of the Rebellion.[4]

Much like the Civil War when the hospital was turned over to the U.S. Army, hospital administrators wore their patriotism with great pride.

The hospital provided services to war veterans through the first quarter of the twentieth century. In its annual report for the period ending on September 30, 1901, it was noted eighty-three soldiers had been admitted for a total of 1,716 days. Since the end of the Civil War, soldiers had spent a total of 79,230 days in the hospital.[5] The pattern continued for many years. In 1924, it was reported that fifty-six veterans had been admitted.

Early in the Spanish-American War, Dr. Daly was named Surgeon-in-Chief of the Volunteer Army of Pennsylvania and appointed major and chief surgeon of the U.S. Volunteers under his old friend, General Nelson A. Miles. He served in various capacities, including field surgeon in charge of a camp, and surgeon-in-charge of bringing a shipload of sick and wounded home from Cuba. Daly showed himself to be in the vanguard of public sentiment when he took on the beef industry at the turn of the century. Six years before the nation passed The Pure Food and Drug Act, Daly became enmeshed in a controversy popularly referred to as the "embalmed beef scandal." Having found the purveyors of beef to the military were experimenting on meat by using hazardous preservatives like boracic and salicylic acid, Daly convinced General Miles to take on the Goliaths of the War Department—Secretary of War Russell A. Alger and Commissary General Charles P. Eagan. The ensuing trial attracted national attention and resulted eventually in the forced resignation of Alger and the court-martial of Eagan.[6] Daly's role in bringing attention to the activities of the meatpacking industry cannot be overstated. The sensational outcome of the hearings and subsequent events remained in the news for months and caught the public's attention. It was not long before Upton Sinclair, and others instigated a clarion call for government intervention.

Sinclair's book, *The Jungle*, published in 1906, exposed unsanitary practices and sweatshop working conditions in Chicago meatpacking. Shortly after publication, President Theodore Roosevelt began receiving hundreds of letters a day demanding action. In response, Sinclair was invited to the White House to provide Roosevelt with a firsthand account of his findings. On a parallel track, Samuel Hopkins Adams was busy exposing the fraudulent practices of the country's patent medicine manufacturers through his *The Great American Fraud* series in *Collier's Weekly* magazine. The public outcry was deafening and now loud enough to require action. Roosevelt ordered an investigation resulting in two landmark pieces of legislation.

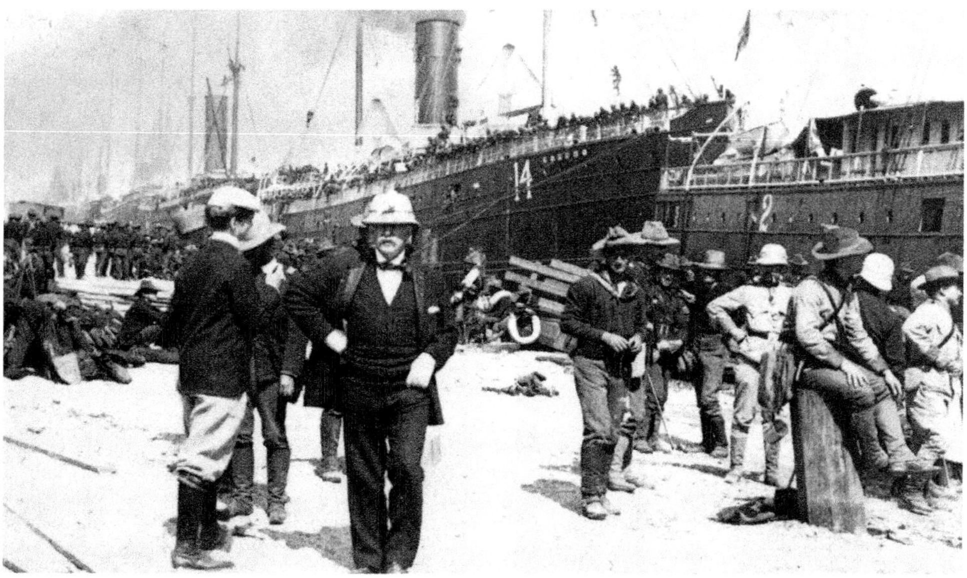

Major General Miles and army transports preparing to sail from Tampa, Florida, 1898. (*Library of Congress*)

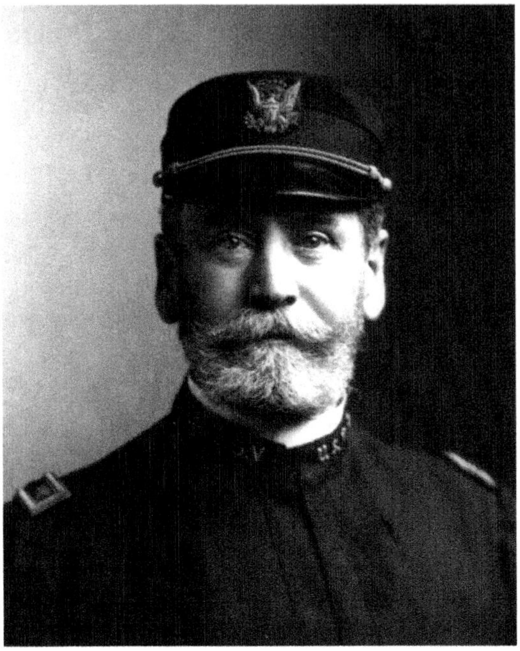

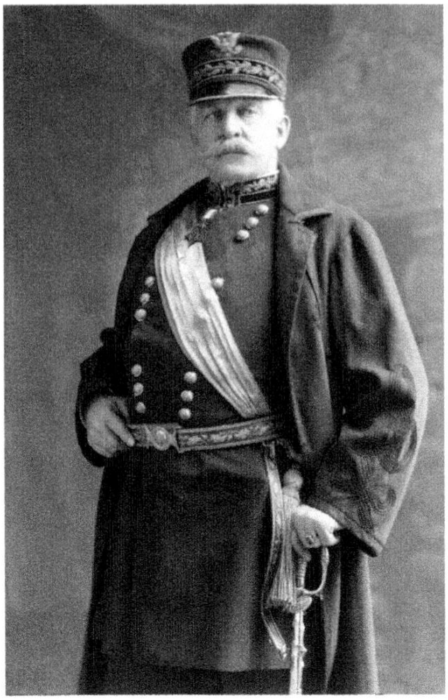

Above left: William Hudson Daly, *c.* 1899. (*National Library of Medicine*)

Above right: General Nelson A. Miles. (*Library of Congress*)

Below left: Secretary of War Russell A. Alger. (*Library of Congress*)

Below right: "Embalmed Beef" investigation report and testimony, 1899. (*National Library of Medicine*)

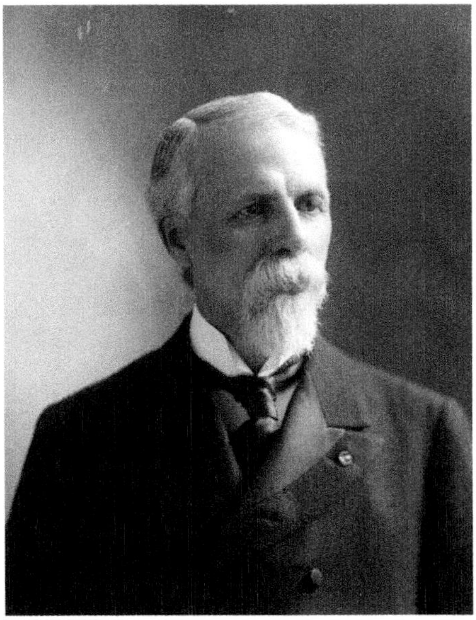

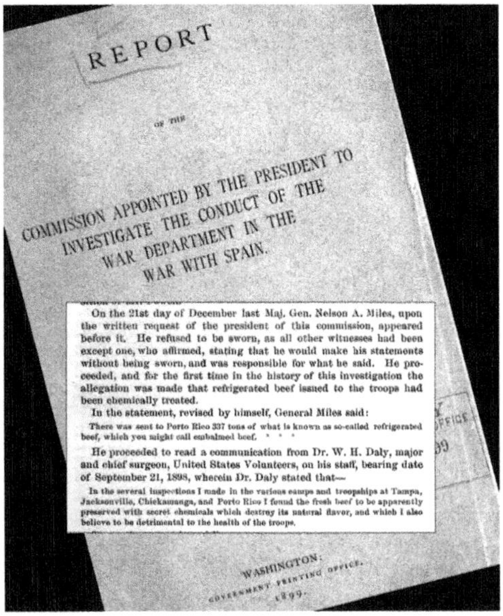

REPORT

OF THE

COMMISSION APPOINTED BY THE PRESIDENT TO INVESTIGATE THE CONDUCT OF THE WAR DEPARTMENT IN THE WAR WITH SPAIN.

On the 21st day of December last Maj. Gen. Nelson A. Miles, upon the written request of the president of this commission, appeared before it. He refused to be sworn, as all other witnesses had been except one, who affirmed, stating that he would make his statements without being sworn, and was responsible for what he said. He proceeded, and for the first time in the history of this investigation the allegation was made that refrigerated beef issued to the troops had been chemically treated.

In the statement, revised by himself, General Miles said:

There was sent to Porto Rico 337 tons of what is known as so-called refrigerated beef, which you might call embalmed beef. * * *

He proceeded to read a communication from Dr. W. H. Daly, major and chief surgeon, United States Volunteers, on his staff, bearing date of September 21, 1898, wherein Dr. Daly stated that—

In the several inspections I made in the various camps and troopships at Tampa, Jacksonville, Chickamauga, and Porto Rico I found the fresh beef to be apparently preserved with secret chemicals which destroy its natural flavor, and which I also believe to be detrimental to the health of the troops.

WASHINGTON:
GOVERNMENT PRINTING OFFICE.
1899.

On 30 June 1906, The Pure Food and Drugs Act and The Meat Inspection Act were enacted. Passage of these laws marked the beginning of determined Federal efforts to assure Americans a safe food and drug supply.

These were exciting times in medicine as improvements continued against a backdrop of war. On a similar trajectory with Daly's campaign against impure food, Major Walter Reed and his team were working to control typhoid fever and eliminate yellow fever in the army. Like Daly, the results of Reed's work would benefit soldiers and civilians alike.

At the dawn of the new century, there was much to be thankful for in Pittsburgh. Over the previous thirty-five years, scientific medicine advanced to such a degree the period might justly be considered the silver age of medicine in the city. With experience gained, lessons learned, and medical infrastructure built, the foundation was laid for what would soon become the twentieth century's golden age of medicine.

Through it all, Pittsburgh's physician-soldiers and their supporters led the charge.

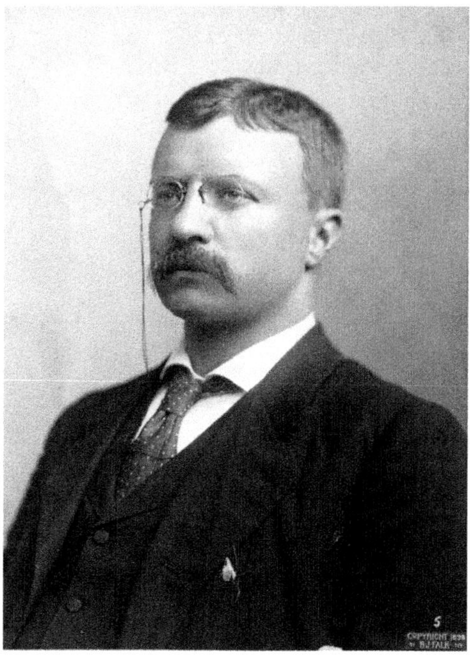

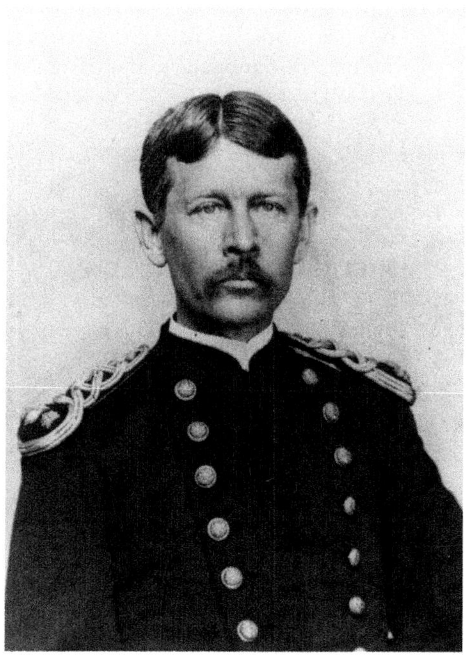

Above left: Colonel Theodore Roosevelt, 1898. (*Library of Congress*)

Above right: Walter Reed. (*National Library of Medicine*)

Endnotes

Introduction

1. The term "forks" is used throughout this book to describe the area of confluence where the Monongahela and Allegheny rivers meet to form the Ohio River in Pittsburgh.

Chapter 1

1. Davis, "Pioneer Physicians of Western Pennsylvania, The President's Address of the Medical Society of the State of Pennsylvania, Delivered at Philadelphia, September 24, 1901" (Reprinted from the *Pennsylvania Medical Journal*, October, 1901), (1901), p. 20.
2. Duffy, John. *The Sanitarians: A History of American Public Health* (1992), p. 9.
3. *Ibid.*
4. *Ibid.*, p.10.
5. Gibson, *Dr. Bodo Otto and the Medical Background of the American Revolution* (1937), pp. 43–52.
6. Smith, *The Indian doctor's dispensatory, or Every man his own physician* (1833), p. 102.
7. *Ibid.*, p. 103.
8. Jones, *Tales of an Indian camp, Vol. 1* (1829), p. 140.
9. Doddridge, *Notes on the Settlement and Indian Wars* (1912), p 24.
10. Gunn, *Gunn's Domestic Medicine or Poor Man's Friend, Thirteenth Edition* (1839), p. 146.
11. Gist, *Instructions given Mr. Christopher Gist by the Committee of the Ohio Company the 11th day of September 1750 [and July 16th 1751. Also, the daily record of Christopher Gist, containing an account of his travels discoveries, transactions with the Indians, etc., from 1750 to 1752* (1880).
12. *Ibid.*
13. Twiss, "Medical Practice in Colonial America," (1960), p 541.

Chapter 2

1. Gibson, *Dr. Bodo Otto and the Medical Background of the American Revolution* (1937), p. 44.
2. Davis, "Pioneer Physicians of Western Pennsylvania, The President's Address of the Medical Society of the State of Pennsylvania, Delivered at Philadelphia, Sept. 24, 1901" (Reprinted from the *Pennsylvania Medical Journal*, October, 1901). (1901), pp. 43–44.
3. Duffy, *From Humors to Medical Science* (1993), p. x.
4. *Ibid*, p. 80.
5. Gibson, *Dr. Bodo Otto and the Medical Background of the American Revolution* (1937), p. 51.
6. Wilson, *Standard History of Pittsburgh Pennsylvania* (1898), p. 604.
7. Buchan, *A Treatise On The Prevention And Cure Of Diseases, By Regimen And Simple Medicines* (1841), p. iv.
8. Rush, *Medical Inquiries and Observations* (1809), p. 446.
9. Duffy, *From Humors to Medical Science* (1993), p. 2.
10. Blanco, "Medicine in the Continental Army, 1775-1781" (1981), p. 677.
11. Doddridge, *Notes on the Settlement and Indian Wars* (1912), pp. 116–120.
12. *Ibid.*, p. 117.
13. *Ibid.*
14. Buchan, *A Treatise On The Prevention And Cure Of Diseases, By Regimen And Simple Medicines* (1841), p. 65.
15. *Ibid.*, p. 81.
16. Nichols, *The Organization of Braddock's Army* (1947), p. 143.

Chapter 3

1. "From George Washington to James Craik, 26 April 1777" (Founders Online, National Archives, last modified February 1, 2018, founders.archives.gov/documents/Washington/03-09-02-0256, [Original source: Chase, Philander D., ed., *The Papers of George Washington, Revolutionary War Series, vol. 9, 28 March 1777–10 June 1777* (1999), pp. 272–273.
2. The British, under General Forbes, captured the ground that Fort Duquesne was built on in November 1758. The French destroyed the fort before evacuating the area. The British built Fort Pitt between 1759 and 1761.
3. Fitzpatrick, *The Last Will and Testament of George Washington and Schedule of his Property, to which is appended the Last Will and Testament of Martha Washington* (1939), p. 17.
4. Davis, "Pioneer Physicians of Western Pennsylvania, The President's Address of the Medical Society of the State of Pennsylvania, Delivered at Philadelphia, Sept. 24, 1901" (Reprinted from the *Pennsylvania Medical Journal*, October, 1901). (1901), p. 15.
5. Baldwin, *Pittsburgh: The Story of a City 1750-1865*, (1937), p. 62.
6. Davis, "Pioneer Physicians of Western Pennsylvania, The President's Address of the Medical Society of the State of Pennsylvania, Delivered at Philadelphia, Sept. 24, 1901" (Reprinted from the *Pennsylvania Medical Journal*, October, 1901). (1901), pp. 21–22.
7. Pontiac's War (also known as Pontiac's Rebellion or Guyasutha's War) took place shortly after the end of the French and Indian War in 1763. Pontiac was the chief of the Ottawa tribe who formed an alliance among many of the tribes along the

Allegheny and Ohio rivers extending to the Great Lakes area. Once the French fortifications and lands were ceded to the British, the American Indian tribes banded together to prevent British settlers from spreading to their lands. It is estimated that from May 1763 until the end of the war in the fall of 1764, Chief Pontiac and his warriors killed or captured more than 600 soldiers and settlers. Many of the participating Indian tribes surrendered to British forces by that time. However, Chief Pontiac remained defiant and did not surrender until the summer of 1766.

8. *Report of the Commission to Locate the Site of the Frontier Forts of Pennsylvania, v2.* (1896), p. 115.
9. Lawrence, "An Account Book of Baynton, Wharton, and Morgan at Fort Pitt, 1765–1767" (1946), p. 144.
10. Dexter, *Diary of David McClure* (1899), p. 29.
11. *Ibid.*, p. 49.
12. Davis, "Pioneer Physicians of Western Pennsylvania, The President's Address of the Medical Society of the State of Pennsylvania, Delivered at Philadelphia, Sept. 24, 1901" (Reprinted from the *Pennsylvania Medical Journal*, October, 1901). (1901), pp. 37–38.
13. Buchan, *A Treatise On The Prevention And Cure Of Diseases, By Regimen And Simple Medicines* (1841), p. 35.
14. Gibson, *Dr. Bodo Otto and the Medical Background of the American Revolution*, (1937), p. 83
15. *Ibid.*, p. 82.
16. Rush, *Medical Inquiries And Observations, The Result Of Observations Made Upon The Diseases Which Occurred In The Military Hospitals Of The United States, During The Revolutionary War Between Great Britain And The United States, Vol. I.* (1818), pp. 147–150.

Chapter 4

1. Davis, "Pioneer Physicians of Western Pennsylvania, The President's Address of the Medical Society of the State of Pennsylvania, Delivered at Philadelphia, Sept. 24, 1901" (Reprinted from the *Pennsylvania Medical Journal*, October, 1901). (1901), p. 39.
2. Twiss, "Medical Practice in Colonial America" (1960), p. 543.
3. Douds, "Merchants And Merchandising In Pittsburgh, 1759–1800" (1937), p. 132.
4. Davis, "Pioneer Physicians of Western Pennsylvania, The President's Address of the Medical Society of the State of Pennsylvania, Delivered at Philadelphia, Sept. 24, 1901" (Reprinted from the *Pennsylvania Medical Journal*, October, 1901). (1901), p. 42.
5. *Ibid.*
6. *Ibid.*, p. 44.
7. Mowry, "The Medical Profession: An Historical Sketch of the Physicians of Allegheny County, During the Last One Hundred Years" (1889), p. 94.
8. Conservative surgery meant operating in a manner that used the least aggressive surgical technique possible in order to preserve the most tissue.
9. *The Pittsburgh Medical Review*, Vol. IV. (1890), p. 207.
10. Grom, "Homeopathy in Pittsburgh: A Historical Perspective" (1995), p. 823.
11. Wilson, *Standard History of Pittsburg Pennsylvania.* (1898), p. 620.

Chapter 5

1. Dix, *Memorial soliciting a state hospital for the insane submitted to the House of Representatives of the Commonwealth of Pennsylvania, February 3, 1845.* (1845), pp. 22–23.
2. *Ibid.*, p. 23.

3. *Ibid.*, p. 24.
4. *Ibid.*, p. 24.
5. *Ibid.*, p. 3.
6. *Pittsburgh Daily Gazette and Advertiser*, 14 July 1857, p. 3.
7. Diller, *Pioneer Medicine in Western Pennsylvania* (1927), p. 185.
8. Riddle, *The Pittsburgh Directory for 1815* (1815), p. 122.
9. *Ibid.*, pp. 185–187.
10. Wilson, *Standard History of Pittsburgh Pennsylvania* (1898), p. 693.
11. Thurston, *Pittsburgh and Allegheny City in the Centennial Year* (1876), p. 30.
12. Boucher, *A Century and a Half of Pittsburgh and Her People, Vol. II.* (1908), pp. 152–153.
13. *Ibid.*, p. 152.
14. *Pittsburgh Daily Gazette and Advertiser*, Thursday, December 27, 1860, p. 2.
15. Mackenzie, *History of the Gazzam Family* (1894), pp. 40–41.
16. *The Rebellion Record of Allegheny County from April 1861 to October 1862* (1862), pp. 11–12.
17. Thurston, *Pittsburgh and Allegheny City in the Centennial Year* (1876), p. 30.
18. *Ibid.*, p. 34.
19. *Ibid.*
20. *The Rebellion Record of Allegheny County from April 1861 to October 1862* (1862), pp. 41–42
21. *The 28th National Encampment of the Grand Army of the Republic, Official Program*, (1894), no page numbers.
22. Killikelly, *The History of Pittsburgh, Its Rise and Progress*, (1906), p. 479.
23. *The Rebellion Record of Allegheny County from April 1861 to October 1862* (1862), p. 41.
24. *The 28th National Encampment of the Grand Army of the Republic, Official Program*, (1894), no page numbers.
25. Miller, "Social Services in a Civil War Hospital in Baltimore" (1945), p. 442.
26. *The 28th National Encampment of the Grand Army of the Republic, Official Program*, (1894), no page numbers.
27. *Ibid.*
28. *Pittsburgh Daily Gazette and Advertiser*, Saturday, April 12, 1862, p. 3. The term "city" refers to the city of Pittsburgh.
29. Fleming, *History of Pittsburgh and Environs, Vol. II.* (1922), p. 235.
30. *Pittsburgh Daily Gazette and Advertiser* (Saturday, 12 April 1862), p. 3.
31. Bakewell, *First Report, Address and Proceedings of the Pittsburgh Sanitary Committee, February 1863* (1863), p. 6.
32. *Pittsburgh Daily Gazette and Advertiser* (Monday, April 28, 1862), p. 3.
33. *Pittsburgh Daily Gazette and Advertiser* (Monday August 4, 1862), p. 1.
34. *A Report to the Secretary of War of the Operations of the Sanitary Commission*, (1861), p. 5.
35. Bakewell, *First Report, Address and Proceedings of the Pittsburgh Sanitary Committee, February 1863* (1863), pp. 11–12.
36. An American Citizen, *The Philanthropic Results of The War in America* (1864), pp. 46–47.
37. *A Report to the Secretary of War of the Operations of the Sanitary Commission*, (1861), p. 11.
38. *Pittsburgh Daily Gazette and Advertiser* (Saturday, April 30, 1864), p. 1.
39. Dorothy, Daniel. "The Sanitary Fair" (1958), p. 146.
40. "Abraham Lincoln papers: Series 1, Image 4. General Correspondence. 1833–1916: Felix R. Brunot, *et al.* to Abraham Lincoln, Friday, April 15, 1864 (Pittsburgh Sanitary Fair)", Library of Congress (1864).

41. Wilson, *Standard History of Pittsburgh Pennsylvania* (1898), p. 601.
42. "Abraham Lincoln papers, Series 1. General Correspondence, 1833–1916: Felix R. Brunot, et al. to Abraham Lincoln, Friday, April 15, 1864, (Pittsburgh Sanitary Fair)", Library of Congress (1864).
43. "Abraham Lincoln papers: Series 1. General Correspondence, 1833–1916: Pittsburgh Sanitary Commission to Abraham Lincoln, Monday, May 02, 1864 (Autograph request)," Library of Congress (1864).
44. "Abraham Lincoln papers: Series 1. General Correspondence. 1833–1916: Felix R. Brunot to Abraham Lincoln, Thursday, June 02, 1864 (Telegram announcing opening of Pittsburgh Sanitary Fair)," Library of Congress (1864).
45. *The Pittsburgh Commercial*, Thursday, June 2, 1864, (1864) p. 2.
46. *The Pittsburgh Commercial*, Thursday, June 2, 1864, (1864) p. 1.
47. Slattery, *Felix Reville Brunot 1820–1898*. (1901), p. 100.
48. Daniel, "The Sanitary Fair" (1958), p. 145.

Chapter 6

1. Brooks, *Civil War Medicine* (1966), p. 12.
2. *Ibid*, p. 41.
3. Flint, *Sanitary Memoirs of the War of the Rebellion* (1867), pp. 43–44.
4. *Ibid.*
5. *Ibid.*
6. Smith, *Volunteer Surgical Aid* (1862), pp. 135–136
7. *Pittsburgh Daily Gazette and Advertiser*, Monday, 23 May 1864, (1864) p. 2.
8. *Revised United States Army regulations of 1861 with an Appendix Containing the Changes and Laws Affecting Army Regulations and Articles of War to June 25, 1863*, (1863), pp. 313–314.
9. "Civil War Army Organization," The Civil War Trust. From www.civilwar.org/learn/articles/civil-war-army-organization (Retrieved April 24, 2018).
10. Brooks, *Civil War Medicine* (1966), p. 127.
11. Barnes, *The Medical and Surgical History of the War of the Rebellion (1861–65), Part III, Volume I, Medical History*, (1888), p. 685.
12. *Ibid.*, (1888), p. 827.
13. Brooks, *Civil War Medicine* (1966), p. 47.
14. *Ibid.*
15. *Ibid.*, p. 48.
16. Barnes, *The Medical and Surgical History of the War of the Rebellion (1861–65), Part III, Volume I, Medical History*, (1888), p. 944.
17. *Ibid.*, (1888), p. 960.
18. *Annual Report of the Managers of the Western Pennsylvania Hospital for 1862*, (1863), p. 8.
19. Medical Staff, U.S.A. General Hospital, Pittsburgh, U.S. Adjutant General's Office. Personnel papers of medical officers and physicians, Record Group 94. National Archives and Records Administration, Washington, D.C.
20. *Revised United States Army regulations of 1861 with an Appendix Containing the Changes and Laws Affecting Army Regulations and Articles of War to June 25, 1863*, (1863), pp. 310–312.
21. "Military surgery, ancient and modern," *United States Service Magazine* (1864), p. 133.

Chapter 7

1. Unless cited otherwise, military and general biographical information for this chapter was drawn from the following sources: *Allegheny County Medical Society Membership History* (internal publication *c.* 1904), Allegheny County Medical Society, Pittsburgh (1904); Mowry, "The Medical Profession", *Cities of Pittsburgh and Allegheny and Their Resources, A Souvenir of Pittsburgh Chronicle Telegraph* (1889); Fleming, *History of Pittsburgh and Environs, Vol. II.* (1922); *Official Army Register of the Volunteer Force of the United States Army for the Years 1861–1865, Part III* (1865); *Pittsburgh Daily Gazette and Advertiser*, Monday, May 1, 1864, p. 3; "Roster of Post and General Hospital Surgeons, Western Pennsylvania Hospital," (Washington, D.C.: Adjutant General's Office, Record Group 94, National Archives and Records Administration, Washington, D.C); Strait, *Roster of all Regimental Surgeons and Assistant Surgeons in the Late War* (1882); Swetnam, *The First Hundred Years, Allegheny County Medical Society*, (1965); *Under the Maltese Cross* (The 155th Regimental Association), (1910).
2. Western Pennsylvania Hospital was turned over to the U.S. Army in 1862. It became known as U.S.A. General Hospital Pittsburgh. In 1865, after the end of the Civil War, it was returned to civilian control, and its former name was reinstated.
3. *Pittsburgh Daily Gazette and Advertiser:* "The Expedition To The Tennessee River—Two Steamers To Be Sent—Volunteer Surgeons and Nurses," Saturday, April 12, 1862, (1862) p. 3.
4. *Railroad Gazette, Volume 22* (1890), p. 247.
5. *Pittsburgh Daily Gazette and Advertiser*, Monday, May 1, 1864, (1864) p. 3.
6. McKenna, Charles F., (ed.), *Under the Maltese Cross, Antietam to Appomattox, Campaigns 155th Pennsylvania Regiment*, (The 155th Regimental Association), (1910), p. 199.
7. *Pittsburgh Daily Gazette and Advertiser,* Monday, May 1, 1864, (1864) p. 3.
8. McKenna, Charles F., (ed.), *Under the Maltese Cross, Antietam to Appomattox, Campaigns 155th Pennsylvania Regiment*, (The 155th Regimental Association) (1910), p. 593.
9. Killikelly, *The History of Pittsburgh* (1906), p. 477.
10. Boucher, *A Century and a Half of Pittsburg and Her People, Vol. 2* (1908), p. 153. (Note: In 1891, Pittsburgh's name was changed by dropping the final -h in response to a requirement of the U.S. Board on Geographic Names. The -h was restored in 1911.
11. *The Press* (Philadelphia, Pennsylvania), Saturday June 27, 1863, (1863), p. 1.
12. *Pittsburgh Daily Gazette and Advertiser*, Monday, October 26, 1863, (1863) p. 3.
13. *Pittsburgh Daily Gazette and Advertiser*, Tuesday, December 22, 1863, (1863) p. 4.

Chapter 8

1. Pittsburgh Chapter Daughters of the American Revolution, *Fort Duquesne and Fort Pitt, Early Names of Pittsburgh Streets* (1899), p. 26.
2. *Ibid.*
3. Fleming, *History of Pittsburgh and Environs, Vol. II*, (1922), p. 272.
4. *Pittsburgh Daily Morning Post,* April 30, 1844, (1844) p. 2.
5. *Pittsburgh Daily Morning Post*, April 1, 1845, (1845) p. 3.
6. Wilson, *Standard History of Pittsburgh Pennsylvania* (1898), p. 602
7. *Daily Morning Post* (Pittsburgh), Wednesday, November 16, 1842, (1842), p. 1.
8. Fleming, *History of Pittsburgh and Environs, Vol. II* (1922), p. 79.
9. *Daily Morning Post* (Pittsburgh), December 16, 1848, (1848), p. 2.

10. *Daily Morning Post* (Pittsburgh), December 2, 1846, (1846), p. 2.
11. *Daily Morning Post* (Pittsburgh), August 4, 1847, (1847), p. 1.
12. *Daily Morning Post* (Pittsburgh), June 9, 1847, (1847), p. 2.
13. Cushing, *History of Allegheny County, Pennsylvania* (1889), p. 712.
14. *Daily Morning Post* (Pittsburgh), October 12, 1847, (1847) p. 2.
15. Boucher, *A Century and a Half of Pittsburg and Her People, Vol. II* (1908), p. 132.
16. *Memoirs of the Pittsburgh Sisters of Mercy*, (1918), p. 256.
17. *Ibid.*
18. *Annual Report of the Managers of the Western Pennsylvania Hospital for 1867* (1868), p. 5.
19. *Ibid.*
20. *Daily Morning Post* (Pittsburgh), March 4, 1847, (1847) p. 2.
21. Cushing, *History of Allegheny County, Pennsylvania, Part I* (1889), p. 417.
22. *Annual Report of the Managers of the Western Pennsylvania Hospital for 1867* (1868), p. 6.
23. *Daily Morning Post* (Pittsburgh), June 25, 1847, (1847), p. 2.
24. *First Annual Report of the Managers of the Western Pennsylvania Hospital, Together with the Act of Incorporation* (1848), p. 3.
25. Wilson, "The Western Pennsylvania Hospital Site" (1989), p. 11.
26. *Daily Morning Post* (Pittsburgh), July 6, 1848, (1848), p. 2.
27. *Daily Morning Post* (Pittsburgh), December 21, 1848, (1848), p. 2.
28. *Annual Reports of the Managers of the Western Pennsylvania Hospital for the years 1850 and 1851* (1851), p. 4.
29. *First Annual Report of the Managers of the Western Pennsylvania Hospital, Together with the Act of Incorporation* (1848), p. 4.
30. Mylin, *Hospitals, Soldiers' Homes and Orphan Schools controlled by the Commonwealth of Pennsylvania, Vol. 1*, (1897), p. 30.
31. Greenawalt, "Public Institutional Care for the Mentally Ill in Allegheny County, Pennsylvania, 1850 to 1900" (1956), p. 55.
32. *Annual Report of the Managers of the Western Pennsylvania Hospital for the Years 1852 and 1853–54* (1854), p. 9.
33. *Ibid.*
34. *Annual Report of the Managers of the Western Pennsylvania Hospital, 1852 and 1853–4* (1854), pp. 22–24.
35. *Ibid.*, p. 6.
36. *Annual Report of the Managers of the Western Pennsylvania Hospital for 1867*, (1868), pp. 6–7.
37. Killikelly, *The History of Pittsburgh, Its Rise and Progress*, (1906), pp. 387–388.
38. *Annual Report of the Managers of the Western Pennsylvania Hospital for 1862* (1863), p. 8.
39. Jolly, *Nuns of the Battlefield* (1977), pp. 200–201.
40. *Ibid.*, p. 199.
41. *Ibid.*, p. 205.
42. *The Daily Pittsburgh Gazette,* August 13, 1864, (1864), p. 1.
43. *Pittsburgh Daily Post*, July 28, 1864, (1864), p. 2.
44. Boucher, *A Century and a Half of Pittsburg and Her People* (1908), p. 132.
45. *Annual Report of the Managers of the Western Pennsylvania Hospital for 1865* (1866), p. 6.
46. *Pittsburgh Daily Gazette*, July 20, 1865, (1865) p. 3.
47. Trombley, "Pennsylvania's Role in the Mexican American War" (2013), p. 117.
48. *Ibid.*, p. 15.
49. The Pittsburgh Infirmary was renamed Passavant Hospital in 1899. To avoid confusion, it should be noted that from 1844–46, Albert G. Walter, M.D., a prominent

Pittsburgh physician, operated a small hospital called the "Pittsburgh Infirmary for the Restoration of Deformities of the Human Fame." Dr. Walter repeatedly ran newspaper advertisements offering to treat "Club or Reeled feet, contracted joints, wry-neck, and Strabismus or Squinting, and Diseases of the Eye, such as Cataract, etc." The hospital was located on Liberty Avenue near the corner of Fourth Street.

50. *Pittsburgh Daily Gazette and Advertiser*, Saturday, May 5, 1849, (1849), p. 3.
51. *Pittsburgh Daily Gazette and Advertiser*, Friday, May 4, 1849, (1849), p. 3.
52. *The Story of Pittsburgh, Volume Number One* (1919), pp. 556–557
53. *Ibid.*, p. 556.
54. *Pittsburgh Daily Gazette and Advertiser*, Monday, May 12, 1862, (1862), p. 3.
55. Glazier, *Peculiarities of American Cities* (1886), p. 333.

Chapter 9

1. Fleming, *Blood Stains in Clinical Trials* (1861), p. 7. Republished from the American Journal of the Medical Sciences, Vol. XXXVII (1859), pp. 84–119.
2. *Ibid.*, dedication page.
3. *Presbyterian Banner* (Pittsburgh), May 11, 1864, (1864), p. 3.
4. Jordan, *Encyclopedia of Pennsylvania Biography* (1914), p. 401.
5. *Pittsburgh Daily Gazette and Advertiser*, May 2, 1864, (1864), p. 3.
6. *Presbyterian Banner* (Pittsburgh), May 11, 1864, (1864), p. 3.
7. Dorwart, "Essential Civil War Curriculum—Civil War Hospitals," essentialcivilwarcurriculum.com/civil-war-hospitals.html. Retrieved April 27, 2018.
8. Wilson and Grom, *Pittsburgh: A City And Its Medicine* (1990), p. 15.
9. Paull, *A Century of Medical Excellence: The History of the University of Pittsburgh School of Medicine* (1986), p. 10.
10. *Ibid.*, p. 17. See also: Mowry, "The Medical Profession: An Historical Sketch of the Physicians of Allegheny County, During the Last One Hundred Years. Cities of Pittsburgh and Allegheny and Their Resources" (Pittsburgh: *Pittsburgh Chronicle Telegraph*, (1889), p. 96. NOTE: List is compiled from both sources. Mowry adds two additional names with titles.
11. Paull, *A Century of Medical Excellence: The History of the University of Pittsburgh School of Medicine* (1986), p. 16.
12. Wilson, and Grom, *Pittsburgh: A City And Its Medicine* (1990), p. 16.
13. Koenig, "Address Before the Pittsburgh Obstetrical and Gynecological Society, January 9th, 1890, By The Retiring President, R. Stansbury Sutton, M.D., LL.D." (1890) pp. 1–5.
14. Adam Reineman was the first president of the Third National Bank of Pittsburgh. He married Emma E. Hechelman on May 1, 1873. Her father was a prominent Pittsburgh physician who had served as a surgeon during the Civil War. Her father was also professor of Diseases of the Eye and Ear at the Medical College.
15. Fleming, *History of Pittsburgh and Environs, Vol. II*, (1922), p. 284.
16. Grom, *No Ordinary Man*, Pittsburgh History, (1991), p. 3.
17. Wilson, "A Historical Review of West Penn's Staff And Departmental Development," (1977), p. 19.
18. Grom, *No Ordinary Man*, Pittsburgh History (1991), p. 5.
19. Mowry, "The Medical Profession: An Historical Sketch of the Physicians of Allegheny County, During the Last One Hundred Years. Cities of Pittsburgh and Allegheny and Their Resources" (Pittsburgh: *Pittsburgh Chronicle Telegraph*, (1889), p. 105.
20. Walter, *Conservative Surgery* (1867), pp. v–vi.
21. *Daily Morning Post* (Pittsburgh), June 18, 1844, (1844), p. 2.
22. *Daily Morning Post* (Pittsburgh), January 18, 1845, (1845), p. 3.

23. Baldwin, *Pittsburgh The Story of a City* (1937), pp. 261–262.
24. *The Hahnemannian Monthly, Vol. 1, No. 1* (1865), p. 4.
25. Grom, *Pittsburgh's Homeopathic Experience,* (1991), p. 25.
26. Wilson and Grom, *Pittsburgh: A City and Its Medicine.* (1990), p. 15.
27. Koenig, "Homeopathy and Medical Progress," (1890), p. 17.
28. Koenig, "Druggists As Agents For Quack Medicines," (1890), pp. 17–18.

Conclusion

1. Engelman and Joy, *Two Hundred Years of Military Medicine,* (1975), p. 12.
2. Swetnam, *Century of Medical Progress 1865–1965* (1965), p. 28.
3. Grom, *Pittsburgh's Homeopathic Experience* (1991), p. 19–20.
4. *Annual Report of the Managers of the Western Pennsylvania Hospital for 1898* (1899), p. 7.
5. *Annual Report of the Managers of the Western Pennsylvania Hospital for 1901* (1902), pp. 5–6.
6. Grom, *No Ordinary Man,* (1991), p. 7.

Bibliography

Abraham Lincoln papers: Series 1. General Correspondence, 1833–1916: Felix R. Brunot, et al. to Abraham Lincoln, Friday, April 15, 1864 (Pittsburgh Sanitary Fair), (Washington, D.C.: Library of Congress).

Abraham Lincoln papers: Series 1. General Correspondence. 1833–1916: Felix R. Brunot to Abraham Lincoln, Thursday, June 02, 1864 (Telegram announcing opening of Pittsburgh Sanitary Fair), (Washington, D.C.: Library of Congress).

Abraham Lincoln papers: Series 1. General Correspondence, 1833–1916: Pittsburgh Sanitary Commission to Abraham Lincoln, Monday, May 02, 1864 (Autograph request), (Washington, D.C.: Library of Congress).

Allegheny County Medical Society Membership History (Pittsburgh: Allegheny County Medical Society, 1904).

An American Citizen, *The Philanthropic Results of The War in America* (New York: Sheldon & Co., 1864).

Annual Reports of the Managers of the Western Pennsylvania Hospital for the years 1850 and 1851 (Pittsburgh: R. C. Stockton, 1851); *Annual Reports of the Managers of the Western Pennsylvania Hospital for the years 1852 and 1853-54* (Pittsburgh: W. S. Haven, 1854); *Annual Reports of the Managers of the Western Pennsylvania Hospital for the years 1862* (Pittsburgh: W. S. Haven & Co., 1863); *Annual Reports of the Managers of the Western Pennsylvania Hospital for the years 1865* (Pittsburgh: W. S. Haven & Co., Pittsburgh, 1866); *Annual Reports of the Managers of the Western Pennsylvania Hospital for the years 1867* (Pittsburgh: W. S. Haven, 1868); *Annual Reports of the Managers of the Western Pennsylvania Hospital for the years 1898* (Pittsburgh: The Meyers & Shinkle Company, 1899); *Annual Reports of the Managers of the Western Pennsylvania Hospital for the years 1901* (Pittsburgh: The Meyers & Shinkle, Co., 1902).

A Report to the Secretary of War of the Operations of the Sanitary Commission (Washington, D.C.: McGill & Withrow, 1861).

Bakewell, T., *First Report, Address, and Proceedings of the Pittsburgh Sanitary Committee* (Pittsburgh: W.S. Haven, 1863).

Baldwin, L. D., *Pittsburgh: The Story of a City 1750–1865*, (Pittsburgh: University of Pittsburgh Press, 1937).

Barnes, J. K., (ed.), *The Medical and Surgical History of the War of the Rebellion (1861–65)* (Washington, D.C.: Government Printing Office, 1870–1888).

Blanco, R. L., "Medicine in the Continental Army, 1775–1781," (New York: *Bulletin New York Academy of Medicine*, Vol. 57, No. 8, October 1981).

Bollet, A. J., *Civil War Medicine: Challenges and Triumphs* (Arizona: Galen Press, Ltd., 2002).

Boucher, J. N., *A Century and a Half of Pittsburgh and Her People, Vol. II* (New York: The Lewis Publishing Company, New York, 1908).

Brooks, S., *Civil War Medicine* (Springfield: Charles C. Thomas, 1966).

Buchan, M.D., W., *A Treatise On The Prevention And Cure Of Diseases, By Regimen And Simple Medicines* (Cincinnati: J. A. James, 1841).

"Civil War Army Organization," The Civil War Trust, www.civilwar.org/learn/articles/civil-war-army-organization, Retrieved April 24, 2018.

Cushing, T., *History of Allegheny County, Pennsylvania* (Chicago: A. Warner & Co., 1889).

Cushing, T., (ed.), *A Genealogical and Biographical History of Allegheny County, Pennsylvania* (excerpted from *History of Allegheny County, Part II,* Chicago, 1889) (Baltimore: Genealogical Publishing, Co., Inc., 1975).

Daniel, D., "The Sanitary Fair" (Pittsburgh: *The Western Pennsylvania Historical Magazine, Vol. 41, No. 2, summer 1958*).

Davis, T. D., "Pioneer Physicians of Western Pennsylvania, The President's Address of the Medical Society of the State of Pennsylvania, Delivered at Philadelphia, Sept. 24, 1901," (Philadelphia: Reprinted from the *Pennsylvania Medical Journal*, October, 1901).

Der Marderosian, A. H., "Colonial drugs and medicine," *Drug Therapy*, July 1976.

Dexter, F. B., *Diary of David McClure* (New York: The Knickerbocker Press, 1899).

Diller, T., *Pioneer Medicine in Western Pennsylvania* (New York: Paul B. Hoeber, Inc., 1927).

Dix, D. L., *Memorial soliciting a state hospital for the insane submitted to the House of Representatives of the Commonwealth of Pennsylvania, February 3, 1845*. (Printed by order of the Legislature of Pennsylvania, February 3, 1845, U.S. National Library of Medicine).

Doddridge, J., *Notes on the Settlement and Indian Wars* (Pittsburgh: John S. Ritenour and Wm. T. Lindsey, 1912).

Douds, H. C., "Merchants And Merchandising In Pittsburgh, 1759–1800," (Pittsburgh: *The Western Pennsylvania Historical Magazine*, Volume 20, Number 2, June 1937).

Dorwart, B. B., "Essential Civil War Curriculum—Civil War Hospitals," essentialcivilwarcurriculum.com/civil-war-hospitals.html. Retrieved April 27, 2018.

Duffy, J., *From Humors to Medical Science* (Urbana: University of Illinois Press, 1993); *The Sanitarians: A History of American Public Health* (Urbana: University of Illinois Press, 1992).

Engelman, R. C., and Joy, R. J. T., *Two Hundred Years of Military Medicine* (Maryland: U.S. Army Medical Department, 1975).

First Annual Report of the Managers of the Western Pennsylvania Hospital, Together with the Act of Incorporation (Pittsburgh: Geo. Parkin & Co., 1848).

First Report, Address and Proceedings of the Pittsburgh Sanitary Committee, February 1863 (Pittsburgh: W.S. Haven, 1863).

Fitzpatrick, J. C., (ed.), *The Last Will and Testament of George Washington and Schedule of his Property, to which is appended the Last Will and Testament of Martha Washington* (Mount Vernon: The Mount Vernon Ladies' Association of the Union, 1939).

Fleming, A., *Blood Stains in Clinical Trials* (Pittsburgh: W. S. Haven, 1861). Republished from the American Journal of the Medical Sciences, Vol. XXXVII, Blanchard and Lea, Philadelphia, 1859.

Fleming, G. T., *History of Pittsburgh and Environs, Vol. II*. (New York: The American Historical Society, Inc., 1922).

Flint, A., (ed.), *Sanitary Memoirs of the War of the Rebellion. Collected and Printed by the United States Sanitary Commission* (New York: H.O. Houghton and Company, 1867).

Fort Duquesne and Fort Pitt, Early Names of Pittsburgh Streets, Pittsburgh Chapter Daughters of the American Revolution (Pittsburgh: The Eichbaum Press, 1899).

"From George Washington to James Craik, 26 April 1777" (Washington, D.C.: Founders Online, National Archives and Records Administration, Washington, D.C., last modified February 1, 2018, founders.archives.gov/documents/Washington/03-09-02-0256. [Original source: Chase, Philander D., ed. *The Papers of George Washington, 28 March 1777–10 June 1777* (Charlottesville: University Press of Virginia, Revolutionary War Series, vol. 9., 1999).

Gibson, J. E., *Dr. Bodo Otto and the Medical Background of the American Revolution* (Springfield: Charles C. Thomas, 1937).

Gist, C., *Instructions given Mr. Christopher Gist by the Committee of the Ohio Company the 11th day of September 1750 [and July 16th 1751]. Also, the daily record of Christopher Gist, containing an account of his travels discoveries, transactions with the Indians, etc., from 1750 to 1752]*, (Publisher unknown, 1880).

Glazier, W., *Peculiarities of American Cities* (Philadelphia: Hubbard Brothers, 1886).

Greenawalt, J. C., "Public Institutional Care for the Mentally Ill in Allegheny County, Pennsylvania, 1850 to 1900," (Pittsburgh: Doctor of Philosophy Dissertation, University of Pittsburgh, 1956).

Griffith, C. E., *The African Dream: Martin R. Delany and the Emergence of Pan-African Thought (University Park:* The Pennsylvania State University Press, 1975).

Grom, R. M., "Homeopathy in Pittsburgh: a Historical Perspective" (Pittsburgh: *Bulletin of the Allegheny County Medical Society*, December 23, 1995); *Pittsburgh's Homeopathic Experience* (Pittsburgh: The West Penn Hospital Foundation, 1991); "No Ordinary Man", *Pittsburgh History* (Pittsburgh: Historical Society of Western Pennsylvania, spring 1991).

Gunn, J. C., *Gunn's Domestic Medicine or Poor Man's Friend, Thirteenth Edition* (Pittsburgh: J. Edwards & J. J. Newman, 1839).

Jolly, E. R., *Nuns of the Battlefield* (Providence: The Providence Visitor Press, 1977).

Jones, J. A., *Tales of an Indian camp*, Vol. 1, (London: Henry Colburn and Richard Bentley, 1829).

Jordan, J. W., *Encyclopedia of Pennsylvania Biography* (New York: Lewis Historical Publishing Company, 1914).

Killikelly, S. H., *The History of Pittsburgh, Its Rise and Progress* (Pittsburgh: B. C. & Gorgon Montgomery Co., 1906).

Mackenzie, A. DeB, *History of the Gazzam Family* (Reading: Charles F. Haage, 1894).

McKenna, C. F., (ed.), *Under the Maltese Cross Antietam to Appomattox, Campaigns 155th Pennsylvania Regiment* (Pittsburg: The 155th Regimental Association, 1910).

"Medical Staff, U.S.A. General Hospital, Pittsburgh," U.S. Adjutant General's Office. Personnel papers of medical officers and physicians, Record Group 94. National Archives and Records Administration, Washington, D.C.

Memoirs of the Pittsburgh Sisters of Mercy (new York: Devin-Adair Company, 1918).

Miller, G., "Social Services in a Civil War Hospital in Baltimore," (Baltimore: *Bulletin of the History of Medicine*, Vol. 17, No. 5, May 1945).

"Military surgery, ancient and modern," *United States Service Magazine*, Vol. 1, (London: Charles B. Richardson, 1864).

Mowry, M.D., R. B., "The Medical Profession: An Historical Sketch of the Physicians of Allegheny County, During the Last One Hundred Years" (Pittsburgh: *Cities of Pittsburgh and Allegheny and Their Resources, Souvenir of the Pittsburgh Chronicle Telegraph*, 1889).

Mylin, A. H., *Hospitals, Soldiers' Homes and Orphan Schools controlled by the Commonwealth of Pennsylvania, Vol. 1* (Harrisburg: Clarence M. Busch, State Printer of Pennsylvania, 1897).

Nichols, F. T., "The Organization of Braddock's Army," (Williamsburg: *The William and Mary Quarterly*, Third Series, Vol. 4, No. 2, April 1947).

Official Army Register of the Volunteer forces of the United States Army for the Years 1861, 1862, 1863, 1864, and 1865, Part III—Pennsylvania, Delaware, Maryland, District of Columbia (Washington, D.C.: Published by Order Of The Secretary of War, in Compliance with the Joint Resolution of the Senate and House of Representatives, Approved March 2, 1865).

Paull, B. I., *A Century of Medical Excellence: The History of the University of Pittsburgh School of Medicine* (Pittsburgh: University of Pittsburgh Medical School Alumni Association, 1986.

Railroad Gazette, Volume 22, New York, 1890.

Reilly, R. F., "Medical and surgical care during the American Civil War, 1861–1865." *Proceedings*, 29 (2). (Dallas: Baylor University Medical Center, 2016).

Report of the Commission to Locate the Site of the Frontier Forts of Pennsylvania, v2. (Pennsylvania: Clarence M. Busch, State printer, 1896).

Revised United States Army regulations of 1861 with an Appendix (Containing the Changes and Laws Affecting Army Regulations and Articles of War to June 25, 1863) (Washington, D.C.: Government Printing Office, 1863).

Riddle, J., (ed.), *The Pittsburgh Directory for 1815*, (Pittsburgh: James Riddle, 1815).

Rush, M.D., B., *Medical Inquiries and Observations*, (Philadelphia: Mathew Carey, *et al.*, 1809); *Medical Inquiries And Observations, The Result Of Observations Made Upon The Diseases Which Occurred In The Military Hospitals Of The United States, During The Revolutionary War Between Great Britain And The United States, Vol. I.* (Philadelphia: M. Carey & Son, 1818).

Slattery, C. L., *Felix Reville Brunot 1820–1898* (New York: Longmans, Green, and Co., 1901).

Smith, A. F., and Merwin, J., *The Indian doctor's dispensatory, or Every man his own physician*, (Ohio: J. Hogan, 1833).

Smith, S., (ed.), "Volunteer Surgical Aid," (New York: *American Medical Times*, Vol. V., 1862).

Strait, N. A., *Roster of all Regimental Surgeons and Assistant Surgeons in the Late War, with their Service, and Last-known Post-Office Address* (Washington, D.C.: United States Pension Office, 1882).

Swetnam, G., *The First Hundred Years: A Century of Medical Progress* (Pittsburgh: Allegheny County Medical Society, 1965).

The Hahnemannian Monthly, Vol. 1, No. 1, August 1865 (Philadelphia: Homeopathic Medical College of Pennsylvania and Hahnemann Medical College and Hospital of Philadelphia, 1865).

The Pittsburgh Medical Review, Vol. IV. (Pittsburgh: Murdoch, Kerr & Co., 1890).

The Rebellion Record of Allegheny County from April 1861 to October 1862. (Pittsburgh: W. A. Lare and W. M., Hartze, 1862).

The Story of Pittsburgh, Volume Number One (Pittsburgh: First National Bank of Pittsburgh, August 1919).

The 28th National Encampment of the Grand Army of the Republic Official Program (Pittsburgh: Grand Army of the Republic, 1894).

Thurman, L. S., "An Account Book of Baynton, Wharton, and Morgan at Fort Pitt, 1765–1767," (Pittsburgh: *The Western Pennsylvania Historical Magazine*, Volume 29, Number 3–4, September–December 1946).

Thurston, G. H., *Pittsburgh and Allegheny City in the Centennial Year* (Pittsburgh: A.A. Anderson & Son, 1876).

Trombley, R. V., "Pennsylvania's Role in the Mexican American War." (Edinboro: Master's Thesis, Edinboro University, Pennsylvania, 2013).

Twiss, J. R., "Medical Practice in Colonial America," (New York: *Bulletin New York Academy of Medicine*, Vol. 36, No. 8, August 1960).

Walter, A. G., *Conservative Surgery* (Pittsburgh: W.G. Johnston & Co., 1867).

Wilson, C. A., "The Western Pennsylvania Hospital Site," (Pittsburgh: Masters thesis, University of Pittsburgh, 1989).

Wilson, Jr., C. R., and Grom, R. M., *Pittsburgh—A City And Its Medicine* (Pittsburgh: The West Penn Hospital Foundation, 1990).

Wilson, Jr., C. R., "A Historical Review of West Penn's Staff And Departmental Development," *WPH Medical Bulletin* Vol. 10, No. 1. (Pittsburgh: The Western Pennsylvania Hospital, 1977).

Wilson, E., (ed.), *Standard History of Pittsburgh Pennsylvania* (Chicago: H.R. Cornell & Company, 1898).

Newspapers

Daily Morning Post (Pittsburgh)
Pittsburgh Daily Gazette and Advertiser
Pittsburgh Daily Morning Post
Presbyterian Banner (Pittsburgh)
The Pittsburgh Commercial
The Daily Pittsburgh Gazette
The Press (Philadelphia, Pennsylvania)

Index